Oxidative Stress Modulators and Functional Foods

Oxidative Stress Modulators and Functional Foods

Editor

Junsei Taira

MDPI • Basel • Beijing • Wuhan • Barcelona • Belgrade • Manchester • Tokyo • Cluj • Tianjin

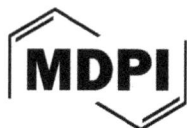

Editor
Junsei Taira
NIT, Okinawa College or
National Institute of Technology,
Okinawa College
Japan

Editorial Office
MDPI
St. Alban-Anlage 66
4052 Basel, Switzerland

This is a reprint of articles from the Special Issue published online in the open access journal *Antioxidants* (ISSN 2076-3921) (available at: https://www.mdpi.com/journal/antioxidants/special_issues/Oxidative_Modulators_Functional_Foods).

For citation purposes, cite each article independently as indicated on the article page online and as indicated below:

LastName, A.A.; LastName, B.B.; LastName, C.C. Article Title. *Journal Name* **Year**, *Volume Number*, Page Range.

ISBN 978-3-0365-0938-9 (Hbk)
ISBN 978-3-0365-0939-6 (PDF)

© 2021 by the authors. Articles in this book are Open Access and distributed under the Creative Commons Attribution (CC BY) license, which allows users to download, copy and build upon published articles, as long as the author and publisher are properly credited, which ensures maximum dissemination and a wider impact of our publications.

The book as a whole is distributed by MDPI under the terms and conditions of the Creative Commons license CC BY-NC-ND.

Contents

About the Editor vii

Preface to "Oxidative Stress Modulators and Functional Foods" ix

Junsei Taira
Oxidative Stress Modulators and Functional Foods
Reprinted from: *Antioxidants* **2021**, *10*, 191, doi:10.3390/antiox10020191 1

Eun-Nam Kim, Hyun-Su Lee and Gil-Saeng Jeong
Cudratricusxanthone O Inhibits H_2O_2-Induced Cell Damage by Activating Nrf2/HO-1 Pathway in Human Chondrocytes
Reprinted from: *Antioxidants* **2020**, *9*, 788, doi:10.3390/antiox9090788 5

Nuria Boix, Elisabet Teixido, Ester Pique, Juan Maria Llobet and Jesus Gomez-Catalan
Modulation and Protection Effects of Antioxidant Compounds against Oxidant Induced Developmental Toxicity in Zebrafish
Reprinted from: *Antioxidants* **2020**, *9*, 721, doi:10.3390/antiox9080721 19

Jelena Tošović and Urban Bren
Antioxidative Action of Ellagic Acid—A Kinetic DFT Study
Reprinted from: *Antioxidants* **2020**, *9*, 587, doi:10.3390/antiox9070587 33

Bianca-Eugenia Ștefănescu, Lavinia Florina Călinoiu, Floricuța Ranga, Florinela Fetea, Andrei Mocan, Dan Cristian Vodnar and Gianina Crișan
Chemical Composition and Biological Activities of the Nord-West Romanian Wild Bilberry (*Vaccinium myrtillus* L.) and Lingonberry (*Vaccinium vitis-idaea* L.) Leaves
Reprinted from: *Antioxidants* **2020**, *9*, 495, doi:10.3390/antiox9060495 47

Mawalle Kankanamge Hasitha Madhawa Dias, Dissanayaka Mudiyanselage Dinesh Madusanka, Eui Jeong Han, Min Ju Kim, You-Jin Jeon, Hyun-Soo Kim, Ilekuttige Priyan Shanura Fernando and Ginnae Ahn
(−)-Loliolide Isolated from *Sargassum horneri* Protects against Fine Dust-Induced Oxidative Stress in Human Keratinocytes
Reprinted from: *Antioxidants* **2020**, *9*, 474, doi:10.3390/antiox9060474 69

Ji Eun Park, Heaji Lee, Hyunkyung Rho, Seong Min Hong, Sun Yeou Kim and Yunsook Lim
Effect of *Quamoclit angulata* Extract Supplementation on Oxidative Stress and Inflammation on Hyperglycemia-Induced Renal Damage in Type 2 Diabetic Mice
Reprinted from: *Antioxidants* **2020**, *9*, 459, doi:10.3390/antiox9060459 81

Seung-Cheol Jee, Min Kim, Kyeong Seok Kim, Hyung-Sik Kim and Jung-Suk Sung
Protective Effects of Myricetin on Benzo[a]pyrene-Induced 8-Hydroxy-2′-Deoxyguanosine and BPDE-DNA Adduct
Reprinted from: *Antioxidants* **2020**, *9*, 446, doi:10.3390/antiox9050446 99

Junsei Taira and Takayuki Ogi
Nitric Oxide Modulation by Folic Acid Fortification
Reprinted from: *Antioxidants* **2020**, *9*, 393, doi:10.3390/antiox9050393 113

Ilekuttige Priyan Shanura Fernando, Mawalle Kankanamge Hasitha Madhawa Dias, Disanayaka Mudiyanselage Dinesh Madusanka, Eui Jeong Han, Min Ju Kim, You-Jin Jeon, Kyounghoon Lee, Sun Hee Cheong, Young Seok Han, Sang Rul Park and Ginnae Ahn
Human Keratinocyte UVB-Protective Effects of a Low Molecular Weight Fucoidan from *Sargassum horneri* Purified by Step Gradient Ethanol Precipitation
Reprinted from: *Antioxidants* **2020**, *9*, 340, doi:10.3390/antiox9040340 . . . . **125**

Choon Young Lee, Ajit Sharma, Julius Semenya, Charles Anamoah, Kelli N. Chapman and Veronica Barone
Computational Study of *Ortho*-Substituent Effects on Antioxidant Activities of Phenolic Dendritic Antioxidants
Reprinted from: *Antioxidants* **2020**, *9*, 189, doi:10.3390/antiox9030189 . . . . **141**

Adriana Elena Bulboaca, Paul-Mihai Boarescu, Alina Silvia Porfire, Gabriela Dogaru, Cristina Barbalata, Madalina Valeanu, Constantin Munteanu, Ruxandra Mioara Râjnoveanu, Cristina Ariadna Nicula and Ioana Cristina Stanescu
The Effect of Nano-Epigallocatechin-Gallate on Oxidative Stress and Matrix Metalloproteinases in Experimental Diabetes Mellitus
Reprinted from: *Antioxidants* **2020**, *9*, 172, doi:10.3390/antiox9020172 . . . . **155**

Ximeng Lin, Keshan Liu, Sheng Yin, Yimin Qin, Peili Shen and Qiang Peng
A Novel Pectic Polysaccharide of Jujube Pomace: Structural Analysis and Intracellular Antioxidant Activities
Reprinted from: *Antioxidants* **2020**, *9*, 127, doi:10.3390/antiox9020127 . . . . **171**

Junsei Taira and Takayuki Ogi
Induction of Antioxidant Protein HO-1 Through Nrf2-ARE Signaling Due to Pteryxin in *Peucedanum Japonicum* Thunb in RAW264.7 Macrophage Cells
Reprinted from: *Antioxidants* **2019**, *8*, 621, doi:10.3390/antiox8120621 . . . . **187**

Artur Junio Togneri Ferron, Giancarlo Aldini, Fabiane Valentini Francisqueti-Ferron, Carol Cristina Vágula de Almeida Silva, Silmeia Garcia Zanati Bazan, Jéssica Leite Garcia, Dijon Henrique Salomé de Campos, Luciana Ghiraldeli, Koody Andre Hassemi Kitawara, Alessandra Altomare, Camila Renata Correa, Fernando Moreto and Ana Lucia A. Ferreira
Protective Effect of Tomato-Oleoresin Supplementation on Oxidative Injury Recoveries Cardiac Function by Improving β-Adrenergic Response in a Diet-Obesity Induced Model
Reprinted from: *Antioxidants* **2019**, *8*, 368, doi:10.3390/antiox8090368 . . . . **197**

Han-A Park and Amy C. Ellis
Dietary Antioxidants and Parkinson's Disease
Reprinted from: *Antioxidants* **2020**, *9*, 570, doi:10.3390/antiox9070570 . . . . **209**

About the Editor

Junsei Taira, Professor, holds an M.S. in Environmental Science (University of Tsukuba, Japan 1987) and Ph.D. from Kyoto Institute of Technology (Japan) attained in 1992. He has been employed as researcher at Kanebo Ltd. (currently Kanebo Cosmetics Inc., Japan) since 1987. In 1995, he was employed as a Fellowship Researcher at National Institutes of Health (NIH), National Cancer Institute (NCI) (USA), and in 1997, he was appointed Principal Investigator at Institute of Health and Environment/Industrial Technology Center in Okinawa Prefectural Government (Japan). He was Visiting Researcher at the Institute of Medical Science, University of Tokyo (Japan), in 2006. In 2007, he was appointed Associate Professor in Department of Bioresources Technology, National Institute of Technology, Okinawa College (Japan), where he was later appointed Professor in 2011. He is current serving on the editorial board of Marine Drugs and as Guest Editor of *Marine Drugs* and *Antioxidants* (MDPI). His research interests cover the field of oxidative stress in cells and the cellular protective/preventive mechanisms of natural product, which have been explored in terrestrial plants and marine natural products.

Preface to "Oxidative Stress Modulators and Functional Foods"

Many years of research have elucidated the role of natural antioxidants and dietary supplements as functional foods with the potential to prevent oxidative stress due to the suppressing of reactive oxygen species (ROS) and reactive nitrogen species (RNS). Recent studies have also revealed that cell signalling pathways, such as Nrf2-ARE, signalling with antioxidant protein (heme oxygenase-1, HO-1) expression and coexisting anti-apoptotic cell signaling, play significant roles to avoid cell damage by the excessive production of ROS, RNS, or electrophiles. Therefore, natural products extending beyond the traditional antioxidant role are gaining a great deal of attention in functional foods, which can protect against various diseases related to oxidative stress. This book of "Oxidative Stress Modulators and Functional Foods" consists of 16 articles including 1 review article related to the antioxidant role of natural products and their ability to modulate oxidative stress and/or reverse disease both in vitro and in animal models. Additionally, the molecular mechanisms of these actions and the modulation of the signalling pathways in the redox system by natural products are included.

I would like to thank all the authors for their valuable contributions and all the reviewers for their availability to review the papers involving their useful suggestions to elevate scientific quality. Appreciate also to the journal's publishing team for their help in disseminating the call for papers and in every step of the publishing process.

Junsei Taira
Editor

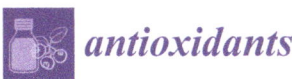

Editorial

Oxidative Stress Modulators and Functional Foods

Junsei Taira

Department of Bioresources Technology, Okinawa College, National Institute of Technology, 905 Henoko, Okinawa, Nago 905-2192, Japan; taira@okinawa-ct.ac.jp

Citation: Taira, J. Oxidative Stress Modulators and Functional Foods. *Antioxidants* 2021, 10, 191. https://doi.org/10.3390/antiox10020191

Received: 26 January 2021
Accepted: 27 January 2021
Published: 29 January 2021

Publisher's Note: MDPI stays neutral with regard to jurisdictional claims in published maps and institutional affiliations.

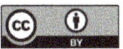

Copyright: © 2021 by the author. Licensee MDPI, Basel, Switzerland. This article is an open access article distributed under the terms and conditions of the Creative Commons Attribution (CC BY) license (https://creativecommons.org/licenses/by/4.0/).

Many years of research have seen the investigation of natural antioxidants and dietary supplements as functional foods with the potential to prevent oxidative stress due to the scavenging of reactive oxygen species (ROS) and reactive nitrogen species (RNS). Recent studies have also revealed that cell signalling pathways, such as Nrf2-ARE, signalling with antioxidant protein (heme oxygenase-1, HO-1) expression, play significant roles in the cell's survival response to avoid cell damage by the excessive production of ROS, RNS, or electrophiles. Therefore, natural products extending beyond the traditional antioxidant role are gaining a great deal of attention in functional foods, which can protect against various diseases related to oxidative stress. This Special Issue consists of 15 articles related to the antioxidant role of natural products, but also their ability to modulate oxidative stress and/or reverse disease both in vitro and in animal models. Additionally, the molecular mechanisms of these actions and the modulation of the signalling pathways in the redox system by natural products are included.

Folic acid (FA) is known as a dietary supplement that can prevent neural tube defects (NTDs), involving the failure of neural tube (NT) closure in the developing embryo, especially spina bifida and anencephaly in the periconceptional period. Previous study indicated that moderate levels of nitric oxide (NO) and nitric oxide synthase (NOS) play a critical role in normal embryonic development. NO inhibits methionine synthase (MS), involving the interference transfer of the methyl group from the methyl donor, 5-methyltetrahydrofolate through the FA metabolite system (Folate pathway), to homocysteine during methionine production. Taira et al. [1] elucidated that FA can directly scavenge NO, suggesting that NO modulation, due to FA, may contribute to alleviation from failure in neural tube formation, causing the high level of NO production.

Understanding the structure–activity relationships of antioxidants and their mechanisms of action is important for designing more potent antioxidants for potential use as therapeutic agents as well as preservatives. The kinetic studies of antioxidative action of ellagic acid (EA) under physiological conditions elucidated that the hydroxyl radical (•OH) with EA conforms to hydrogen atom transfer and radical adduct formation mechanisms, whereas the sequential proton loss electron transfer mechanism is responsible for the scavenging of the $CCl_3OO•$ radical, generating in the organism during the metabolism of CCl_4. In addition, compared to trolox, EA was found to be more reactive toward •OH, but less reactive toward $CCl_3OO•$ in which their calculated rate constants are in very good agreement with the corresponding experimental values [2]. From another viewpoint of antioxidant mechanisms, the computational study for antioxidant mechanisms was carried out using total enthalpy values on the electronic effects of ortho-substituents in dendritic tri-phenolic antioxidants, comprising a common phenol moiety and two other phenol units with electron-donating or electron-withdrawing substituents. As the preferred antioxidant mechanism, in sequential proton loss electron transfer (SPLET) it was found that electron-donating groups, such as the OCH_3 group, are useful for designing potent dendritic antioxidants, while the nitro and halogens do not add value to the radical scavenging antioxidant activity [3]. Furthermore, to predict the antioxidant potentiality in vivo, Boix et al. [4] proposed that the zebrafish model assay has the capability to predict in vivo protective activity or to determine their underlying mechanisms of action. This article showed a useful experimental system to evaluate the in vivo protective effects of different antioxidant compounds, based on the zebrafish embryo test under oxidative stress conditions using tert-butyl hydroperoxide, tetrachlorohydroquinone and lipopolysaccharide chemicals. This system was also applied to the study of the effects of well-known antioxidants, such as vitamin E, quercetin, and lipoic acid, and confirmed the zebrafish model as a useful in vivo tool to test the protective effects of antioxidant compounds.

Recent studies have revealed that cell signalling pathways, such as Nrf2-ARE signalling with HO-1 expression play significant roles to avoid cell damage causing oxidative-related various diseases. Taira et al. [5] focused on exploring the Nrf2 active compound and over five hundred various edible medicinal herbs were evaluated by a reporter assay, and the highest Nrf2 activity was found in the ethanol extract of *Peucedanum japonicum* leaves. The active compound in the extract was identical to pteryxin based on ^{1}H, ^{13}C-NMR spectra and liquid chromatography/time-of-fright/mass spectrometry (LC/TOF/MS). Pteryxin accumulated the transcription factor Nrf2 in the nucleus and resulted in the expression of the HO-1. This study also suggested that the electrophilicity, due to α,β-carbonyl and/or substituted acyl groups in the molecule, modulates the cysteine residue in Keap1 via the Michel reaction, at which point the Nrf2 is dissociated from the Keap1. Furthermore, the Nrf2 activator in bioresource reported the function in relation to disease. Osteoarthritis (OA) is a common joint degenerative disease induced by oxidative stress in chondrocytes. Kim et al. [6] demonstrated the inhibitory effects of cudratricusxanthone O (CTO), isolated from the *Maclura tricuspidata* Bureau (Moraceae), on the H_2O_2-induced damage of SW1353 chondrocytes. CTO induced HO-1 expression, involving the translocation of Nrf2 into the nucleus. Pretreatment with CTO in H_2O_2-treated cells regulated ROS production by inducing, expression of antioxidant enzymes (SOD, catalase, glutathione peroxidase (GSH-Px), glutathione reductase, and HO-1, and also prevented H_2O_2-induced apoptosis by regulating the expression of anti-apoptotic proteins, such as Bcl-2 and Bax. Environmental stress, involving oxidative stress, due to Ultraviolet (UV) and air pollutants contributing fine dust (FD) containing hazardous chemicals, induces triggering allergic reactions and inflammation of the skin, which lead to thickening of the epidermis, discoloration, skin wrinkling, loss of elasticity and skin-cell growth retardation [7,8]. Fernando et al. [7] reported that a low molecular weight fucoidan fraction (SHC4, 60 kDa, with 37.43% fucose and 28.01% sulfate), isolated from *Sargassum horneri*, reduced intracellular ROS levels and increased the cell viability on UVB (280–320 nm) exposed HaCaT keratinocytes and inhibited UVB-induced apoptotic body formation, sub-G1 accumulation of cells through the mitochondria-mediated pathway. The UVB protective effect of SHC4 was facilitated by enhancing intracellular antioxidant defence via Nrf2-HO-1 signalling. The FD in air pollutants also produced the ROS in human HaCaT keratinocytes. (–)-loliolide (HTT), isolated from *Sargassum horneri*, has the potential to increase cell viability by reducing the ROS production in FD-stimulated keratinocytes, involving the mitochondria-mediated apoptosis pathway. HTT suppressed FD-stimulated DNA damage and the formation of apoptotic bodies, and it reduced the population of cells in the sub-G1 apoptosis phase. The cytoprotective effects of the HTT against FD-stimulated oxidative damage is mediated through squaring the Nrf2-HO-1 pathway involved in increasing HO-1 and NAD(P)H dehydrogenase (quinone) 1 in the cytosol [8].

In this Special Issue, the approach to find new biological activities of antioxidants in relation to various diseases and the different bioactivities, due to habitat-derived conditions, were reported by the following: (1) Type 2-diabetes mellitus (T2-DM) is caused by hyperglycaemic abnormalities in controlling blood glucose and insulin resistance. This article showed the mechanism of ameliorative effects due to quamoclit angulata (QA) on diabetes. QA supplementation (5 or 10 mg/kg/day) for 12 weeks reduced homeostasis model assessment insulin resistance, kidney malfunction, and glomerular hypertrophy in T2-DM. Moreover, the QA treatment significantly attenuated renal NLRP3 inflammasome-dependent hyper-inflammation and the consequential renal damage caused by oxidative stress, apoptosis, and fibrosis in T2-DM [9]. (2) In a similar model animal experiment, the high sugar-fat

(HSF) diet induced obesity, insulin resistance, cardiac dysfunction, and oxidative damage. When tomato-oleoresin supplementation (containing 10 mg lycopene/kg body weight (BW) per day) was given orally every morning for a 10-week period, the insulin resistance, cardiac remodelling, and dysfunction were improved by regulating the β-adrenergic response. [10]. (3) The antioxidant properties of epigallocatechin-gallate (EGCG), a green tea compound, have been already studied in various diseases. To improve the bioavailability of EGCG, this article demonstrated the result of the comparative effect of liposomal EGCG (L-EGCG) with EGCG solution in experimental DM induced by streptozotocin in rats. L-EGCG indicated a better efficiency regarding the improvement of oxidative stress parameters for malondialdehyde (MDA), NO, and total oxidative status; antioxidant status for total antioxidant capacity of plasma, thiols, and catalase and matrix-metalloproteinase-2 were also significantly reduced in the L-EGCG-treated group, compared with the EGCG group [11]. (4) Myricetin is present in many natural foods with various biological activities, such as anti-oxidative and anti-cancer activities. Benzo[a]pyrene (B[a]P), a group 1 carcinogen, induces mutagenic DNA adducts. B[a]P is metabolized by phase I enzymes, cytochrome P450 (CYP), and CYP1A1 also produces the metabolites conjugated with the DNA-BPDE (B[a]P-7,8-dihydrodiol-9,10-epoxide) adduct and 8-hydroxy-2′-deoxyguanosine formation. This article showed that myricetin reduces B[a]P-induced toxicity by inhibiting those metabolites by the reduction of the B[a]P metabolism via reduced CYP1A1 expression, and the elimination of B[a]P metabolites via enhanced GST expression [12]. (5) The variations in the phenolic profile for 21 compounds and bioactivities for antioxidant and antimutagenic activities between bilberry and lingonberry leaves different from three locations due to different altitude, solar exposure and temperature range were investigated. As a result, flavonols, hydroxycinnamic acids, and anthocyanins, due to habitat-derived conditions, could be clearly distinguished in these species [13].

As a large molecule antioxidant, a novel pectic polysaccharide, SAZMP4 (M.W, 28.94 kDa), mainly containing 1,4-linked galacturonic acid (GalA, 93.48%), with side chains of various neutral sugars, such as rhamnose, arabinose was isolated from Jujube pomace and the structure was determined by GC, FI-IR, GC-MS, NMR for molecule analysis, and SEM (scanning electron microscope) and AFM (atomic force microscope) for molecular morphological analysis. In addition, the antioxidant activity of SAZMP4 against H_2O_2-induced oxidative stress in Caco-2 cells demonstrated SOD activity and GSH-Px, MDA. Additionally, a better water retention capacity and the thermal stability of SAZMP4 indicated a potential application in the food industry as an additive [14].

The review article in this Special Issue discussed cellular and genetic factors that increase oxidative stress in Parkinson's disease (PD). PD is a neurodegenerative disorder caused by the depletion of dopaminergic neurons in the basal ganglia, the movement centre of the brain. The accumulation of oxidative stress-induced neuronal damage, due to the increased production of ROS or impaired intracellular antioxidant defences, invariably occurs at the cellular levels. The dopaminergic prodrugs and agonists can alleviate some of the symptoms of PD, but they could not be completely prohibited by the progression of PD pathology. The progress of PD takes a long time for the neurodegenerative process; therefore, the authors proposed that strategies to prevent or delay PD pathology may be well suited to lifestyle changes, such as dietary modification with antioxidant-rich foods, including vitamin C, vitamin E, carotenoids, selenium, and polyphenols [15].

Funding: This research received no external funding.

Conflicts of Interest: The author declares no conflict of interest.

References

1. Taira, J.; Ogi, T. Nitric Oxide Modulation by Folic Acid Fortification. *Antioxidants* **2020**, *9*, 393. [CrossRef] [PubMed]
2. Tošović, J.; Bren, U. Antioxidative Action of Ellagic Acid—A Kinetic DFT Study. *Antioxidants* **2020**, *9*, 587. [CrossRef] [PubMed]
3. Lee, C.Y.; Sharma, A.; Semenya, J.; Anamoah, C.; Chapman, K.N.; Barone, V. Computational Study of Ortho-Substituent Effects on Antioxidant Activities of Phenolic Dendritic. *Antioxidants* **2020**, *9*, 189. [CrossRef] [PubMed]

4. Boix, N.; Teixido, E.; Pique, E.; Llobet, J.M.; Gomez-Catalan, J. Modulation and Protection Effects of Antioxidant Compounds against Oxidant Induced Developmental Toxicity in Zebrafish. *Antioxidants* **2020**, *9*, 721. [CrossRef] [PubMed]
5. Taira, J.; Ogi, T. Induction of Antioxidant Protein HO-1 Through Nrf2-ARE Signaling Due to Pteryxin in *Peucedanum Japonicum* Thunb in RAW264.7 Macrophage Cells. *Antioxidants* **2019**, *8*, 621. [CrossRef] [PubMed]
6. Kim, E.-N.; Lee, H.-S.; Jeong, G.-S. Cudratricusxanthone O Inhibits H_2O_2-Induced Cell Damage by Activating Nrf2/HO-1 Pathway in Human Chondrocytes. *Antioxidants* **2020**, *9*, 788. [CrossRef]
7. Fernando, I.P.S.; Dias, M.K.H.M.; Madusanka, D.M.D.; Han, E.J.; Kim, M.J.; Jeon, Y.-J.; Lee, K.; Cheong, S.H.; Han, Y.S.; Park, S.R.; et al. Human Keratinocyte UVB-Protective Effects of a Low Molecular Weight Fucoidan from *Sargassum horneri* Purified by Step Gradient Ethanol Precipitation. *Antioxidants* **2020**, *9*, 340. [CrossRef]
8. Dias, M.K.; Madusanka, D.M.; Han, E.J.; Kim, M.J.; Jeon, Y.-J.; Kim, H.S.; Fernando, I.P.; Ahn, G. (−)-Loliolide Isolated from Sargassum horneri Protects against Fine Dust-Induced Oxidative Stress in Human Keratinocytes. *Antioxidants* **2020**, *9*, 474. [CrossRef] [PubMed]
9. Park, J.E.; Lee, H.; Rho, H.; Hong, S.M.; Kim, S.Y.; Lim, Y. Effect of *Quamoclit angulata* Extract Supplementation on Oxidative Stress and Inflammation on Hyperglycemia-Induced Renal Damage in Type 2 Diabetic Mice. *Antioxidants* **2020**, *9*, 459. [CrossRef]
10. Ferron, A.J.T.; Aldini, G.; Francisqueti-Ferron, F.V.; Silva, C.C.V.d.A.; Bazan, S.G.Z.; Garcia, J.L.; Campos, D.H.S.d.; Ghiraldeli, L.; Kitawara, K.A.H.; Altomare, A.; et al. Protective Effect of Tomato-Oleoresin Supplementation on Oxidative Injury Recoveries Cardiac Function by Improving β-Adrenergic Response in a Diet-Obesity Induced Model. *Antioxidants* **2019**, *8*, 368. [CrossRef] [PubMed]
11. Bulboaca, A.E.; Boarescu, P.-M.; Porfire, A.S.; Dogaru, G.; Barbalata, C.; Valeanu, M.; Munteanu, C.; Râjnoveanu, R.M.; Nicula, C.A.; Stanescu, I.C. The Effect of Nano-Epigallocatechin-Gallate on Oxidative Stress and Matrix Metalloproteinases in Experimental Diabetes Mellitus. *Antioxidants* **2020**, *9*, 172. [CrossRef] [PubMed]
12. Jee, S.-C.; Kimm, M.; Kim, K.S.; Kim, H.-S.; Sung, J.-S. Protective Effects of Myricetin on Benzo[a]pyrene-Induced 8-Hydroxy-20-Deoxyguanosine and BPDE-DNA Adduct. *Antioxidants* **2020**, *9*, 446. [CrossRef]
13. Ștefănescu, B.-E.; Călinoiu, L.F.; Ranga, F.; Fetea, F.; Mocan, A.; Vodnar, D.C.; Cris, G. Chemical Composition and Biological Activities of the Nord-West Romanian Wild Bilberry (*Vaccinium myrtillus* L.) and Lingonberry (*Vaccinium vitis-idaea* L.) Leaves. *Antioxidants* **2020**, *9*, 495. [CrossRef]
14. Lin, X.; Liu, K.; Yin, S.; Qin, Y.; Shen, P.; Peng, Q. A Novel Pectic Polysaccharide of Jujube Pomace: Structural Analysis and Intracellular Antioxidant Activities. *Antioxidants* **2020**, *9*, 127. [CrossRef] [PubMed]
15. Park, H.-A.; Ellis, A.C. Dietary Antioxidants and Parkinson's Disease. *Antioxidants* **2020**, *9*, 570. [CrossRef] [PubMed]

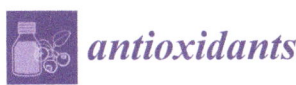

Article

Cudratricusxanthone O Inhibits H_2O_2-Induced Cell Damage by Activating Nrf2/HO-1 Pathway in Human Chondrocytes

Eun-Nam Kim [†], Hyun-Su Lee [†] and Gil-Saeng Jeong *

College of Pharmacy, Keimyung University, 1095 Dalgubeol-daero, Daegu 42601, Korea; enkimpharm@gmail.com (E.-N.K.); hyunsu.lee@kmu.ac.kr (H.-S.L.)
* Correspondence: gsjeong@kmu.ac.kr; Tel.: +82-53-580-6649
† These two authors contributed equally to this work.

Received: 24 July 2020; Accepted: 23 August 2020; Published: 25 August 2020

Abstract: Osteoarthritis (OA) is a common joint degenerative disease induced by oxidative stress in chondrocytes. Although induced-heme oxygenase-1 (HO-1) has been found to protect cells against oxygen radical damage, little information is available regarding the use of bioactive compounds from natural sources for regulating the HO-1 pathway to treat OA. In this study, we explored the inhibitory effects of cudratricusxanthone O (CTO) isolated from the *Maclura tricuspidata* Bureau (*Moraceae*) on H_2O_2-induced damage of SW1353 chondrocytes via regulation of the HO-1 pathway. CTO promoted HO-1 expression by enhancing the translocation of nuclear factor erythroid 2-related factor 2 (Nrf2) into the nucleus without inducing toxicity. Pretreatment with CTO-regulated reactive oxygen species (ROS) production by inducing expression of antioxidant enzymes in H_2O_2-treated cells and maintained the functions of H_2O_2-damaged chondrocytes. Furthermore, CTO prevented H_2O_2-induced apoptosis by regulating the expression of anti-apoptotic proteins. Treatment with the HO-1 inhibitor tin-protoporphyrin IX revealed that these protective effects were exerted due to an increase in HO-1 expression induced by CTO. In conclusion, CTO protects chondrocytes from H_2O_2-induced damages—including ROS accumulation, dysfunction, and apoptosis through activation of the Nrf2/HO-1 signaling pathway in chondrocytes and, therefore, is a potential therapeutic agent for OA treatment.

Keywords: cudratrixanthone O; reactive oxygen species; nuclear transcription factor erythroid-2-like factor 2; hemeoxygenase-1; apoptosis

---

1. Introduction

Osteoarthritis (OA) is a chronic joint degenerative disease that affects normal movements due to loss of articular cartilage, particularly in older adults [1,2]. OA is accompanied by decomposition and destruction of the mesochondrium and cartilage, as well as synovial inflammation, but the main pathological reasons include oxidative stress, aging, and expression of inflammation-related genes [3]. A previous study showed that the degradation of the extracellular matrix (ECM) by the inflammatory response is essential for OA progression, and the damaged joint tissues produce severe cytokines and ECM degradation by-products [4]. Chondrocytes play an important role in maintaining the function of the joints and can generate tissue ECM—including collagen II and proteoglycan—to maintain tissue homeostasis and joint movement [5]. Reactive oxygen species (ROS)—such as hydrogen peroxide (H_2O_2)—are crucial modulators of the redox-sensitive cell signaling pathway, and involved in biological processes—such as host defense, oxygen sensing, proliferation, and apoptosis. However, from a pathological point of view, the overproduction of ROS is associated with inflammation, atherosclerosis, diabetes, high blood pressure, tumor formation, and OA [6]. Therefore, suppressing cell damage to chondrocytes by regulating ROS production in osteoarthritis is an important treatment strategy.

To eliminate cell damage caused by excessive ROS production, most cells, including chondrocytes, have endogenous defense strategies that protect cells from oxidative stress through the nuclear factor erythroid-2-related factor 2 (Nrf2) pathway [7,8]. The defense system activated by Nrf2 leads to induction of superoxide dismutase (SOD), glutathione peroxidase (GPx), glutathione (GSH), and heme oxygenase-1 (HO-1) [9]. Heme oxygenases (HOs) are a group of enzymes that catalyze heme breakdown, and four metabolites have been identified: iron, carbon monoxide (CO), and biliverdin. Three types of HO have been discovered, including HO-1, HO-2, and HO-3. HO-1 plays a key role in the defense mechanism against oxidative damage [10–12]. Although activation of Nrf2 and HO-1 as endogenous defense mechanisms in chondrocytes is important, little is known about whether bioactive small molecules isolated from natural products promote the Nrf2/HO-1 pathway to defend cells from oxidative damage.

Maclura tricuspidata Bureau (Moraceae) is a deciduous broad-leaved tree that is common in China, Korea, and Japan. It has been used in Korean traditional medicine to treat inflammation, gastritis, cancer, and liver damage [13–15]. The major components of *M. tricuspidata* are xanthones, flavonoids, isoflavonoids, and benzylated flavonoids. Among them, prenylated xanthones exhibit antioxidative, anti-inflammatory, antiatherosclerotic, and neuroprotective activities [16–18]. Moreover, prenylated xanthones have shown anti-inflammatory effects in RAW264.7 cells stimulated with lipopolysaccharides (LPS) by inhibiting the expression of pro-inflammatory mediators through HO-1 expression [19]. However, despite these various biological activities, prenylated xanthones have not been studied for OA. Previous studies have shown that hypoxia or inflammatory induction of SW1353 chondrocytes stimulated by IL-1β, monosodium iodoacetate (MIA), and H_2O_2 is known as a representative in vitro model for OA studies [20–23]. In this study, we investigated the role of prenylated xanthones, cudratricusxanthone O (CTO), isolated from *M. tricuspidata*, on the suppression of H_2O_2-induced cell damage by promoting the Nrf2/HO-1 pathway in SW1353 cells.

2. Materials and Methods

2.1. Chemicals and Reagents

Dulbecco's Modified Eagle Medium (DMEM), fetal bovine serum (FBS), penicillin, and streptomycin were purchased from Welgene Inc. (Korea). 3-(4,5-Dimethylthiazol-2-yl)-2,5-diphenyltetrazoliumbromide (MTT) was purchased from Amresco Inc. (Solon, OH, USA). The primary antibodies of Nrf2, HO-1, β-actin, Bcl-2, superoxide dismutase (SOD) and catalase (CAT) were purchased from Santa Cruz Biotechnology Inc. (Santa Cruz, CA, USA), Bax and Caspase-3 were purchased from Cell Signaling Technology (Danvers, MA, USA). Hydrogen peroxide solution (H_2O_2), Protoporphyrin IX (SnPP), Cobalt protoporphyrin (CoPP) and DCF-DA (2′, 7′-dichlorofluorescin diacetate) were bought from Sigma Aldrich (St. Louis, MO, USA). RIPA buffer and ECL Western blotting detection reagents were purchased from Fisher Scientific Inc. (Waltham, MA, USA).

2.2. Plant Materials and Isolation of Compounds

A voucher specimen (accession number KMU 002019-0116) was deposited at the College of Pharmacy, Keimyung University, Daegu, Korea. Cudratrixanthone O (CTO) was isolated from the bark extract of *M. tricuspidata*, and the structure of CTO was identified using nuclear magnetic resonance (NMR) and electrospray ionization mass spectrometry (ESIMS) compared with previously reported literature [24].

2.3. Cell Culture

The human chondrosarcoma cell line SW1353 was purchased from the American Type Culture Collection (ATCC, Manassas, VA, USA) and cultured in Dulbecco's modified Eagle medium (DMEM)

(Welgene, Gyeongsangbuk-do, Korea) containing 10% (v/v) fetal bovine serum, 10 µg/mL streptomycin, and 100 U/mL penicillin (Gibco BRL, Grand Island, NY, USA) in incubated on at 37 °C in 5% CO_2.

2.4. Cell Viability and Coefficient Assays

SW1353 cells (5×10^3 cells/well) were seeded in 96-well plates for 24 h, and cultured with or without CTO (1, 2, 5 µM) for 24 h. Then, 50 µL of MTT (5 mg/mL in PBS, Sigma-Aldrich) was treated to each well for 4 h. Four hours later, supernatant was aspirated, and 150 µL of DMSO was added to each well. The absorbance values were measured at 540 nm on a microplate reader (TECAN, Austria), and for confluency assays cells were seeded in 24-well plates for 24 h, after then, with CTO (1, 2, 5 µM), and the cells counted with Incucyte® Live-Cell analysis systems (Göttingen, Germany).

2.5. Western Blot Analysis

Western blot analysis was performed to examine the expression levels of indicated proteins in SW1353 chondrocytes. Cells were lysed in RIPA buffer containing protease inhibitors and centrifuged at 14,000 rpm for 30 min and quantitate by Bradford assay using a Bio-Rad Bradford assay reagent (Hercules, CA, USA). Then, proteins were separated using 8–12% SDS/polyacrylamide gel electrophoresis and transferred on to PVDF membranes, After blocking with TBS-T buffer containing skim milk (5%), The membranes were incubated with the primary antibodies overnight at 4 °C, after with a secondary antibody. PVDF membrane was detected with Healthcare Life Science ECL-plus (Tokyo, Japan), the images were taken by ImageQuant LAS 4000 (GE Healthcare Life Science, Tokyo, Japan). The expressional value of cytosolic proteins was normalized to the intensity level of β-actin and proteins compared with the untreated cells (control) using image J software.

2.6. Cytosolic and Nuclear Protein Extraction

SW1353 cells were seeded at 5×10^5 cells/mL in a 6-well plate. The harvested cells were then lysed on ice for 20 min with radioimmunoprecipitation assay (RIPA) buffer (Thermo Fisher Scientific, Waltham, MA, USA) and the isolated cytoplasm and nuclei were removed using the NE-PER nuclear and cytoplasmic extraction reagent kit (Pierce Biotechnology, Rockford, IL, USA) according to the manufacturer's instructions.

2.7. Measurement of ROS Generation

The production of intracellular ROS was assessed using a cell-permeable fluorogenic probe, 2′,7′-dichlorodihydrofluorescein diacetate (DCF-DA). SW-1353 cells were seeded in 6-well plate at 1×10^5 cells/well for 24 h, and after pretreated with different concentrations of CTO for 6 h and then cultured for 2 h in the presence or absence of 0.5 mM H_2O_2. Then, the cells were washed twice with PBS to and DCF-DA was incubated in a dark place at 37 °C for 20 min. After 20 min, cells were washed with PBS and fixed with 4% paraformaldehyde (pH 7.4) for 20 min. After observation, the ROS was detected by a fluorescence Olympus IX microscope 71-F3 2PH (Tokyo, Japan).

2.8. RT-qPCR Analysis

After treatment, total RNA was extracted from the SW-1353 cells using TRIzol/chloroform reagent (Bioneer, Korea) according to the manufacturer's instructions. Total RNA was transcribed into cDNA by PrimeScript-RT reagent kit, then the cDNA was amplified by the SYBR Premix Ex Taq (Sangon). The cycling conditions were 40 cycles at 50 °C for 2 min, 95 °C initial denaturation for 10 min, 95 °C denaturation for 15 s, and 60 °C annealing for 30 s. The mRNA encoding each target was measured using real-time PCR and GAPDH was used as the housekeeping gene. The cycle threshold (Ct) value of the target gene was normalized to GAPDH. The primers and amplification products of each gene used in this study are shown in Table 1.

Table 1. Primer sequences.

Target Gene		Sequence
col2a1	Forward (5'-3')	TGGACGCCATGAAGGTTTTCT
	Reverse (3'-5')	TGGGAGCCAGATTGTCATCTC
aggrecan	Forward (5'-3')	GAAGTGGCGTCCAAACCAA
	Reverse (3'-5')	CGTTCCATTCACCCCTCTCA
timp1	Forward (5'-3')	AATTCCGACCTCGTCATCAG
	Reverse (3'-5')	GTTGTGGGACCTGTGGAAGT
mmp3	Forward (5'-3')	GGT GTG GAG TTC CTG ATG TTG
	Reverse (3'-5')	AGC CTG GAG AAT GTG AGT GG
mmp13	Forward (5'-3')	TCA GGA AAC CAG GTC TGG AG
	Reverse (3'-5')	TGA CGC GAA CAA TAC GGT TA
adamts	Forward (5'-3')	TTCCACGGCAGTGGTCTAAAG
	Reverse (3'-5')	CCACCAGGCTAACTGAATTACG
sod	Forward (5'-3')	GGGAGATGGCCCAACTACTG
	Reverse (3'-5')	CCAGTTGACATCGAACCGTT
cat	Forward (5'-3')	ATGGTCCATGCTCTCAAACC
	Reverse (3'-5')	CAGGTCATCCAATAGGAAGG
bcl2	Forward (5'-3')	AGG CTG GGA TGC CTT TGT GG
	Reverse (3'-5')	GGG CAG GCA TGT TGA CTT CAC
bax	Forward (5'-3')	TTCTGACGGCAACTTCAACTGG
	Reverse (3'-5')	AGGAAGTCCAATGTCCAGCC
caspase3	Forward (5'-3')	GGAATTGATGCGTGATGTT
	Reverse (3'-5')	TGGCTCAGAAGCACACAAAC
gapdh	Forward (5'-3')	ACCCAGAAGACTGTGGATGG
	Reverse (3'-5')	CACATTGGGGGTAGGAACAC

2.9. Annexin V-FITC/PI Apoptosis Assay

SW-1353 cells were seeded in six-well plates for 24 h, then pretreated with CTO (0, 1, 2, 5 µM) for 6 h. The positive control group and the CTO-treated groups were then exposed to H_2O_2 to a final concentration of 0.5 mM for 2 h. Cells were collected by centrifugation and washed twice with PBS, and apoptotic incidence was analyzed by the Annexin V-FITC/PropidiumIodide (PI) detection kit (BD Biosciences, San Diego, CA, USA) according to the manufacturer's instructions. The rate of apoptosis was analyzed using a Incucyte® Live-Cell analysis systems.

2.10. Statistical Analysis

Each experiment was performed in triplicate and expressed as mean value and standard deviation. Statistical analysis was conducted using SPSS Statistics 19.0 software. Differences among groups were analyzed by one-way analysis of variance (ANOVA) followed by Tukey's test or Student's *t*-test. $p < 0.05$ were considered to indicate statistical significance.

3. Results

3.1. CTO Is Not Cytotoxic to SW1353 Chondrocytes

To investigate whether CTO (Figure 1A) showed cytotoxicity in chondrocytes, SW1353 chondrocytes were treated with 0, 1, 2, and 5 µM of CTO for 24 h, and cell viability was examined by MTT analysis. No cytotoxicity was observed in the CTO-treated cells, and no morphological change in CTO-treated SW1353 cells (Figure 1B). Moreover, treatment with CTO (0–5 µM) did not affect cellular confluency in SW1353 cells (Figure 1C). CTO showed no statistically significant changes in cytotoxicity or cellular confluency.

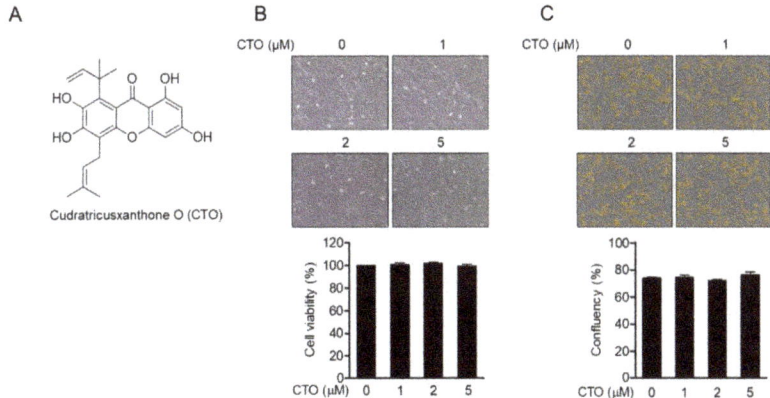

Figure 1. Cudratricusxanthone O (CTO) is not cytotoxic to SW1353 chondrocytes. (**A**) The chemical structure of CTO. (**B**) SW1353 chondrocytes were seeded at a density of 1×10^4 cells/well and treated with CTO at the indicated concentrations (0–5 µM) for 24 h, then after CTO cytotoxicity was evaluated by 3-(4,5-Dimethylthiazol-2-yl)-2,5-diphenyltetrazoliumbromide (MTT) assay. (**C**) The confluency of cells was determined using IncuCyte imaging system. The Student's *t*-test was used for statistical analysis.

3.2. CTO Induces HO-1 Expression by Promotion of Nrf2 Translocation

Nrf2 and HO-1, the major downstream antioxidant signaling pathway, play a major role in regulating oxidative stress. Therefore, the protein expression of HO-1 was measured by Western blot to confirm that CTO activates the Nrf2/HO-1 signaling pathway. After treatment with 5 µM of CTO in SW1353 cells, the expression of HO-1 was induced in a time- and dose-dependent manner. HO-1 was expressed in cells treated with CTO for 6 h and showed the highest expression at 18 h (Figure 2A, top). Concentration-dependent experiments showed that treatment with CTO promoted HO-1 expression in a dose-dependent manner (Figure 2A, bottom). Western blot was used to verify whether Nrf2 translocation into the nucleus was involved in HO-1 expression by CTO. Dose-dependent treatment with 5 µM CTO reduced Nrf2 in the cytosol but enhanced its expression in the nucleus (Figure 2B). HO-1 expression is induced by the activation of MAPK, of which ERK1/2, JNK, and p38 act as upstream regulators of the Nrf2 cascade. We investigated whether CTO promotes Nrf2 translocation and HO-1 induction through activation of the MAPK pathway. Western blotting was performed on SW1353 cells treated with CTO 5 µM in a time-dependent manner for 15, 30, and 60 min. Gradually enhanced phosphorylation of MAPKs was observed after CTO treatment (Figure 2C). These results suggested that CTO was involved in Nrf2 translocation and HO-1 expression by activation of MAPKs in SW1353 cells.

3.3. CTO Suppresses ROS Production by Inducing SOD and CAT in SW1353 Cells

It has been reported that treatment with H_2O_2 of chondrocytes produces ROS, which leads to cell apoptosis. To evaluate the effect of CTO on the production of ROS from cells treated with H_2O_2 in chondrocytes, the production of ROS and the expression of antioxidant enzymes such as SOD and CAT were evaluated in H_2O_2-stimulated SW1353 cells. In DCF-DA fluorescence staining, H_2O_2-stimulated cells showed an increase in ROS, but pretreatment with dose-dependent CTO reduced ROS production (Figure 3A). Expression levels of antioxidant proteins SOD and CAT were inhibited by H_2O_2 treatment but significantly protected by CTO treatment (Figure 3B). Furthermore, the effect of CTO on mRNA levels of SOD and CAT was evaluated by real-time PCR. We confirmed that expression levels of both antioxidant protein and mRNA were protected (Figure 3C). These results suggest that CTO regulates ROS production by preventing H_2O_2-induced apoptosis and retaining the expression of antioxidant proteins in chondrocytes.

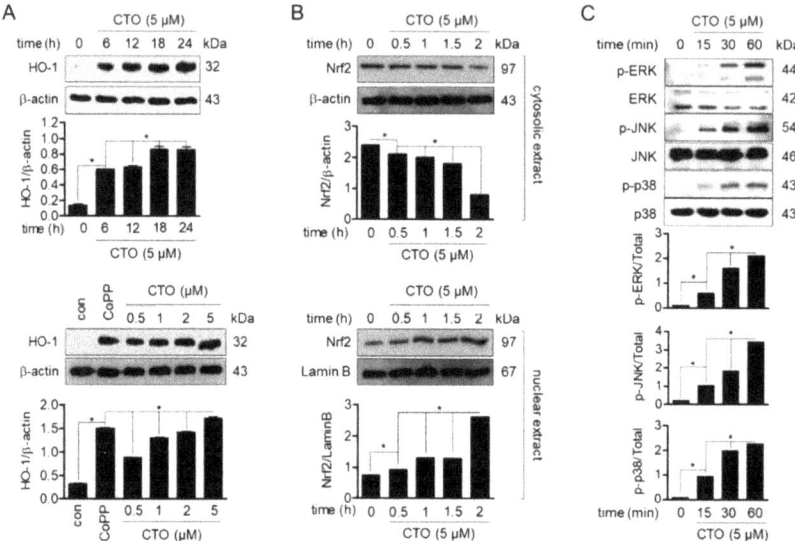

Figure 2. CTO induces heme oxygenase-1 (HO-1) expression by the promotion of Nrf2 translocation. (**A**) The cells (5 × 10^5 cells/mL) were treated with 5 μM for the indicated time (0, 6, 12, 18, 24 h) or with the indicated concentrations of CTO (0.5, 1, 2, and 5 μM) and cobalt protoporphyrin (CoPP) (20 μM) for 18 h. The induced HO-1 expression was detected by Western blot analysis. (**B**) The translocation of Nrf2 was analyzed by Western blot analysis from cells treated with 5 μM of CTO for the indicated time. (**C**) The cells were treated with 5 μM CTO for the indicated times (0–60 min) and phosphorylation of ERK1/2, JNK and p38 were determined by Western blot analysis. * $p < 0.05$ was considered significant differences between groups are indicated.

3.4. CTO Up-Regulates Chondrocytes-Specific Genes but Inhibits the Expression of MMPs in H_2O_2 Treated SW1353 Cells

Accumulating evidence suggests that H_2O_2-induced ROS production degrades the function of chondrocytes. Cartilage-specific genes such as *col2a1* and *aggrecan* play an essential role in the creation and maintenance of cartilage tissue, and proteolytic enzymes such as MMPs induce cartilage tissue loss. Therefore, to explore whether CTO pretreatment prevents functional loss of chondrocytes by H_2O_2, the mRNA levels of essential genes for cartilage tissue formation (*col2a1, aggrecan*), *timps, mmps,* and *adamts* were measured using real-time PCR in H_2O_2-treated SW1353 chondrocytes. We found that the mRNA levels of *col2a1, aggrecan, timp1,* and *timp3* were suppressed by H_2O_2, but protected in a concentration-dependent manner by CTO (Figure 4A). Moreover, we confirmed that the mRNA levels of *mmps* and *adamts* (a group of secreted proteinases and proteolytic enzymes), which suppressed the functions of chondrocytes, were increased by H_2O_2 treatment but significantly decreased by CTO treatment (Figure 4B). These results suggest that CTO protects the function of chondrocytes by upregulating essential genes for cartilage tissue formation as well as downregulating *mmps* and *adamts* upon H_2O_2 treatment.

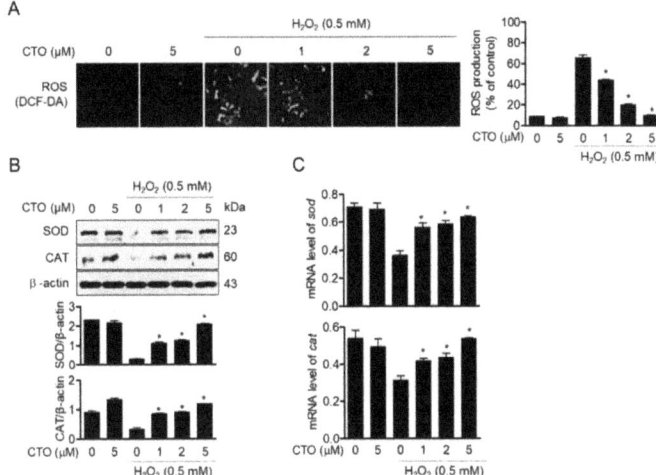

Figure 3. CTO suppresses ROS production by inducing superoxide dismutase (SOD) and catalase (CAT) in SW1353 cells. (**A**) The cells were pre-treated with the indicated concentrations of CTO for 6 h, and then stimulated with or without 0.5 mM H_2O_2 for 2 h. The cells were incubated at 37 °C in the dark for 20 min with culture medium containing 2 µM 2′, 7′-dichlorofluorescin diacetate (DCF-DA) to monitor reactive oxygen species (ROS) production. The degree of ROS production was measured by fluorescence microscope. (**B**) The expression of SOD and CAT proteins were measured by Western blot analysis from cells pre-treated with CTO and stimulated by 0.5 mM H_2O_2. (**C**) The mRNA level of these genes was measured by real-time PCR. * $p < 0.05$ was considered significant compared to only H_2O_2 treat group.

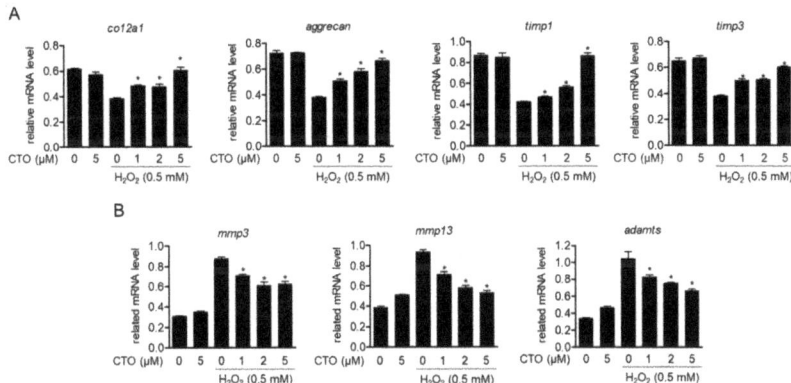

Figure 4. CTO up-regulates chondrocytes-specific genes but inhibits the expression of *mmps* in H_2O_2 treated SW1353 cells. (**A,B**) SW1353 cells were pre-treated with the indicated concentration of CTO (0, 1, 2, and 5 µM) for 6 h, and then incubated with 0.5 mM H_2O_2 for 2 h. The mRNA levels of cartilage-specific core genes and *timps* (**A**) and *mmps* genes (**B**) were determined by real-time PCR analysis. The results were normalized to *gapdh* expression. * $p < 0.05$ was considered significant compared only to H_2O_2 treat group.

3.5. CTO Inhibits Apoptotic Pathway Induced by Treatment with H_2O_2 in SW1353 Cells

To evaluate whether pretreatment with CTO of chondrocytes prevents H_2O_2-induced apoptosis, we measured the confluency of H_2O_2-stimulated cells. Cellular confluency revealed that pretreatment with CTO protected cells from the cytotoxicity of H_2O_2 in chondrocytes in a concentration-dependent manner (Figure 5A). To confirm whether pretreatment with CTO prevents cells to undergo apoptosis, Annexin V and caspase 3/7 from SW1353 cells pretreated with CTO and stimulated with H_2O_2 were detected by IncuCyte imaging system. In the CTO-pretreated cells, the previously increased intensity of Annexin V by H_2O_2 was then significantly reduced, and the previously decreased intensity of caspase 3/7 by H_2O_2 was then enhanced. (Figure 5B). To examine whether CTO pretreatment affected the mRNA levels of anti-apoptotic genes such as *bcl2* and *caspases3* or pro-apoptotic genes including *bax* in H_2O_2-treated conditions, we performed real-time PCR for SW1353 cells incubated with the indicated condition. The expression of *bcl2* and *caspases3* was reduced by H_2O_2 treatment, but retained by CTO pretreatment. On the other hand, the enhanced expression of the pro-apoptotic gene *bax* by H_2O_2 treatment decreased in a concentration-dependent manner by CTO pretreatment (Figure 5C). Protein levels of these genes were confirmed through Western blotting (Figure 5D). These results suggest that CTO pretreatment effectively prevents chondrocytes from H_2O_2-induced apoptosis by regulating the expression of apoptosis-related genes.

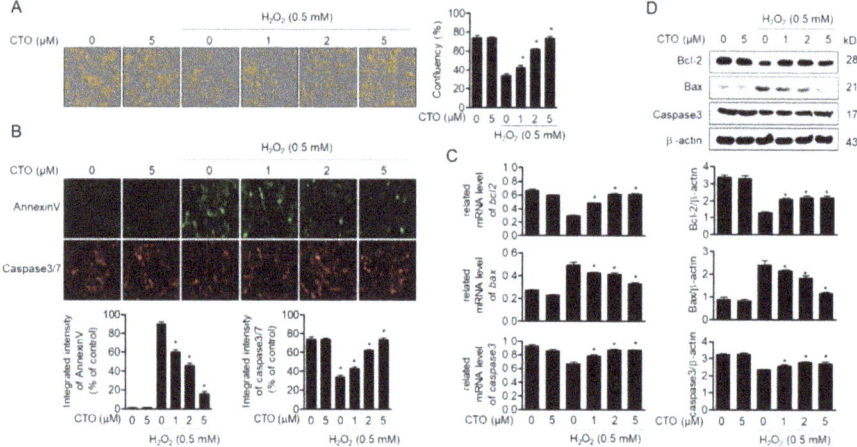

Figure 5. CTO inhibits the apoptotic pathway induced by treatment with H_2O_2 in SW1353 cells. (**A, B**) The cells were pre-treated with or without the indicated concentration of CTO (0, 1, 2, and 5 μM) for 6 h and then incubated with 0.5 mM H_2O_2 for 2 h. The confluency of cells was measured by IncuCyte imaging system (**A**), and apoptotic cells were evaluated by staining with Annexin V and caspase-3/7 (**B**). (**C, D**) The mRNA levels of *bcl-2*, *bax* and *caspase3* were measured by real-time PCR (**C**) and protein expressions were confirmed by Western blot analysis (**D**). The results were normalized to *gapdh* (**C**) or β–actin (**D**) expression. * $p < 0.05$ was considered significant compared to only H_2O_2 treat group.

3.6. Upregulated HO-1 by Pre-Treatment with CTO Protects SW1353 Cells from ROS Production Induced by H_2O_2

In Section 3.2, we showed that CTO effectively induces HO-1 expression by promoting Nrf2 translocation in SW1353 cells. We next investigated the effect of CTO on ROS production and antioxidant enzymes induced by H_2O_2 treatment in suppressing the expression of HO-1 by treatment with tin protoporphyrin IX (SnPP), an inhibitor of heme oxygenase enzyme. CTO treatment suppressed ROS generated by H_2O_2 stimulation in a concentration-dependent manner; however, the inhibitory effect of CTO on ROS production was reversed in the presence of SnPP (Figure 6A). Moreover, the recovery of SOD and CAT expression by pretreatment with CTO in H_2O_2-treated cells was inhibited in the SnPP-treated group (Figure 6B) and mRNA (Figure 6C). These results suggested that HO-1 induced by CTO pretreatment in H_2O_2-stimulated SW1353 cells is involved in the regulation of ROS production and recovery of antioxidant enzymes.

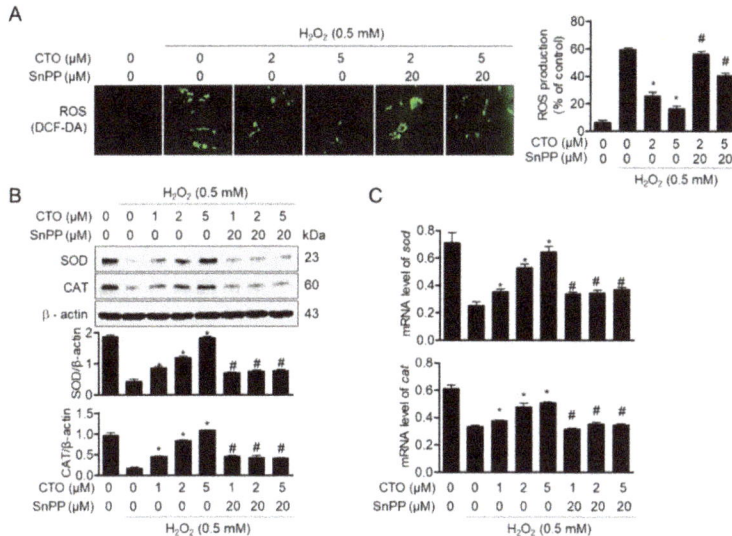

Figure 6. Upregulated HO-1 by pre-treatment with CTO protects SW1353 cells from ROS production induced by H_2O_2. (**A**) SW1353 cells were seeded at a density of 5×10^4 cell/well and pre-treated with or without 20 µM Protoporphyrin IX (SnPP) for 1 h. Then cells were treated with the indicated concentrations of CTO (0, 1, 2, and 5 µM) for 6h, and incubated with 0.5 mM of H_2O_2 for 2h. The cells were incubated with culture medium containing 20 µM DCF-DA to monitor ROS production at 37 °C in the dark for 20 min. The images were obtained by fluorescent microscope system. (**B, C**) Protein expressions and mRNA levels of *sod* and *cat* were detected by Western blot analysis (**B**) and real-time PCR (**C**) from cells cultured with the indicated conditions. The results were normalized with β–actin (**B**) or *gapdh* (**C**) expression. $^*p < 0.05$ vs. only H_2O_2 treat group; $^\#p < 0.05$ vs. only CTO treated group.

3.7. Induced HO-1 by CTO Regulates Chondrocytes-Specific Genes and Expression of mmps in H_2O_2 Treated SW1353 Cell

We evaluated the effects of CTO on the specific genes and its function regulation of chondrocytes. Therefore, we additionally evaluated whether HO-1 expression by pretreatment with CTO protects chondrocyte-specific genes and functions in SW1353 cells in H_2O_2-treated conditions. CTO dose-dependently recovered the mRNA levels of *col2a1, aggrecan, timp1* and *timp3*; however, SnPP-treated cells did not show recovery of *col2a1, aggrecan, timp1* and *timp3* in H_2O_2-treated conditions (Figure 7A). We subsequently evaluated the effect of HO-1 expression by CTO treatment in H_2O_2-stimulated SW1353 cells on the mRNA levels of *mmps* and *adamts*, components of the extracellular matrix. We confirmed that the enhanced mRNA levels of *mmp3, mmp13*, and *adamts* by H_2O_2 were significantly blocked by CTO treatment, but recovered by treatment with SnPP (Figure 7B). These results suggest that the CTO-induced HO-1 protects SW1353 cells against dysfunction caused by H_2O_2 treatment, such as restoring cartilage-specific core proteins and inhibiting proteolytic enzymes.

3.8. Enhanced HO-1 by CTO Shows Protective Effect from Apoptosis Induced by H_2O_2 in SW1353 Cells

In Section 3.7, we confirmed that CTO protected SW1353 cells H_2O_2-induced apoptosis. To investigate whether induced HO-1 expression by CTO pretreatment plays a protective role in apoptosis induced by H_2O_2 treatment, the expression of annexin V and caspase 3/7 were assessed in cells treated with SnPP. Suppression of Annexin V by CTO pretreatment was significantly increased by SnPP treatment. The level of caspase-3/7 upregulated by CTO treatment was re-inhibited by SnPP treatment (Figure 8). These results suggest that the induction of HO-1 by CTO pretreatment prevents H_2O_2-induced apoptosis in SW1353 cells.

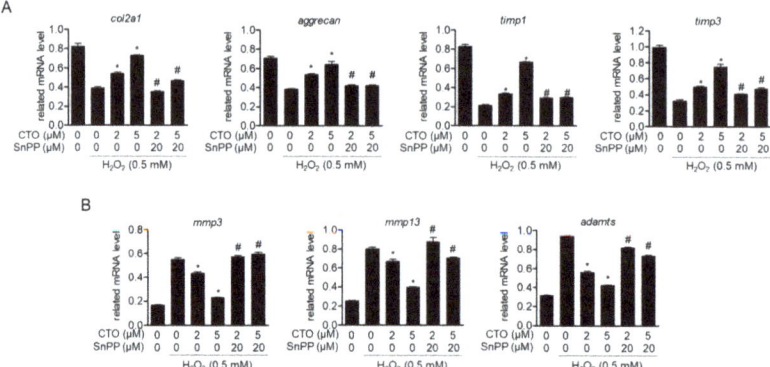

Figure 7. Induced HO-1 by CTO regulates chondrocytes-specific genes and expression of MMPs in H_2O_2 treated SW1353 cells. (**A**, **B**) SW1353 cells were pre-treated with or without 20 µM SnPP for 1h. Then cells were treated with the indicated concentration of CTO (2 or 5 µM) for 6 h, and incubated with 0.5 mM H_2O_2 for 2 h. The mRNA levels of cartilage-specific core genes and *timps* (**A**) and *mmps* genes (**B**) were determined by real-time PCR analysis. The results were normalized to *gapdh* expression. * $p < 0.05$ vs. only H_2O_2 treat group; # $p < 0.05$ vs. only CTO treated group.

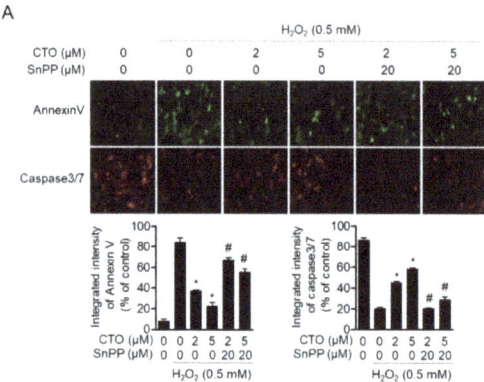

Figure 8. Enhanced HO-1 by CTO shows a protective effect from apoptosis induced by H_2O_2 in SW1353 cells. (**A**) SW1353 cells were pre-treated with or without 20 µM SnPP for 1h. Then cells were treated with the indicated concentration of CTO (2 or 5 µM) for 6 h, and incubated with 0.5 mM H_2O_2 for 2 h. Apoptotic cells were evaluated by staining with caspase 3/7. Reagents using IncuCyte imaging system. * $p < 0.05$ vs. only H_2O_2 treat group; # $p < 0.05$ vs. only CTO treated group.

4. Discussion

Promoting the expression of antioxidant enzymes in articular chondrocytes and inhibiting oxidative stress has been considered as a potential therapeutic approach in OA [25,26]. Hydrogen peroxide (H_2O_2) is a general type of ROS, and enzymes such as SOD, CAT, GPX, glutathione reductase (GR), and HO-1 protect the oxides caused by oxidative stress [27]. Nrf2 is a nuclear transcription factor that promotes the expression of antioxidant-related enzymes, such as HO-1, through binding to antioxidant response elements (AREs) and shows a protective role against cellular damages [28].

The MAPK pathway is involved in the translocation of Nrf2 to regulate oxidative stress [29]. Western blot analysis showed that CTO increased HO-1 expression depending on the concentration and time of translocation of Nrf2 to the nucleus. Moreover, CTO enhanced the phosphorylation of MAPKs in a time-dependent manner. These results suggest that CTO defends the cells against oxidative damage by up-regulating HO-1 expression via the MAPK pathway.

As one of several antioxidant mechanisms to prevent ROS-induced damage, SOD and CAT play vital roles in reducing oxidative stress by removing H_2O_2 [30]. In these mechanisms, CTO down-regulated the level of ROS stimulated by H_2O_2, and Western blot analysis showed the recovery of expression levels of antioxidant enzymes previously inhibited by H_2O_2. Reduced expression of Col2A1 and Aggrecan in chondrocytes is an important feature of cartilage degeneration; MMP-3 and MMP-13 are responsible for the degradation of the extracellular matrix that damages cartilage structures and properties, and TIMPs inhibit activities of these MMPs [31,32]. Inhibition of MMPs is recognized as a major treatment strategy to block joint cartilage loss in OA, and H_2O_2 promotes the expression and secretion of enzymes such as MMP-3, MMP-13, and ADAMTS [33]. CTO effectively inhibited the MMP-3, MMP-13, and ADAMTS enzymes secreted from H_2O_2 stimulated chondrocytes, and recovered Col2A1, Aggrecan, and TIMP mRNA, which play an essential role in cartilage degeneration caused by H_2O_2. From the previous results, CTO is an HO-1 inducer. Therefore, to investigate the protective effect of CTO-induced HO-1 expression on the H_2O_2-stimulated chondrocytes, we reversed the protective effect of chondrocytes by treatment with SnPP, an HO-1 inhibitor.

H_2O_2 causes apoptosis by increasing the production of ROS and destroying the mitochondrial membrane potential, which activates Bax of apoptosis and inactivates antiapoptosis Bcl-2 [34,35]. It also sequentially activates stimulators of apoptosis, such as caspase-3 and 7 [36]. In this study, CTO recovered the mRNA and protein expression levels of the anti-apoptotic protein BCL-2 in H_2O-treated conditions and further inhibited those of apoptotic stimulants, such as BAX, induced by H_2O_2. The protein and mRNA levels of caspase-3 were also reversed. Previous studies showed that hypoxia leads to the formation of ROS, which induces oxidative stress and partially activates the transcription factor Nrf2, resulting in HO-1 expression and hypoxia-inducible factors through the phosphoinositide 3-kinase (PI3K)/Akt signaling pathway [37]. In this study, H_2O_2-stimulated SW1353 chondrocytes were treated with SnPP, an HO-1 inhibitor, to suppress HO-1 expression induced by CTO. Therefore, the ROS inhibitory and anti-apoptotic effects of CTO as shown above, and the expression of antioxidant enzymes, were reversed. These results suggest that the protective effect on chondrocytes appears through HO-1 expression by the activity of Nrf2 by CTO rather than by Nrf2 activity by H_2O_2. These results suggest that, through activation of Nrf2 and HO-1, CTO could suppress ROS production and apoptosis as well as regulate antioxidant enzyme expression stimulated by H_2O_2 in SW1353 cells.

5. Conclusions

In this study, we investigated the effects of CTO on apoptotic, antioxidant enzymes and cartilage-specific proteins caused by ROS, a major cause of osteoarthritis in H_2O_2 stimulated SW1353 cells. We found that CTO effectively regulated ROS generation by H_2O_2 and apoptosis of SW1353 through Nrf2/HO-1 activity, and recovered lost antioxidant enzymes. This study revealed a new pharmacological effect of prenylated xanthones CTO, isolated from *M. tricuspidata*, and suggests its potential as a novel natural treatment for osteoarthritis.

Author Contributions: E.-N.K. and H.-S.L. performed the experiments and wrote the manuscript, performed the statistical analysis. G.-S.J. participated in study design and coordination as well as drafting the manuscript. All authors have read and agreed to the published version of the manuscript.

Funding: This work was supported by Basic Science Research Program through the National Research Foundation of Korea (NRF) funded by the Ministry of Education (NRF-2016R1A6A1A03011325).

Conflicts of Interest: The authors declare no conflict of interest.

References

1. Chen, D.; Shen, J.; Zhao, W.; Wang, T.; Han, L.; Hamilton, J.L.; Im, H.J. Osteoarthritis: Toward a comprehensive understanding of pathological mechanism. *Bone Res.* **2017**, *5*, 16044. [CrossRef] [PubMed]
2. Felson, D.T.; Anderson, J.J.; Naimark, A. The prevalence of knee osteoarthritis in the elderly. The framingham osteoarthritis study. *Arthritis Rheum.* **1987**, *30*, 914–918. [CrossRef] [PubMed]
3. Kapoor, M.; Martel-Pelletier, J.; Lajeunesse, D. Role of proinflammatory cytokines in the pathophysiology of osteoarthritis. *Nat. Rev. Rheumatol.* **2011**, *7*, 33–42. [CrossRef] [PubMed]
4. Hayami, T.; Funaki, H.; Yaoeda, K. Expression of the cartilage derived anti-angiogenic factor chondromodulin-I decreases in the early stage of experimental osteoarthritis. *J. Rheumatol.* **2003**, *30*, 2207–2217.
5. Pacifici, M.; Koyama, E.; Iwamoto, M.; Gentili, C. Development of articular cartilage: What do we know about it and how may it occur? *Connect Tissue Res.* **2000**, *41*, 175–184. [CrossRef]
6. Mendes, A.F.; Carvalho, A.P.; Caramona, M.M.; Lopes, M.C. Diphenyleneiodonium inhibits NF-kappaB activation and iNOS expression induced by IL-1beta: Involvement of reactive oxygen species. *Mediators Inflamm.* **2001**, *10*, 209–215. [CrossRef]
7. Ndisang, J.F. Synergistic interaction between heme oxygenase (HO) and nuclear-factor E2-related factor-2 (Nrf2) against oxidative stress in cardiovascular related diseases. *Curr. Pharm. Des.* **2017**, *23*, 1465–1470. [CrossRef]
8. Lee, D.H.; Park, J.S.; Lee, Y.S.; Sung, S.H.; Lee, Y.H.; Bae, S.H. The hypertension drug, verapamil, activates Nrf2 by promoting p62-dependent autophagic Keap1 degradation and prevents acetaminophen-induced cytotoxicity. *BMB Rep.* **2017**, *50*, 91–96. [CrossRef]
9. Jaramillo, M.C.; Zhang, D.D. The emerging role of the Nrf2-Keap1 signaling pathway in cancer. *Genes Dev.* **2013**, *27*, 2179–2191. [CrossRef]
10. Ryter, S.W.; Tyrrell, R.M. The heme synthesis and degradation pathways: Role in oxidant sensitivity. Heme oxygenase has both pro- and antioxidant properties. *Free Radic. Biol. Med.* **2000**, *28*, 289–309. [CrossRef]
11. Takahashi, T.; Morita, K.; Akagi, R.; Sassa, S. Heme oxygenase-1: A novel therapeutic target in oxidative tissue injuries. *Curr. Med. Chem.* **2004**, *11*, 1545–1561. [CrossRef] [PubMed]
12. Zhou, H.; Lu, F.; Latham, C.; Zander, D.S.; Visner, G.A. Heme oxygenase-1 expression in human lungs with cystic fibrosis and cytoprotective effects against Pseudomonas aeruginosa in vitro. *Am. J. Respir. Crit. Care Med.* **2004**, *170*, 633–640. [CrossRef] [PubMed]
13. Hiep, N.T.; Kwon, J.; Kim, D.W.; Hwang, B.Y.; Lee, H.J.; Mar, W.; Lee, D. Isoflavones with neuroprotective activities from fruits of *Cudrania tricuspidata*. *Phytochemistry* **2015**, *111*, 141–148. [CrossRef] [PubMed]
14. Lee, H.; Ha, H.; Lee, J.K.; Seo, C.s.; Lee, N.h.; Jung, D.Y.; Park, S.J.; Shin, H.K. The fruits of *Cudrania tricuspidata* suppress development of atopic dermatitis in NC/Nga mice. *Phytother. Res.* **2012**, *26*, 594–599. [CrossRef]
15. Han, X.H.; Hong, S.S.; Jin, Q.; Li, D.; Kim, H.K.; Lee, J.; Kwon, S.H.; Lee, D.; Lee, C.K.; Lee, M.K. Prenylated and benzylated flavonoids from the fruits of *Cudrania tricuspidata*. *J. Nat. Prod.* **2008**, *72*, 164–167. [CrossRef]
16. Tian, Y.H.; Kim, H.C.; Cui, J.M.; Kim, Y.C. Hepatoprotective constituents of *Cudrania tricuspidata*. *Arch. Pharm. Res.* **2005**, *28*, 44–48. [CrossRef]
17. Jeong, G.S.; An, R.B.; Pae, H.O.; Chung, H.T.; Yoon, K.H.; Kang, D.G.; Lee, H.S.; Kim, Y.C. Cudratricusxanthone A protects mouse hippocampal cells against glutamate-induced neurotoxicity via the induction of heme oxygenase-1. *Planta Med.* **2008**, *74*, 1368–1373. [CrossRef]
18. Quang, T.H.; Ngan, N.T.; Yoon, C.S.; Cho, K.H.; Kang, D.G.; Lee, H.S.; Kim, Y.C.; Oh, H. Protein tyrosine phosphatase 1B inhibitors from the roots of *Cudrania tricuspidata*. *Molecules* **2015**, *20*, 11173–11183. [CrossRef]
19. Jeong, G.S.; Lee, D.S.; Kim, Y.C. Cudratricusxanthone A from Cudrania Tricuspidata suppresses pro-Inflammatory mediators through expression of anti-inflammatory Heme oxygenase-1 in RAW264.7 macrophages. *Int. Immunopharmacol.* **2009**, *9*, 241–246. [CrossRef]
20. Xiaolei, X.; Xudan, L.; Yingchun, Y.; Jianyi, H.; Mengqi, J.; Yue, H.; Xiaotong, L.; Li, L.; Hailun, G. Resveratrol Exerts Anti-Osteoarthritic Effect by Inhibiting TLR4/NF-κB Signaling Pathway via the TLR4/Akt/FoxO1 Axis in IL-1β-Stimulated SW1353 Cells. *Drug Des. Dev. Ther.* **2020**, *14*, 2079–2090.
21. Huang, T.C.; Chang, W.T.; Hu, Y.C.; Hsieh, B.S.; Cheng, H.L.; Yen, J.H.; Chiu, P.R.; Chang, K.L. Zinc Protects Articular Chondrocytes through Changes in Nrf2-Mediated Antioxidants, Cytokines and Matrix Metalloproteinases. *Nutrients* **2018**, *10*, 471. [CrossRef] [PubMed]

22. Park, C.; Jeong, J.W.; Lee, D.S.; Yim, M.J.; Lee, J.M.; Han, M.H.; Kim, S.; Kim, H.S.; Kim, G.Y.; Park, E.K.; et al. *Sargassum serratifolium* Extract Attenuates Interleukin-1_-Induced Oxidative Stress and Inflammatory Response in Chondrocytes by Suppressing the Activation of NF-kB, p38 MAPK, and PI3K/Akt. *Int. J. Mol. Sci.* **2018**, *19*, 2308. [CrossRef] [PubMed]
23. Hong, G.U.; Lee, J.Y.; Kang, H.; Kim, T.Y.; Park, J.Y.; Hong, E.Y.; Shin, Y.H.; Jung, S.H.; Chang, H.B.; Kim, Y.H.; et al. Inhibition of Osteoarthritis-RelatedMolecules by Isomucronulatol 7-O-β-D-glucoside and Ecliptasaponin A in IL-1β-Stimulated Chondrosarcoma Cell Model. *Molecules* **2018**, *23*, 2807. [CrossRef] [PubMed]
24. Lee, W.H.; Ku, S.K.; Kim, T.I.; Kim, E.N.; Park, E.K.; Jeong, G.S.; Bae, J.S. Inhibitory effects of cudratricusxanthone O on particulate matter-induced pulmonary injury. *Int. J. Environ. Health Res.* **2019**, 1–14. [CrossRef]
25. Cai, D.; Yin, S.; Yang, J.; Jiang, Q.; Cao, W. Histone deacetylase inhibition activates Nrf2 and protects against osteoarthritis. *Arthritis Res. Ther.* **2015**, *17*, 269. [CrossRef] [PubMed]
26. Takada, T.; Miyaki, S.; Ishitobi, H.; Hirai, Y.; Nakasa, T.; Igarashi, K.; Lotz, M.K.; Ochi, M. Bach1 deficiency reduces severity of osteoarthritis through upregulation of heme oxygenase-1. *Arthritis Res. Ther.* **2015**, *17*, 285. [CrossRef] [PubMed]
27. Jakus, V. The role of free radicals, oxidative stress and antioxidant systems in diabetic vascular disease. *Bratislavské Lekárske Listy* **2000**, *101*, 541–551.
28. Kang, K.W.; Lee, S.J.; Kim, S.G. Molecular mechanism of Nrf2 activation by oxidative stress. *Antioxid. Redox. Sign.* **2005**, *7*, 1664–1673. [CrossRef]
29. Wu, P.S.; Yen, J.H.; Kou, M.C.; Wu, M.J. "Luteolin and apigenin attenuate 4-hydroxy-2-nonenal-mediated cell death through modulation of UPR, Nrf2-ARE and MAPK pathways in PC12 cells. *PLoS ONE* **2015**, *10*. [CrossRef]
30. Okamoto, O.K.; Robertson, D.L.; Fagan, T.F. Different regulatory mechanisms modulate the expression of a dinoflagellate iron-superoxide dismutase. *J. Biol. Chem.* **2001**, *276*, 19989–19993. [CrossRef]
31. Poole, A.R.; Kobayashi, M.; Yasuda, T.; Laverty, S.; Mwale, F.; Kojima, T.; Sakai, T.; Wahl, C.; El-Maadawy, S.; Webb, G.; et al. Type II collagen degradation and its regulation in articular cartilage in osteoarthritis. *Ann. Rheum. Dis.* **2002**, *61*, 78–81. [CrossRef] [PubMed]
32. Sandya, S.; Achan, M.A.; Sudhakaran, P.R. Multiple matrix metalloproteinases in type II collagen induced arthritis. *Indian J. Clin. Biochem.* **2009**, *24*, 42–48. [CrossRef] [PubMed]
33. Mancini, F.; Nannarone, S.; Buratta, S.; Ferrara, G.; Stabile, A.M.; Vuerich, M. Effects of xylazine and dexmedetomidine on equine articular chondrocytes *in vitro*. *Vet. Anaesth. Analg.* **2017**, *44*, 295–308. [CrossRef] [PubMed]
34. Ott, M.; Robertson, J.D.; Gogvadze, V.; Zhivotovsky, B.; Orrenius, S. Cytochrome c release from mitochondria proceeds by a two-step process. *Proc. Natl. Acad. Sci. USA* **2002**, *99*, 1259–1263. [CrossRef] [PubMed]
35. Gogvadze, V.; Orrenius, S.; Zhivotovsky, B. Multiple pathways of cytochrome c release from mitochondria in apoptosis. *Biochim. Biophys. Acta.* **2006**, *1757*, 639–647. [CrossRef]
36. Kiraz, Y.; Adan, A.; Kartal Yandim, M.; Baran, Y. Major apoptotic mechanisms and genes involved in apoptosis. *Tumour Biol.* **2016**, *37*, 8471–8486. [CrossRef]
37. Zhao, R.; Feng, J.; He, G. Hypoxia increases Nrf2-induced HO-1 expression via the PI3K/Akt pathway. *Front. Biosci.* **2016**, *21*, 385–396.

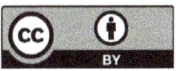

© 2020 by the authors. Licensee MDPI, Basel, Switzerland. This article is an open access article distributed under the terms and conditions of the Creative Commons Attribution (CC BY) license (http://creativecommons.org/licenses/by/4.0/).

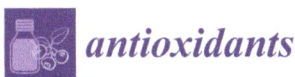

Article

Modulation and Protection Effects of Antioxidant Compounds against Oxidant Induced Developmental Toxicity in Zebrafish

Nuria Boix [1,2,*], Elisabet Teixido [1,2], Ester Pique [1,2], Juan Maria Llobet [1,2] and Jesus Gomez-Catalan [1,2]

1. Toxicology Unit, Pharmacology, Toxicology and Therapeutical Chemistry Department, Pharmacy School, University of Barcelona, Avda Joan XXIII s/n 08028 Barcelona, Spain; eteixido1511@ub.edu (E.T.); esterpique@ub.edu (E.P.); jmllobet@ub.edu (J.M.L.); jesusgomez@ub.edu (J.G.-C.)
2. INSA-UB Nutrition and Food Safety Research Institute, University of Barcelona, Food and Nutrition Torribera Campus, Prat de la Riba 171, 08921 Santa Coloma de Gramenet, Spain
* Correspondence: nuriaboix@ub.edu; Tel.: +34-934-020-277

Received: 22 July 2020; Accepted: 4 August 2020; Published: 8 August 2020

Abstract: The antioxidant effect of compounds is regularly evaluated by in vitro assays that do not have the capability to predict in vivo protective activity or to determine their underlying mechanisms of action. The aim of this study was to develop an experimental system to evaluate the in vivo protective effects of different antioxidant compounds, based on the zebrafish embryo test. Zebrafish embryos were exposed to tert-butyl hydroperoxide (tBOOH), tetrachlorohydroquinone (TCHQ) and lipopolysaccharides from *Escherichia coli* (LPS), chemicals that are known inducers of oxidative stress in zebrafish. The developmental toxic effects (lethality or dysmorphogenesis) induced by these chemicals were modulated with N-acetyl L-cysteine and Nω-nitro L-arginine methyl ester hydrochloride, dimethyl maleate and DL-buthionine sulfoximine in order to validate the oxidant mechanism of oxidative stress inducers. The oxidant effects of tBOOH, TCHQ, and LPS were confirmed by the determination of significant differences in the comparison between the concentration–response curves of the oxidative stress inducers and of the modulators of antioxidant status. This concept was also applied to the study of the effects of well-known antioxidants, such as vitamin E, quercetin, and lipoic acid. Our results confirm the zebrafish model as an in vivo useful tool to test the protective effects of antioxidant compounds.

Keywords: oxidative stress; zebrafish embryo; in vivo model; antioxidant effect

---

1. Introduction

Reactive oxygen species (ROS) and reactive nitrogen species (RNS) are products of cellular metabolism, which play a dual role in beneficial and deleterious effects over different organs [1]. Aerobic organisms have antioxidant defenses to protect cells from oxidative damage. These defenses can be enzymatic (antioxidant enzymes) or non-enzymatic (antioxidant compounds) [2]. The imbalance between reactive metabolite production and antioxidant defenses in the organism is denominated oxidative stress (OS) and can produce potential detrimental effects in the organisms [3]. The consequences of OS can be very variable depending on the reactive species implicated, the subcellular structure where they are generated, the organs or tissues implicated in the effect, the genetic characteristics of the organism or developmental stage, among other factors. It is a phenomenon which has been related to different processes (aging, cancer, diabetes, cardiovascular and neurodegenerative diseases, etc.) as it can damage and inhibit the normal function of lipids, proteins, and DNA [4].

Antioxidants are chemicals that can inhibit or prevent oxidation processes. Such compounds can be produced within the human body or absorbed from dietary intake [5]. The antioxidant capacity of compounds is usually evaluated by in vitro techniques as the oxygen radical absorbance capacity (ORAC) or the total radical-trapping antioxidant parameter (TRAP), which are useful for the high-throughput screening of the antioxidative or radical-scavenging capacities of the compounds [6]. There are also cell-culture approaches, such as the cell-based antioxidant assay (CAA), which uses Caco-2 cells that allow for the study of intracellular influence of antioxidant chemicals [7]. These in vitro assays and biological techniques, which are regularly used to evaluate antioxidant capacity, do not have predictive capability for the protective activity that natural compounds have in vivo, or to determine their underlying mechanisms of action [8]. In vivo assays of antioxidant capacity of natural compounds have been performed in mice [9], in rats [10], and using other animal models, such as *Caenorhabditis elegans* [11] and adult zebrafish [12]. However, until now none of these in vivo models have been established and validated to systematically evaluate the protective effects of natural compounds.

Zebrafish (*Danio rerio*, ZF) is a tropical fish of the *Cyprinidae* family. The ZF embryo is considered a potential tool for investigating environmental exposures with direct relation to human health [13]. The ZF embryo presents multiple advantages, from which it can be highlighted that it is an in vivo model which studies the whole organism, with the main characteristics of an in vitro model: easy maintenance, large number of offspring, rapid embryonic development, possibility to combine with other biochemical, cellular and molecular techniques, screening of compounds, application to high-throughput methods, etc. [14–16]. The ZF embryo has been used as a model to study alterations and diseases related to OS mechanisms: inflammation [17], senescence [18], teratogenicity [19], neurodegenerative [20], and cardiovascular diseases [21]. Furthermore, ZF presents antioxidant genes and enzymes to protect them against OS effects. These defenses are analogous to mammalian antioxidant systems [22,23]. The protective effects of some antioxidants against exposure to OS inducers in ZF embryos have been studied with the objective to investigate the antioxidant mechanisms of action and demonstrate the usefulness of these antioxidants against oxidative damage [19,24,25].

The aim of the present work was to design an experimental system based on the ZF embryo test, which could be the basis for the study of in vivo protective effects of chemicals with antioxidant activity against oxidant-induced developmental toxicity in ZF embryos.

2. Materials and Methods

2.1. Chemicals and Solution Preparation

Tetrachlorohydroquinone (TCHQ, CAS number 87-87-6), lipopolysaccharides from *Escherichia coli* 0111:B4 (LPS), Nω–nitro L-arginine methyl ester hydrochloride (L-NAME, CAS number 51298-62-5), DL-buthionine sulfoximine (BSO, CAS number 5072-26-4), (±)-α-tocopherol (vitamin E, CAS number 10191-41-0), (±)-α-lipoic acid (lipoic acid, CAS number 1077-28-7), and quercetin hydrate (quercetin, CAS number 337951) were obtained from Sigma-Aldrich, Madrid, Spain. Tert-butyl hydroperoxide (tBOOH, CAS number: 75-91-2) was acquired from TCI Europe and N-acetyl-L-cysteine (NAC, CAS number 616-91-1) and diethyl maleate (DEM, CAS number 141-05-9) were obtained from Cymit Química, Barcelona, Spain.

tBOOH, LPS, NAC, and DEM were directly dissolved in 0.3X Danieau's buffer (17.4 mM NaCl; 0.23 mM KCl; 0.12 mM $MgSO_4 \cdot 7 H_2O$; 0.18 mM $Ca(NO_3)_2$; 1.5 mM HEPES (N-(2-hydroxyethyl) piperazine-N'-(2-ethanesulfonic acid); pH 7.4). TCHQ, vit. E, quercetin, and lipoic acid were dissolved in 100% dimethyl sulfoxide (DMSO, Sigma-Aldrich, Madrid, Spain) and subsequently diluted in 0.3× Danieau's buffer to a final DMSO concentration of 0.05 % (*v/v*).

Our previous experience with 0.05 % DMSO in 0.3× Danieau's buffer clearly indicates that it does not produce any effects in lethality or dysmorphogenesis in ZF embryos, and it was not expected to modify the toxicity of the compounds. Moreover, DMSO is only expected to modify the permeability of chemicals if used at higher concentrations > 0.1% [26].

Concentrations of all chemicals are expressed in molarity, except for LPS that is given as µg/mL, due to the variable molecular mass of LPS, as it is part of the outer membrane of bacteria—in this case, *Escherichia coli*.

2.2. Animals and Embryo Production

Adult wild type ZF (BCN Piscicultura Iberica; Terrassa, Spain) were kept in aquariums with a closed flow-through system at 26 ± 1 °C and 10–14 h constant dark–light cycle. Females and males were housed separately and fed with commercial flakes and brine shrimp (Ocean Nutrition, San Diego, USA). The day before the experiments, females and males were transferred to a breeding tank (10 females; 8 males). ZF embryos were collected within 1 h after the onset of lights in the morning. They were extensively cleaned, and fertilized eggs were staged according to [27] and selected for subsequent exposure under a dissection stereomicroscope (Motic SMZ168, Motic China Group, LTD., Luwan, Shanghai, China). The study was approved by the Ethic Committee for Animal Experimentation of the University of Barcelona and by the Department of Environment and Housing of the Generalitat de Catalunya with license number DAAM 7971.

2.3. Exposure of Zebrafish Embryos to Oxidative Stress Related Compounds

To characterize the effects on embryonic development produced by compounds related to OS, ZF embryos were exposed to OS inducers, modulators of antioxidant status and antioxidants. For compounds which were dissolved in DMSO and diluted with Danieau's buffer, a vehicle negative control group with 0.05% DMSO in 0.3× Danieau's buffer was assayed.

Exposures to antioxidants and to modulators were performed from 2 to 26 h post-fertilization (hpf) in order to select, for each of the compounds of study, the highest concentration at which any effect in lethality or in embryonic development was observed (maximum tolerable concentration, MTC). From 26 to 50 hpf, embryos were incubated with 0.3× Danieau's buffer with or without DMSO, depending on the dissolution of the compound of study.

Exposure to OS inducers was conducted from 26 to 50 hpf to select the working concentrations of these compounds for the experimental design. In this case, from 2 to 26 hpf, embryos were incubated with Danieau's buffer with or without DMSO, depending on the dissolution of the compound of study.

Exposure of ZF embryos was semi-static and was carried out in 6-well plates (Greiner Bio-one, Frickenhausen, Germany). Ten embryos per group were selected and randomly distributed into the wells and filled with 5mL of the corresponding solution of the compound. Embryos were incubated at 26 ± 1 °C with a dark–light cycle of 10–14 h. Renewal of the medium and of the solutions was made every 24 h. Evaluation of the embryos was performed at different time points. Lethality was determined at 8, 26, and 50 hpf based on egg coagulation, the absence of tail detachment, or somite formation and the absence of heartbeat [28]. Dysmorphogenic effects were evaluated at 50 hpf by the total morphological score system described by [29]. For each compound of study, at least three independent experiments were performed using embryos from different spawning events ($n = 3$).

The percentage of lethality and of dysmorphogenesis was calculated per compound at every tested concentration, and the concentration–response curves for these effects were plotted. From these curves the concentration, which produced mortality to 50% of the embryos (lethal concentration 50, LC_{50}), and the concentration at which 50% of the embryos presented at least one dysmorphogenic feature (effective concentration 50 for dysmorphogenesis, EC_{50}), were calculated.

2.4. Pre-Exposure of the Embryos to Modulators of Antioxidant Status + Exposure to OS Inducers

To elucidate the OS role in the developmental effects produced by OS inducers, another assay was performed by modulating the ZF embryos' OS responses through pre-exposure to the MTC of compounds which can affect OS conditions, and the posterior exposure to the working concentrations of OS inducers. NAC and L-NAME were used to potentiate antioxidant status, as NAC increases glutathione levels [30] and L-NAME inhibits nitric oxide production [31]. On the other hand, DEM and BSO were used to inhibit glutathione synthesis [32] by increasing the sensitivity of the embryos to OS.

At 2 hpf, embryos were pre-exposed to the MTC of modulators of antioxidant status for 24 h, and then washed with 0.3× Danieau's buffer. At 26 hpf, embryos were exposed to OS inducers at the selected working concentrations. Lethality and dysmorphogenesis were evaluated as previously described, and concentration–response curves were plotted. A comparison of the concentration–response curves of pre-exposure to modulators of antioxidant status + exposure to OS inducers with concentration–response curves of OS inducers exposure was performed.

2.5. Pre-Exposure of the Embryos to Antioxidant Compounds + Exposure to OS Inducer

To detect the protective effects of chemicals against oxidant induced developmental toxicity in ZF embryos, different compounds with well determined antioxidant activity were assayed.

A pre-exposure to the MTC of vitamin (vit.) E, lipoic acid and quercetin was performed from 2 to 26 hpf, followed by a washing step with 0.3× Danieau's solution and the exposure to the working concentrations of the selected OS inducer for 24 h. Evaluation of the embryos was performed as described before, and concentration–response curves were graphically represented. A comparison between the concentration–response curves of pre-exposure to antioxidants + exposure to the selected OS inducer with the concentration–response curve of the exposure to the selected OS inducer was performed.

2.6. Data Evaluation

Comparison of categorical variables was performed with the Fisher's exact test. Concentration–response curves for lethality and dysmorphogenesis were fitted to all the data using the Hill model in GraphPad Prism 6 software and compared with the extra sum-of-squares F test, which compares the parameters fit to datasets (GraphPad Software, La Jolla, CA, USA). Confidence intervals were set at 95% and a probability of $p < 0.05$ was considered as statistically significant.

3. Results

3.1. Characterization of the Effects of Oxidative Stress Related Compounds in Zebrafish Embryos

The results of the characterization of the lethal and dysmorphogenic effects produced by ZF embryos exposure to OS inducers, modulators and antioxidants are shown in Table 1.

Table 1. Characterization of lethality and dysmorphogenesis in zebrafish embryos, produced by oxidative stress-related compounds.

Compounds	Range of Concentrations	MTC	LC$_{50}$	EC$_{50}$	Exposure Window
OS Inducers					
Tert-butyl hydroperoxide (tBOOH)	1–4 mM	n.d.[a]	2.4 mM	1.6 mM	26–50 hpf
Tetrachlorohydroquinone (TCHQ)	2.5–20 µM	n.d.[a]	16.0 µM	3.9 µM	26–50 hpf
Lipopolysaccharides from *Escherichia coli* 0111:B4 (LPS)	5–60 µg/mL	25 µg/mL	50.1 µg/mL	35.9 µg/mL	26–50 hpf
Modulators of Antioxidant Status					
N-acetyl-L-cysteine (NAC)	50–2500 µM	250 µM	1874 µM	920.6 µM	2–26 hpf
Diethyl maleate (DEM)	0.1–100 µM	0.5 µM	n.d.[b]	1.5 µM	2–26 hpf
Nω-nitro L-arginine methyl ester hydrochloride (L-NAME)	0.1–100 µM	5 µM	n.d.[c]	44.36 µM	2–26 hpf
DL-buthionine sulfoximine (BSO)	1–5000 µM	50 µM	n.d.[c]	2722 µM	2–26 hpf
Antioxidants					
Vit. E	1–1000 µM	100 µM	n.d.[d]	n.d.[d]	2–26 hpf
Lipoic acid	0.1–1000 µM	5 µM	116.4 µM	n.d.[c]	2–26 hpf
Quercetin	0.1–30 µM [e]	20 µM	n.d.[d]	n.d.[d]	2–26 hpf

Range of tested concentrations, maximum tolerable concentration (MTC), lethal concentration 50 (LC$_{50}$), effective concentration 50 for dysmorphogenesis (EC$_{50}$) and exposure window for each of the studied compounds. n.d.: data were not determined. [a]: MTC was not determined because the compound produced lethal or dysmorphogenic effects at all the studied concentrations. [b]: LC$_{50}$ was not calculated because no lethal effects were observed until the highest concentration, where lethality was of 100%. [c]: LC$_{50}$ or EC$_{50}$ was not calculated because no significant effects in the mortality of the embryos were observed. [d]: LC$_{50}$ and EC$_{50}$ were not calculated because the compounds did not produce lethal or dysmorphogenic effects at any of the tested concentrations. [e]: Quercetin solution precipitated from 30 µM. It was not possible to evaluate the effects at higher concentrations.

OS inducers produced developmental effects in zebrafish embryos (lethality and dysmorphogenic effects), which were concentration-dependent. Modulators of antioxidant status and antioxidants did not produce lethality at the studied concentrations, and the dysmorphogenic effects observed in the embryos exposed to the tested compounds were mainly developmental delay, cardiac oedema, and brain necrosis, which were not specific alterations. The only compound-specific effect was observed in TCHQ exposure, which produced an effect in the pigmentation of the embryos.

3.2. Pre-Exposure to Modulators of Antioxidant Status + Exposure to OS Inducers

We attempted to modulate the embryotoxic and lethal effects produced by OS inducers in zebrafish embryos by pre-exposing them to a set of known modulators of antioxidant status in zebrafish (Table 2), in order to evaluate if the effects produced by OS inducers were caused by an OS mechanism.

Table 2. Lethality and dysmorphogenesis effective concentration values in zebrafish embryos on the modulation of developmental effects produced by OS inducers.

Modulator of Antioxidant Status	OS Inducer	LC_{50} (95% CI)	EC_{50} (95% CI)
None [1]		2.38 mM (2.28–2.48)	1.64 mM (1.44–1.87)
N-acetyl-L-cysteine (NAC)		n.d.	2.28 mM ** (2.11–2.46)
N_ω-nitro L-arginine methyl ester hydrochloride (L-NAME)	Tert-butyl hydroperoxide (tBOOH)	n.d.	3.17 mM *** (2.85–3.52)
Diethyl maleate (DEM)		2.06 mM * (1.78–2.38)	1.17 mM ** (1.07–1.29)
DL-buthionine sulfoximine (BSO)		1.95 mM *** (1.85–2.05)	1.20 mM * (1.07–1.33)
None		15.2 µM (13.8–16.7)	8.84 µM (7.15–10.9)
NAC		19.6 µM * (16.6–23.3)	15.5 µM *** (14.8-16.3)
L-NAME	Tetrachlorohydroquinone (TCHQ)	19.0 µM * (17.3–20.9)	17.1 µM *** (16.9–17.3)
DEM		9.78 µM ** (7.31–13.1)	4.79 µM * (3.88–5.91)
BSO		6.89 µM *** (6.13–7.75)	4.17 µM ** (3.62–4.81)
None [1]		50.1 µg/mL (48.6–51.8)	36.0 µg/mL (28.4–45.6)
NAC		51.6 µg/mL * (48.8–54.5)	39.6 µg/mL (35.0–44.8)
L-NAME	Lipopolysaccharides from *Escherichia coli* 0111:B4 (LPS)	53.4 µg/mL * (51.9–55.0)	51.3 µg/mL ** (49.6–53.0)
DEM		42.1 µg/mL *** (37.9–46.8)	31.1 µg/mL (26.3–36.6)
BSO		45.2 µg/mL ** (43.2–47.4)	36.2 µg/mL (29.4–44.5)

Lethal concentration 50 (LC_{50}), effective concentration 50 for dysmorphogenesis (EC_{50}) and 95% confidence interval. Statistically significant differences with respect to the group, which was not exposed to any modulator: *: $p < 0.05$; **: $p < 0.01$; ***: $p < 0.001$; n.d.: no lethality was observed; [1] A unique tBOOH and LPS concentration–response curve was generated with the dissolution of the compounds in Danieau's buffer without DMSO and compared to all the concentration–response curves of the groups pre-exposed to chemicals (initially dissolved or not in DMSO) due to the lack of effect of DMSO in the embryonic development of ZF.

In embryos which were exposed to tBOOH, a pre-exposure to NAC and L-NAME significantly drifted the tBOOH concentration–response curves to higher concentrations (Figure 1), the fact that, at the NAC and L-NAME pre-exposure group, no significant effects in mortality of the embryos were observed being of special importance. On the contrary, when ZF embryos where pre-exposed to DEM and BSO, a significant shift in the concentration–response curves to lower concentrations of tBOOH was observed (Figure 1). As described before, the tBOOH concentration–response curve was generated after a pre-incubation of the embryos for 24 h in 0.3× Danieau's buffer without DMSO, due to the lack of effects of DMSO in ZF development.

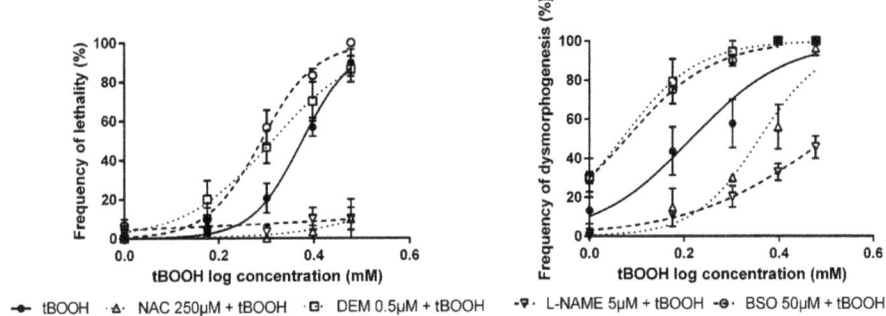

Figure 1. Concetration–response curves for lethality and dysmorphogenesis of tert-butyl hydroperoxide (tBOOH) alone or in combination with modulators of antioxidant status.

The modulation of antioxidant status in embryos exposed to TCHQ presented similar results to tBOOH. When ZF embryos were pre-exposed to NAC and L-NAME, the concentration–response curves for lethality and dysmorphogenesis were significantly shifted to higher concentrations of TCHQ (Figure 2). On the other hand, assays conducted with pre-exposure to DEM and BSO produced a statistically significant drift in the concentration–effect curves for lethality and dysmorphogenesis to lower concentrations of TCHQ (Figure 2).

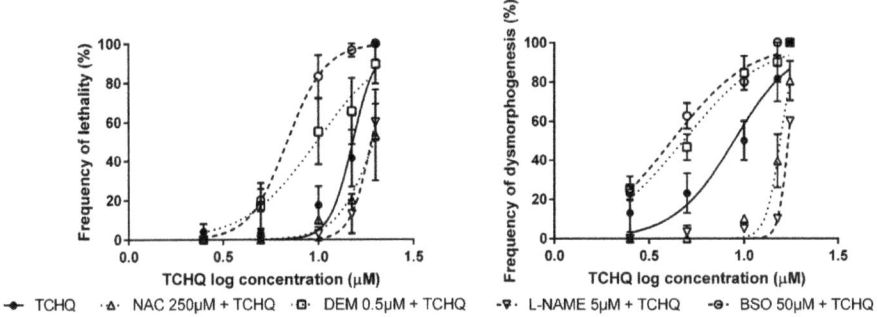

Figure 2. Concentration–response curves for lethality and dysmorphogenesis of tetrachlorohydroquinone (TCHQ) alone or in combination with modulators of antioxidant status.

Pre-exposure of ZF embryos to NAC, DEM, L-NAME, and BSO followed by LPS exposure at the selected working concentrations shifted the lethality concentration–effect curves significantly. In the analysis of dysmorphogenic effects in ZF embryos, no significant effects were observed in embryos pre-exposed to NAC, DEM, and BSO, and subsequently exposed to LPS. Only a significant reduction in dysmorphogenic effects was observed in L-NAME pre-exposed embryos (Figure 3). As described in the previous section, embryos were pre-incubated with 0.3× Danieau's buffer without DMSO, followed by LPS exposure and calculation of the concentration–response curve, due to the lack of effects of DMSO in ZF development.

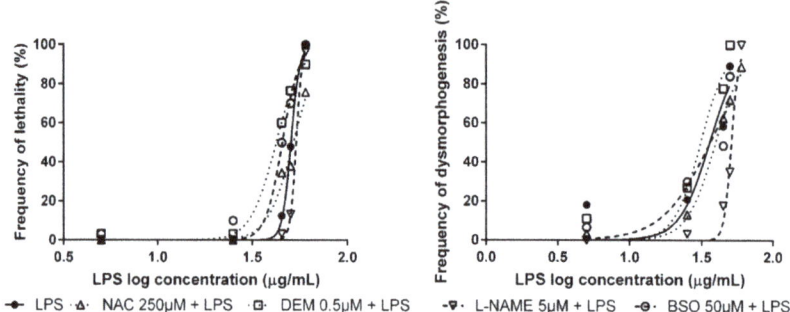

Figure 3. Concentration–response curves for lethality and dysmorphogenesis of lipopolysaccharides of *Escherichia coli* 0111:B4 (LPS) alone or in combination with modulators of antioxidant status.

The modulation of antioxidant status in embryos exposed to tBOOH produced more consistent results than other OS inducers. The observed effects in the embryonic development were general alterations not compound-specific. tBOOH was selected as the general OS inducer for the study of protective effects of antioxidant compounds.

3.3. Detection of Protective Effects of Antioxidant Compounds in Zebrafish Embryos

The second part of the study consisted in the use of tBOOH as a general OS inducer for the detection of compounds with very well-known antioxidant capacity. ZF embryos were exposed from 2 to 26 hpf to antioxidant compounds (vit. E, lipoic acid, and quercetin), before exposing them to tBOOH from 26 to 50 hpf.

In all cases, pre-exposure to the studied compounds produced a significant drift in the concentration–response curves of lethality and dysmorphogenesis to higher concentrations of tBOOH (Figure 4), which may indicate an antioxidant effect.

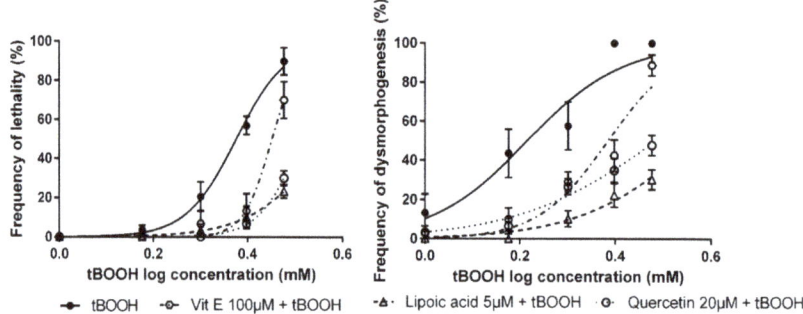

Figure 4. Concentration–response curves for lethality and dysmorphogenesis of tBOOH alone or in combination with different antioxidant compounds.

The LC_{50}, after tBOOH exposure, was 2.38 mM, and values obtained after vit. E, lipoic acid, and quercetin exposure were 2.83 mM, 3.72 mM, and 3.26 mM, respectively. For the EC_{50} values, the situation was similar, from tBOOH exposure, the EC_{50} was 1.64 mM, while pre-exposure to the studied compounds returned an EC_{50} of 2.42 mM for vit. E, 3.70 mM for lipoic acid and 3.05 mM for quercetin (Table 3).

Table 3. Effects of antioxidant compounds in lethality and dysmorphogenesis of zebrafish embryos exposed to tBOOH.

Antioxidant Compounds	OS Inducer	LC_{50} (95% CI)	EC_{50} (95% CI)
None [1]	Tert-butyl hydroperoxide (tBOOH)	2.38 mM (2.28–2.48)	1.64 mM (1.44–1.87)
Vitamin E		2.83 mM *** (2.70–2.69)	2.42 mM *** (2.17–2.70)
Lipoic acid		3.72 mM *** (3.14–4.40)	3.70 mM *** (3.03–4.51)
Quercetin		3.26 mM *** (2.83–3.76)	3.05 mM *** (2.64–3.54)

Lethal concentration 50 (LC_{50}), effective concentration 50 for dysmorphogenesis (EC_{50}) and 95% confidence interval. Statistically significant differences with respect to the group which was not exposed to any antioxidant compound: ***: $p < 0.001$; [1] A unique tBOOH concentration–response curve was generated and compared to all the concentration–response curves of the antioxidants pre-exposure groups (initially dissolved or not in DMSO) due to the lack of effect of DMSO in the embryonic development of ZF.

4. Discussion

Oxygen is an essential element for cell life and, from its metabolism, some toxic derivatives are produced, such as ROS, which are highly reactive to biological molecules and can produce OS [33]. An important factor that could prevent OS effects is the alimentary antioxidants intake. For this reason, the study of antioxidant capacity of compounds has been gaining interest in the past few years. It has been postulated that, in order to evaluate the antioxidant potential, a method which includes in vivo techniques would have more impact on the results because OS implies mechanisms which depend on many system conditions, especially the kinetic part of the reactions [34]. We have proposed the ZF embryo test, which could be a valuable in vivo method to test the antioxidant capacity of compounds, with the main advantages of an in vitro technique.

In the first part of this study, we characterized the embryotoxic and dysmorphogenic effects of several compounds, which have an OS-related mechanism of action on the ZF embryos: tBOOH, TCHQ, and LPS. The induction of OS by tBOOH is due to its capacity to generate butoxyl radicals which deplete antioxidant systems and lead to cell death [35], and it has been previously used in ZF embryos to induce OS [36]. TCHQ can induce OS by producing superoxide radicals, favoring the depletion of the reduced glutathione concentrations [37], and it has also been observed that TCHQ can produce DNA strand breakage in cells [38]. LPS is a microbial product of bacteria and its contribution to ROS production has been studied as a secondary effect to inflammation [39]. It has been used as an OS inducer in different in vitro and in vivo models [40]. All the studied OS inducers produced a significant increase in lethality and in the production of dysmorphogenesis in the exposed ZF embryos.

In order to check if the observed effects in ZF embryos could be produced by an OS mechanism, we performed assays of modulation of the embryos' antioxidants statuses with compounds related to OS. The modulation was carried out through raising or decreasing the antioxidant defenses of the embryos with NAC and L-NAME, and DEM and BSO, respectively. NAC is an antioxidant compound, which is a rate-limiting substrate in glutathione synthesis, and it can also act as a scavenger of free radicals [41]. L-NAME is an inhibitor of nitric oxide synthase, the enzyme responsible for nitric oxide synthesis. As a result of this inhibition, it reduces the production of endogenous nitric oxide, which is a compound that can produce reactive nitrogen species and consequently, OS [30]. DEM is an alkylating agent that can produce a conjugation and depletion of glutathione [42], and it can also activate the nuclear factor (erythroid-derived 2)-like 2 (Nrf2) pathway [22], and BSO is an antioxidant molecule suppressor, which specifically inhibits γ-glutamyl cysteine synthetase, the enzyme for glutathione biosynthesis, and causes the depletion of glutathione levels [43].

In general terms, we have demonstrated that the lethal and dysmorphogenic effects of tBOOH and TCHQ were significantly reduced when the embryos were pre-treated with antioxidant compounds (NAC and L-NAME). From the opposite position, the observed effects in mortality and in dysmorphogenesis were significantly increased when ZF embryos were pre-exposed to compounds which decrease the antioxidant status (DEM and BSO). We could conclude that tBOOH and TCHQ produced their embryolethal and dysmorphogenic effects in ZF embryos by an OS mechanism of action. No significant effects in dysmorphogenesis related to OS were observed in the LPS treatment group. The observed effects in the lethality of ZF embryos exposed to LPS could be more related to its mechanism as an inflammation inducer [44] than as an OS mechanism. Nevertheless, the effects of these compounds, associated with an OS mechanism, should be verified by analyzing parameters directly related to OS, like evaluation of the expression of OS-related genes in the exposed ZF embryos.

Because of its consistent results, tBOOH was selected as the OS inducer to be used to evaluate the antioxidant potential of compounds. To validate the use of tBOOH to detect the protective effects of antioxidant compounds, ZF embryos were pre-exposed to diverse compounds with a well-established antioxidant capacity (vit. E, lipoic acid, and quercetin) and posteriorly exposed to tBOOH. In addition, a statistical analysis was performed by comparing the concentration–effect curves for lethality and for dysmorphogenesis obtained in both experiments: tBOOH alone and antioxidants + tBOOH.

Vit. E is a compound with free-radical scavenging activity, which leads to an antioxidant action that has been demonstrated in vitro [45]. Lipoic acid is a thiol regenerating compound, which increases the level of glutathione. It inhibits the formation of hydroxyl radicals, and it also scavenges ROS [46]. Quercetin is a flavonol found in apples, tea, and onions, and exerts its antioxidant effect through different bioactive effects. Its main antioxidant mechanism of action is through quenching different radicals, such as hydroxyl, peroxyl, and superoxide, as well as nitric oxide and lipid oxidation [5]. Quercetin can induce antioxidant gene expression through the activation of Nrf2 [47]. Among these, quercetin can also modulate mitochondrial biogenesis by reducing ROS production in various cell types [48]. The pre-exposure of the embryos to vit. E, quercetin, and lipoic acid, followed by the exposure to the OS inducer, has confirmed the protective effects of well-known antioxidant compounds against oxidant-induced developmental toxicity in ZF. In all the cases, the pre-exposure of ZF embryos to the compounds followed by the exposure to the selected concentrations of tBOOH produced a significant shift of the concentration–effect curves of lethality and dysmorphogenesis. These results indicated the preventive effect of vit. E, lipoic acid, and quercetin against the toxic effects of tBOOH, which were related to an OS mechanism of action. The antioxidant effect of these compounds versus oxidant effects produced by the OS inducer should be confirmed by the application of antioxidant capacity evaluation methods.

The ZF embryo test has been widely used to study different types of compounds, including OS-related chemicals. Recently, a new stable transgenic line has been developed for the rapid detection of oxidative stress, although it has not been systematically tested to evaluate the antioxidant capacity of chemicals [49]. The results of our study are similar to those observed by the authors in [25], in which they observed the protective effect of vit. E in ZF embryos exposed to PCB126, which causes OS. There are other studies in which they evaluated the effects of compounds, which may have part of its mechanism of action related to oxidative injury, such as ethanol, in ZF embryos [19]. In this case, they analyzed and confirmed the partial prevention of ethanol-induced cardiovascular dysfunction by lipoic acid in ZF embryos. Natural antioxidant compounds, such as quercetin, have demonstrated their antioxidant capacity and their protective activity against different diseases using the ZF embryo test [12], reinforcing the results obtained in our study.

5. Conclusions

The ZF embryo has been established as the basis for the study of the modulative and protective effects of antioxidant compounds in oxidant induced developmental toxicity in ZF. An experimental design using tBOOH as an OS inducer has been developed in the present study. The evaluation of the

OS-related effects produced by tBOOH was estimated by a modulation of the antioxidant status assay with NAC, L-NAME, DEM, and BSO. The study of the protective effects of antioxidant compounds was performed with pre-exposure of ZF embryos to vit. E, lipoic acid, and quercetin, which are compounds with a well-established antioxidant capacity, and the protective effect of these compounds on developmental effects in the embryos was confirmed.

Our experimental system could be used as a valuable in vivo tool for testing compounds with presumable antioxidant activity, with advantages in respect to other techniques used in the evaluation of the antioxidant capacity (analytical or cell-based assays).

Further studies should be done to extensively characterize the effects of tBOOH as an OS inducer, as well as to evaluate the antioxidant capacity of compounds, in order to establish an OS model based on ZF embryos to study new antioxidant compounds and the mechanism of action by which they exert their antioxidant activity.

Author Contributions: Conceptualization, N.B., E.T., E.P., J.M.L., and J.G.-C.; Formal analysis, N.B., E.T., E.P., and J.G.-C.; Funding acquisition, J.M.L.; Investigation, N.B. and J.G.-C.; Methodology, N.B., E.T., and E.P.; Project administration, J.M.L. and J.G.-C.; Resources, J.M.L. and J.G.-C.; Supervision, E.P., J.M.L., and J.G.-C.; Validation, N.B., E.T., E.P., J.M.L., and J.G.-C.; Visualization, N.B., E.T., E.P., J.M.L., and J.G.-C.; Writing—original draft, N.B.; Writing—review and editing, N.B., E.T., E.P., J.M.L., and J.G.-C. All authors have read and agreed to the published version of the manuscript.

Funding: This research received no external funding.

Conflicts of Interest: The authors declare no conflict of interest.

References

1. Valko, M.; Rhodes, C.J.; Moncol, J.; Izakovic, M.; Mazur, M. Free radicals, metals and antioxidants in oxidative stress-induced cancer. *Chem. Biol. Interact.* **2006**, *160*, 1–40. [CrossRef]
2. Gülçin, I. Antioxidant activity of food constituents: An overview. *Arch. Toxicol.* **2012**, *86*, 345–391. [CrossRef]
3. Dröge, W. Free radicals in the physiological control of cell function. *Physiol. Rev.* **2002**, *82*, 47–95. [CrossRef]
4. Valko, M.; Leibfritz, D.; Moncol, J.; Cronin, M.T.D.; Mazur, M.; Telser, J. Free radicals and antioxidants in normal physiological functions and human disease. *Int. J. Biochem. Cell Biol.* **2007**, *39*, 44–84. [CrossRef]
5. Albarracin, S.L.; Stab, B.; Casas, Z.; Sutachan, J.J.; Samudio, I.; Gonzalez, J.; Gonzalo, L.; Capani, F.; Morales, L.; Barreto, G.E. Effects of natural antioxidants in neurodegenerative disease. *Nutr. Neurosci.* **2012**, *15*, 1–9. [CrossRef]
6. Prior, R.L.; Wu, X.; Schaich, K. Standardized methods for the determination of antioxidant capacity and phenolics in foods and dietary supplements. *J. Agric. Food Chem.* **2005**, *53*, 4290–4302. [CrossRef]
7. Becker, K.; Schroecksnadel, S.; Gostner, J.; Zaknun, C.; Schennach, H.; Überall, F.; Fuchs, D. Comparison of in vitro tests for antioxidant and immunomodulatory capacities of compounds. *Phytomedicine* **2014**, *21*, 164–171. [CrossRef] [PubMed]
8. Frankel, E.N.; Finley, J.W. How to standardize the multiplicity of methods to evaluate natural antioxidants. *J. Agric. Food Chem.* **2008**, *56*, 4901–4908. [CrossRef] [PubMed]
9. Chagas, P.M.; Weber Fulco, B.D.C.; Pesarico, A.P.; Roehrs, J.A.; Wayne, N.C. Bis(phenylimidazolselenazolyl) diselenide as an antioxidant compound: An in vitro and in vivo study. *Chem. Biol. Interact.* **2015**, *233*, 14–24. [CrossRef] [PubMed]
10. Speroni, E.; Guerra, M.C.; Minghetti, A.; Crespi-Perellino, N.; Pasini, P.; Piazza, F.; Roda, A. Oleuropein evaluated in vitro and in vivo as an antioxidant. *Phyther. Res.* **1998**, *12*, 14–24. [CrossRef]
11. Phulara, S.C.; Shukla, V.; Tiwari, S.; Pandey, R. Bacopa monnieri promotes longevity in caenorhabditis elegans under stress conditions. *Pharmacogn. Mag.* **2015**, *11*, 410–416. [PubMed]
12. Zhang, Z.J.; Cheang, L.C.V.; Wang, M.W.; Lee, S.M.Y. Quercetin exerts a neuroprotective effect through inhibition of the iNOS/NO system and pro-inflammation gene expression in PC12 cells and in zebrafish. *Int. J. Mol. Med.* **2011**, *27*, 195–203. [PubMed]
13. Bugel, S.M.; Tanguay, R.L.; Planchart, A. Zebrafish: A marvel of high-throughput biology for 21st century. *Toxicol. Curr. Environ. Heal. Rep.* **2014**, *1*, 341–352. [CrossRef]

14. De Esch, C.; Slieker, R.; Wolterbeek, A.; Woutersen, R.; de Groot, D. Zebrafish as potential model for developmental neurotoxicity testing. A mini review. *Neurotoxicol. Teratol.* **2012**, *34*, 545–553. [CrossRef] [PubMed]
15. Rubinstein, A.L. Zebrafish: From disease modeling to drug discovery. *Curr. Opin. Drug Discov. Devel.* **2003**, *6*, 218–223.
16. Scholz, S.; Fischer, S.; Gündel, U.; Küster, E.; Luckenbach, T.; Voelker, D. The zebrafish embryo model in environmental risk assessment—Applications beyond acute toxicity testing. *Environ. Sci. Pollut. Res.* **2008**, *15*, 394–404. [CrossRef]
17. Park, K.H.; Cho, K.H. A zebrafish model for the rapid evaluation of pro-oxidative and inflammatory death by lipopolysaccharide, oxidized low-density lipoproteins, and glycated high-density lipoproteins. *Fish Shellfish Immunol.* **2011**, *31*, 904–910. [CrossRef]
18. Kishi, S.; Bayliss, P.E.; Uchiyama, J.; Koshimizu, E.; Qi, J.; Nanjappa, P.; Imamura, S.; Islam, A.; Neuberg, D.; Amsterdam, A.; et al. The identification of zebrafish mutants showing alterations in senescence-associated biomarkers. *PLoS Genet.* **2008**, *4*, e1000152. [CrossRef]
19. Reimers, M.J.; La Du, J.K.; Periera, C.B.; Giovanini, J.; Tanguay, R.L. Ethanol-dependent toxicity in zebrafish is partially attenuated by antioxidants. *Neurotoxicol. Teratol.* **2006**, *28*, 497–508. [CrossRef]
20. Xi, Y.; Noble, S.; Ekker, M. Modeling neurodegeneration in zebrafish. *Curr. Neurol. Neurosci. Rep.* **2011**, *11*, 274–282. [CrossRef]
21. Bakkers, J. Zebrafish as a model to study cardiac development and human cardiac disease. *Cardiovasc. Res.* **2011**, *91*, 279–288. [CrossRef] [PubMed]
22. Nakajima, H.; Nakajima-Takagi, Y.; Tsujita, T.; Akiyama, S.I.; Wakasa, T.; Mukaigasa, K.; Kaneko, H.; Tamaru, Y.; Yamamoto, M.; Kobayashi, M. Tissue-restricted expression of Nrf2 and its target genes in zebrafish with gene-specific variations in the induction profiles. *PLoS ONE* **2011**, *6*, e26884. [CrossRef] [PubMed]
23. Timme-Laragy, A.R.; Karchner, S.I.; Franks, D.G.; Jenny, M.J.; Harbeitner, R.C.; Goldstone, J.V.; McArthur, A.G.; Hahn, M.E. Nrf2b, novel zebrafish paralog of oxidant-responsive transcription factor NF-E2-related factor 2 (NRF2). *J. Biol. Chem.* **2012**, *287*, 4609–4627. [CrossRef] [PubMed]
24. Cordero, M.D.; Moreno-Fernández, A.M.; Gomez-Skarmeta, J.L.; de Miguel, M.; Garrido-Maraver, J.; Oropesa-Ávila, M.; Rodríguez-Hernández, Á.; Navas, P.; Sánchez-Alcázar, J.A. Coenzyme Q10 and alpha-tocopherol protect against amitriptyline toxicity. *Toxicol. Appl. Pharmacol.* **2009**, *235*, 329–337. [CrossRef] [PubMed]
25. Na, Y.R.; Seok, S.H.; Baek, M.W.; Lee, H.Y.; Kim, D.J.; Park, S.H.; Lee, H.K.; Park, J.H. Protective effects of vitamin E against 3,3′,4,4′,5-pentachlorobiphenyl (PCB126) induced toxicity in zebrafish embryos. *Ecotoxicol. Environ. Saf.* **2009**, *72*, 714–719. [CrossRef] [PubMed]
26. Kais, B.; Schneider, K.E.; Keiter, S.; Henn, K.; Ackermann, C.; Braunbeck, T. DMSO modifies the permeability of the zebrafish (Danio rerio) chorion-Implications for the fish embryo test (FET). *Aquat. Toxicol.* **2013**, *140–141*, 229–238. [CrossRef]
27. Kimmel, C.B.; Ballard, W.W.; Kimmel, S.R.; Ullmann, B.; Schilling, T.F. Stages of embryonic development of the zebrafish. *Dev. Dyn.* **1995**, *203*, 253–310. [CrossRef]
28. Nagel, R. DarT: The embryo test with the Zebrafish *Danio rerio*–a general model in ecotoxicology and toxicology. *ALTEX* **2002**, *19*, 38–48.
29. Teixidó, E.; Piqué, E.; Gómez-Catalán, J.; Llobet, J.M. Assessment of developmental delay in the zebrafish embryo teratogenicity assay. *Toxicol. Vitr.* **2013**, *27*, 469–478. [CrossRef]
30. Chen, T.H.; Lin, C.Y.; Tseng, M.C. Behavioral effects of titanium dioxide nanoparticles on larval zebrafish (*Danio rerio*). *Mar. Pollut. Bull.* **2011**, *63*, 303–308. [CrossRef]
31. Holmberg, A.; Olsson, C.; Holmgren, S. The effects of endogenous and exogenous nitric oxide on gut motility in zebrafish *Danio rerio* embryos and larvae. *J. Exp. Biol.* **2006**, *209*, 2472–2479. [CrossRef] [PubMed]
32. Usenko, C.Y.; Harper, S.L.; Tanguay, R.L. Fullerene C60 exposure elicits an oxidative stress response in embryonic zebrafish. *Toxicol. Appl. Pharmacol.* **2008**, *229*, 44–55. [CrossRef] [PubMed]
33. Halliwell, B.; Gutteridge, J. Free radicals and antioxidant protection: Mechanisms and significance in toxicology and disease. *Hum. Toxicol.* **1988**, *7*, 7–13. [CrossRef] [PubMed]
34. Prieto, M.A.; Murado, M.A. A critical point: The problems associated with the variety of criteria to quantify the antioxidant capacity. *J. Agric. Food Chem.* **2014**, *62*, 5472–5484. [CrossRef]

35. Kanupriya; Prasad, D.; Sai Ram, M.; Sawhney, R.C.; Ilavazhagan, G.; Banerjee, P.K. Mechanism of tert-butylhydroperoxide induced cytotoxicity in U-937 macrophages by alteration of mitochondrial function and generation of ROS. *Toxicol. Vitr.* **2007**, *21*, 846–854. [CrossRef]
36. Timme-Laragy, A.R.; Van Tiem, L.A.; Linney, E.A.; Di Giulio, R.T. Antioxidant responses and NRF2 in synergistic developmental toxicity of PAHs in zebrafish. *Toxicol. Sci.* **2009**, *109*, 217–227. [CrossRef]
37. Wang, Y.J.; Ho, Y.S.; Chu, S.W.; Lien, H.J.; Liu, T.H.; Lin, J.K. Induction of glutathione depletion, p53 protein accumulation and cellular transformation by tetrachlorohydroquinone, a toxic metabolite of pentachlorophenol. *Chem. Biol. Interact.* **1997**, *105*, 1–16. [CrossRef]
38. Wang, Y.J.; Lee, C.C.; Chang, W.C.; Liou, H.B.; Ho, Y.S. Oxidative stress and liver toxicity in rats and human hepatoma cell line induced by pentachlorophenol and its major metabolite tetrachlorohydroquinone. *Toxicol. Lett.* **2001**, *122*, 157–169. [CrossRef]
39. Zhao, L.; Chen, Y.H.; Wang, H.; Ji, Y.L.; Ning, H.; Wang, S.F.; Zhang, C.; Lu, J.W.; Duan, Z.H.; Xu, D.X. Reactive oxygen species contribute to lipopolysaccharide-induced teratogenesis in mice. *Toxicol. Sci.* **2008**, *103*, 149–157. [CrossRef]
40. Kim, Y.S.; Kim, E.K.; Jeon, N.J.; Ryu, B.I.; Hwang, J.W.; Choi, E.J.; Moon, S.H.; Jeon, B.T.; Park, P.J. Antioxidant effect of Taurine-Rich Paroctopus dofleini extracts through inhibiting ROS production against LPS-induced oxidative stress in vitro and in vivo model. *Adv. Exp. Med. Biol.* **2017**, *975*, 1165–1177.
41. Kerksick, C.; Willoughby, D. The antioxidant role of glutathione and N-acetyl-cysteine supplements and exercise-induced oxidative stress. *J. Int. Soc. Sports Nutr.* **2005**, *2*, 38–44. [CrossRef] [PubMed]
42. Priya, S.; Nigam, A.; Bajpai, P.; Kumar, S. Diethyl maleate inhibits MCA+TPA transformed cell growth via modulation of GSH, MAPK, and cancer pathways. *Chem Biol Interact.* **2014**, *219*, 37–47. [CrossRef] [PubMed]
43. Griffith, O.W. Mechanism of action, metabolism, and toxicity of buthionine sulfoximine and its higher homologs, potent inhibitors of glutathione synthesis. *J. Biol. Chem.* **1982**, *257*, 13704–13712. [PubMed]
44. Novoa, B.; Bowman, T.V.; Zon, L.; Figueras, A. LPS response and tolerance in the zebrafish (*Danio rerio*). *Fish Shellfish Immunol.* **2009**, *26*, 326–331. [CrossRef] [PubMed]
45. Davis, S.; Davis, B.M.; Richens, J.L.; Vere, K.A.; Petrov, P.G.; Winlove, C.P.; O'shea, P. α-Tocopherols modify the membrane dipole potential leading to modulation of ligand binding by P-glycoprotein 4. *J. Lipid. Res.* **2015**, *56*, 1543–1550. [CrossRef] [PubMed]
46. Maczurek, A.; Hager, K.; Kenklies, M.; Sharman, M.; Martins, R.; Engel, J.; Carlson, D.A.; Münch, G. Lipoic acid as an anti-inflammatory and neuroprotective treatment for Alzheimer's disease. *Adv. Drug Deliv. Rev.* **2008**, *60*, 13–14. [CrossRef]
47. Miyamoto, N.; Izumi, H.; Miyamoto, R.; Kondo, H.; Tawara, A.; Sasaguri, Y.; Kohno, K. Quercetin induces the expression of peroxiredoxins 3 and 5 via the Nrf2/NRF1 transcription pathway. *Invest. Ophthalmol Vis. Sci.* **2011**, *22*, 1055–1063. [CrossRef]
48. Rayamajhi, N.; Kim, S.-K.; Go, H.; Joe, Y.; Callaway, Z.; Kang, J.-G.; Ryter, S.; Chung, H. Quercetin induces mitochondrial biogenesis through activation of HO-1 in HepG2 cells. *Oxidative Med. Cell. Longev.* **2013**, *2013*, 154279. [CrossRef]
49. Mourabit, S.; Fitzgerald, J.A.; Ellis, R.P.; Takesono, A.; Porteus, C.S.; Trznadel, M.; Metz, J.; Winter, M.J.; Kudoh, T.; Tyler, C.R. New insights into organ-specific oxidative stress mechanisms using a novel biosensor zebrafish. *Environ. Int.* **2019**, *133*, 105138. [CrossRef]

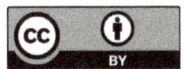

© 2020 by the authors. Licensee MDPI, Basel, Switzerland. This article is an open access article distributed under the terms and conditions of the Creative Commons Attribution (CC BY) license (http://creativecommons.org/licenses/by/4.0/).

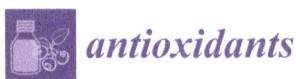

Article

Antioxidative Action of Ellagic Acid—A Kinetic DFT Study

Jelena Tošović [1,2] and Urban Bren [1,3,*]

[1] Faculty of Chemistry and Chemical Engineering, University of Maribor, Smetanova Street 17, SI-2000 Maribor, Slovenia; jelena.tosovic@um.si
[2] Department of Chemistry, Faculty of Science, University of Kragujevac, 12 Radoja Domanovića, 34000 Kragujevac, Serbia
[3] Faculty of Mathematics, Natural Sciences and Information Technologies, University of Primorska, Glagoljaška 8, SI-6000 Koper, Slovenia
* Correspondence: urban.bren@um.si

Received: 8 June 2020; Accepted: 3 July 2020; Published: 6 July 2020

Abstract: Although one can find numerous studies devoted to the investigation of antioxidative activity of ellagic acid (EA) in the scientific literature, the mechanisms of its action have not yet been fully clarified. Therefore, further kinetic studies are needed to understand its antioxidative capacity completely. This work aims to reveal the underlying molecular mechanisms responsible for the antioxidative action of EA. For this purpose, its reactions with $HO^\bullet$ and $CCl_3OO^\bullet$ radicals were simulated at physiological conditions using the quantum mechanics-based test for overall free-radical scavenging activity. The density functional theory in combination with the conductor-like polarizable continuum solvation model was utilized. With $HO^\bullet$ radical EA conforms to the hydrogen atom transfer and radical adduct formation mechanisms, whereas sequential proton loss electron transfer mechanism is responsible for scavenging of $CCl_3OO^\bullet$ radical. In addition, compared to trolox, EA was found more reactive toward $HO^\bullet$, but less reactive toward $CCl_3OO^\bullet$. The calculated rate constants for the reactions of EA with both free radicals are in a very good agreement with the corresponding experimental values.

Keywords: QM-ORSA; antioxidative mechanisms; reaction rate constants; physiological conditions; polyphenols

1. Introduction

In recent years, therapeutic applications of non-drug substances such as functional foods, are progressively increasing. Therefore, studies on functional foods represent a cutting-edge topic among nutritional scientists. The significance of bioactive compounds as functional supplements of foods has been well established due to their effectiveness in health promotion by disease prophylaxis or treatment. Special attention has been devoted to investigations of polyphenolic compounds, known for their various nutritional, biologic, and pharmacological effects. In order to provide the health benefits to the consumers, functional foods and nutraceuticals have been supplemented with these compounds in recent years [1].

Among polyphenolic compounds, ellagic acid (EA) attracts an ever-increasing interest due to its great potential in food technology, as well as in pharmaceutical, medical and cosmetic industries [2]. EA, a dimeric derivative of gallic acid, arises from acidic hydrolysis of ellagitannins. It represents a planar molecule which contains four hydroxyl and two lactone groups (see Figure 1). This dietary polyphenol can be found in a wide variety of fruits. Raspberries, cranberries, strawberries, grapes, as well as pomegranate seeds, are known for example for their high content of EA [3]. Other sources include pecans, walnuts and distilled beverages [4].

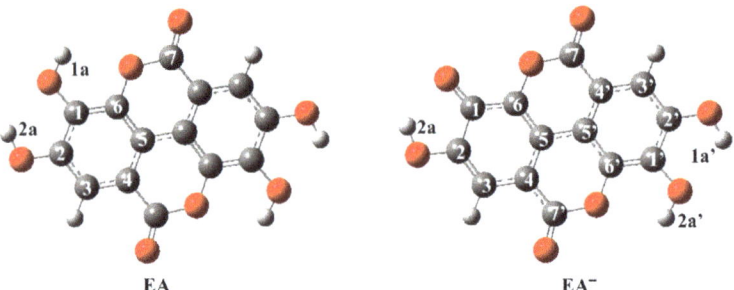

Figure 1. Optimized structures of neutral ellagic acid and its monoanion. Carbon atoms are depicted in gray, oxygen atoms in red, chlorine atoms in green and hydrogen atoms in white color. The atom labeling scheme and color coding are applied throughout the study.

Like other dietary polyphenols, EA possesses a wide range of biological activities suggesting that it can exert strong beneficial effects on human health. In many epidemiological and experimental studies, anticarcinogenic, anti-inflammatory, antiviral, antibacterial, anti-atherosclerosis, antihypertensive, antihyperglycemic, cardioprotective and anti-fibrosis actions of EA have been demonstrated [5–11]. It can inhibit carcinogenesis by occupying sites (i.e., microsomal *P*-450 enzymes, glutathione-S -transferase or DNA), that would normally interact with ultimate carcinogens, through several mechanisms [12,13]. The anticarcinogenic effect of ellagic acid has been studied in various cancer cells. There it exhibits antiproliferative activity, combined with the ability to cause cell cycle arrest and to induce apoptosis [14]. The anticarcinogenic effects of ellagic acid have been observed in several cancer types: prostate, skin, esophageal and colon cancers [15]. Moreover, EA causes cell-specific responses, meaning that tumor cells are more susceptible to EA than normal cells [10]. In addition, EA prevents metabolic activation of aflatoxin B1, polycyclic aromatic hydrocarbons (PAHs) and nitroso compounds into ultimate carcinogens that cause DNA damage [12]. Due to its beneficial effects against a wide range of diseases, EA represents a great candidate for a therapeutic and chemopreventive agent, especially in the form of functional food supplements [16].

It has been shown that the high free radical scavenging activity of EA may be at least partially responsible for the observed in vivo biologic effects [14]. The presence of four hydroxyl groups enables EA to scavenge numerous reactive oxygen and nitrogen species and makes this compound a powerful antioxidant [17,18]. EA represents also a very efficient inhibitor of lipid peroxidation even at micromolar concentrations [19]. Furthermore, studies of Hassoun et al. showed that EA exhibits a better antioxidative efficacy against oxidative stress and lipid peroxidation than vitamin E [19]. Finally, besides numerous beneficial effects on human health, EA as a strong antioxidant can prolong shelf life and preserve the quality of foods [1].

In scientific literature, one can find a few theoretical studies devoted to the examination of the antioxidative activity of EA through thermodynamic and kinetic approaches. Marković et al. have shown that the thermochemical viability of different antioxidative mechanisms depends on the deprotonated portion of EA, the polarity of reaction media, as well as on the properties of the free radical [20]. Based on the calculated thermodynamic parameters, they have suggested that the hydrogen atom transfer (HAT) is the most favorable mechanism in nonpolar media, whereas sequential proton loss electron transfer (SPLET) is preferred in polar media, which is in agreement with results reported by Mazzone et al. [21]. Utilizing the transition state theory, Tiwari and Mishra have determined the rate constants for the reactions of EA (as well as its monomethyl and dimethyl derivatives) with hydroxyl (HO$^\bullet$), methoxy (CH$_3$O$^\bullet$) and nitrogen dioxide (NO$_2$$^\bullet$) radicals [22]. However, the calculated rate constants of HO$^\bullet$ and CH$_3$O$^\bullet$ radicals have been overestimated by several orders of magnitude in comparison with the experimentally obtained values [17,18]. Galano et al. have also investigated several aspects related to the antioxidant activity of EA [17]. They have demonstrated that the free radical scavenging activity of EA does not decrease upon metabolism and provides continuous protection against oxidative stress. To the best of our knowledge, the results of Tiwari and Mishra and Galano et al. represent the only theoretical studies dedicated to kinetic investigations of antioxidative activity of EA [17,22].

However, one can find numerous experimental studies devoted to the examination of EA as an important component of various foods and beverages, its antioxidative mechanisms have not been fully clarified. Elucidation of the mechanisms by which dietary polyphenols prevent and suppress various diseases represents an important step in understanding their effects in vivo and may help the design of novel strategies for disease prophylaxis and treatment. Therefore, further kinetic investigations are needed to reveal and to fully understand the underlying molecular mechanisms responsible for the antioxidative action of EA. Consequently, the hydrogen atom transfer (HAT), radical adduct formation (RAF), sequential proton loss electron transfer (SPLET) and single electron transfer (SET) mechanisms [23–25] were studied by simulating the reactions of EA with two free radicals, HO$^\bullet$ and CCl$_3$OO$^\bullet$, at physiological conditions (pH = 7.4 in aqueous solution) using quantum-chemical methods. An additional goal was to determine the relative antioxidative activity of EA, using trolox (6-hydroxy-2,5,7,8-tetramethylchroman-2-carboxylic acid, Tx) as a reference compound.

2. Materials and Methods

2.1. Computational Methods

All results were obtained from calculations using the density functional theory (DFT) approach. Full geometry optimizations and subsequent frequency calculations were performed using the hybrid meta M06-2X functional in conjunction with flexible 6-311++G(d,p) basis set and conductor-like polarizable continuum model (CPCM) [26], as implemented in the Gaussan 09, Revision D.01, software package [27]. Implicit water solution (dielectric constant, ε = 78.3553) was employed to mimic the physiological aqueous environment. The M06-2X functional was developed for studying main-group thermochemistry and kinetics [28,29]. In addition, this theoretical model has recently demonstrated robustness and very good overall performance in investigations of several related polyphenolic systems [30–34]. Restricted and unrestricted calculations were applied for the closed-shell and open-shell structures, respectively. The nature of the reactive species was confirmed by analyzing the results of the subsequent frequency calculations in the harmonic approximation: only real frequencies for equilibrium geometries and exactly one imaginary frequency for transition states (TSs) were obtained. The intrinsic reaction coordinate (IRC) calculations were additionally performed to verify each transition state. IRC represents the minimum energy reaction pathway (MERP) in mass-weighted cartesian coordinates between the transition state and the corresponding reactants and products. Moreover, the natural bond orbital (NBO) analysis was applied for all structures to obtain the corresponding partial atomic charges [35]. The IRC and NBO analyses were performed using default settings.

2.2. Quantum Mechanics-Based Test for Overall, Free-Radical Scavenging Activity

Four antioxidative mechanisms—HAT, RAF, SPLET and SET—were examined following the quantum mechanics-based test for overall free-radical scavenging activity (QM-ORSA) protocol [36], which was designed for studying free-radical reactions in solutions of different polarities. QM-ORSA represents a universal and quantitative method of evaluating the free radical scavenging activity of chemical compounds, that is, their primary antioxidant activity. This methodology involves revealing of all thermodynamically feasible reaction pathways included in the antioxidative process, which are subjected to subsequent kinetic investigations. By calculating the reaction pathways for all present acid–base forms of the investigated compound, QM-ORSA takes into account also the influence of pH. Namely, at a particular pH, the antioxidant can be present in different acid–base forms (cationic, neutral, monoanionic, dianionic, etc.) depending on its *pKa* values. The reliability of the QM-ORSA protocol was confirmed on the set of test reactions, where the correlation between the logarithms of the calculated and experimental rate constants was excellent (the R value is very close to one (0.99), the slope is very close to one (0.99), and the intercept is very close to zero (0.06) [36]. Moreover, the absolute error of the Gibbs activation free energies of 1.213 kJ mol^{-1} was significantly lower than the accepted computational accuracy of 4.184 kJ mol^{-1}. Finally, this protocol has been successfully applied for several investigations of antioxidative activity in the scientific literature [31,32,34,37–42].

2.2.1. Thermodynamic Considerations

The thermochemical viability of all possible reaction pathways and reaction sites included in the antioxidative process was investigated in terms of the reaction Gibbs free energies (ΔG_r). The free energies of the examined reactions were determined at T = 298.15 K and P = 101,325 Pa. The exergonic ($\Delta G_r < 0$) and isoergonic ($\Delta G_r \approx 0$) reaction paths were subjected to further kinetic calculations.

2.2.2. Kinetic Considerations

Depending on the type of the mechanism, the reaction rate constants were obtained in two different ways. In the case of HAT and RAF mechanisms, where the transformation of reactants to products occurs over energy barriers, the Eckart method [43] also known as zero-tunneling method (ZCT-0) was applied. This method uses the Eckart function for generating the ground-state potential energy function based on information on the stationary points (reactants, transition state and products) along MERP. To perform the Eckart method calculations TheRate program [44] was utilized. For the electron transfer reactions involved in SPLET and SET mechanisms, the Marcus theory [45] was applied.

The overall reaction rate constants ($k_{overall}$), which correspond to experimentally observed reaction rates of specific free-radical reactions, were calculated. The $k_{overall}$ values were obtained as a sum over all acid–base species (*i*) present at the physiological pH (7.4) of the total reaction rate constant values (k_{TOT}) multiplied by the corresponding molar fractions (*f*):

$$k_{overall} = \sum_{i = \{acid-base\ species\}} f(i) \times k_{TOT}(i) \quad (1)$$

The k_{TOT} values for all acid–base species were obtained as sums of the reaction rate constants corresponding to each antioxidative mechanism (*j*):

$$k_{TOT} = \sum_{j = \{antioxidative\ mechanism\}} k_{mech}(j) \quad (2)$$

The k_{mech} is defined as a sum of reaction rate constants (*k*) belonging to the same antioxidative mechanism calculated at different reactive sites (*l*):

$$k_{mech} = \sum_{l = \{antioxidative\ pathway\}} k(l) \quad (3)$$

The antioxidative pathway belongs to a specific antioxidative mechanism at a specific reactive site. To determine the relative contribution of an antioxidative pathway (*l*), the branching ratio, $\Gamma(l)$, was calculated using the following relation:

$$\Gamma(l) = \frac{k(l)}{k_{overall}} \quad (4)$$

2.2.3. Relative Antioxidative Activity

The relative antioxidative activity of **EA** (r^T) was calculated by dividing $k_{overall}$ of EA with $k_{overall}$ of **Tx**:

$$r^T = \frac{k^{EA}_{overall}}{k^{Tx}_{overall}} \tag{5}$$

3. Results and Discussion

3.1. Thermodynamic Considerations

In the previous study of Galano at al. it was found that the dominant species of EA present at physiological conditions (pH = 7.4) are neutral (~10.7%) and monoanionic (EA$^-$, ~89.3%) forms, which is also in accordance with the reported *pKa* values (Figure 1) [17].

To select favorable mechanistic pathways for further kinetic investigations of the antioxidative action of EA the Gibbs free energies of the following reactions of neutral species:

$$\text{HAT}: \text{EA} + \text{R}^\bullet \rightarrow \text{EA}^\bullet + \text{RH} \tag{6}$$

$$\text{RAF}: \text{EA} + \text{R}^\bullet \rightarrow [\text{EA} - \text{R}]^\bullet \tag{7}$$

$$\text{SPLET (I step)}: \text{EA} + \text{HO}^- \rightarrow \text{EA}^- + \text{H}_2\text{O} \tag{8}$$

$$\text{SPLET (II step)}: \text{EA}^- + \text{R}^\bullet \rightarrow \text{EA}^\bullet + \text{R}^- \tag{9}$$

$$\text{SET}: \text{EA} + \text{R}^\bullet \rightarrow \text{EA}^{\bullet+} + \text{R}^- \tag{10}$$

as well as of monoanionic species:

$$\text{HAT}: \text{EA}^- + \text{R}^\bullet \rightarrow \text{EA}^{\bullet-} + \text{RH} \tag{11}$$

$$\text{RAF}: \text{EA}^- + \text{R}^\bullet \rightarrow [\text{EA} - \text{R}]^{\bullet-} \tag{12}$$

$$\text{SPLET (I step)}: \text{EA}^- + \text{HO}^- \rightarrow \text{EA}^{2-} + \text{H}_2\text{O} \tag{13}$$

$$\text{SPLET (II step)}: \text{EA}^{2-} + \text{R}^\bullet \rightarrow \text{EA}^{\bullet-} + \text{R}^- \tag{14}$$

$$\text{SET}: \text{EA}^- + \text{R}^\bullet \rightarrow \text{EA}^\bullet + \text{R}^- \tag{15}$$

had to be examined first. In reactions (6)–(15) R$^\bullet$ stands for HO$^\bullet$ or CCl$_3$OO$^\bullet$. The HO$^\bullet$ represents the most electrophilic among the oxygen-centered radicals capable of reacting immediately after its formation with almost any molecule in the vicinity. It is responsible for 60% to 70% of the tissue damage caused by ionizing radiations and most oxidative damage to DNA [23]. CCl$_3$OO$^\bullet$ is generated in the organism during the metabolism of CCl$_4$, a well-known liver toxin. As most of the oxygen radicals, CCl$_3$OO$^\bullet$ reacts with various biomolecules such as proteins, DNA and lipids [46,47]. In addition, CCl$_3$OO$^\bullet$ was specifically selected because it is often used in experimental studies to imitate larger peroxyl radicals [48]. A wide variety of experimental studies have been indeed conducted in order to elucidate an effective scavenger of this radical, especially among the naturally occurring antioxidants. However, to the best of our knowledge, computational investigations regarding the reactivity of CCl$_3$OO$^\bullet$ remain surprisingly scarce.

Structures of EA and its monoanion employed in the present study are consistent with the structures published in previous papers [17,20]. The calculated reaction free energies are summarized in Table 1. In the case of the neutral species, only half of the positions in the molecule must be considered explicitly due to the symmetry, whereas in the case of the monoanion the symmetry is broken and all the sites must be considered explicitly.

Table 1. Gibbs energies ΔG_r (kJ mol^{-1}) of the reactions of ellagic acid (EA) and its monoanion (EA$^-$) with HO$^\bullet$ and Cl$_3$COO$^\bullet$; HAT, RAF, SPLET and SET denote hydrogen atom transfer, radical adduct formation, sequential proton loss electron transfer and single electron transfer mechanisms, respectively.

Mechanism	Position	EA		EA$^-$	
		HO$^\bullet$	Cl$_3$COO$^\bullet$	HO$^\bullet$	Cl$_3$COO$^\bullet$
HAT	1a	−144.0	−36.3		
	2a	−144.2	−36.4	−167.5	−59.7
	1a'			−150.7	−42.9
	2a'			−151.8	−44.0
RAF	1	−62.6	32.8	−16.9	/
	2	−47.4	39.7	−66.4	8.5
	3	−47.9	32.9	−43.4	33.7
	4	−7.6	78.3	−24.5	49.7
	5	−11.2	66.1	0.5	66.7
	6	−39.9	45.9	−66.8	10.8
	1'			−61.8	31.0
	2'			−47.8	42.0
	3'			−45.9	48.0
	4'			−6.0	75.1
	5'			−6.1	65.8
	6'			−40.0	50.8
SPLET	1a	−161.6		−145.1	
	/	17.6	0.7	−5.6	−22.5
SET	/	127.6	110.72	17.6	0.7

According to the highly exergonic ΔG_r values, EA and EA$^-$ can scavenge both free radicals through HAT reaction pathways. In the case of EA, all four positions (1a = 1a' and 2a = 2a') are equally feasible, whereas in the case of EA$^-$ the reaction pathway at position 2a' becomes the most favorable. In the case of the RAF mechanism, the reaction pathways at positions 7 and 7' are excluded from the examination. Namely, the significant partial positive charge of carbonyl carbons, makes these positions unsuitable for the attack of the studied electrophilic free radicals (Figure S1). All remaining reactive positions with HO$^\bullet$ radical are exergonic or isoergonic ($\Delta G_r \approx 0$), suggesting that the RAF mechanism is thermodynamically favorable. As for CCl$_3$OO$^\bullet$ radical, we were unable to locate the corresponding radical adduct for the reaction with EA$^-$ at position 1 and all remaining positions are endergonic. These findings imply that RAF mechanism cannot be responsible for the antioxidative action of EA in the case of CCl$_3$OO$^\bullet$ radical.

The basic environment provides conditions for proton loss from EA and EA$^-$, to form EA$^-$ and EA^{2-}, respectively, which is reflected in the negative ΔG_r values for the first step of the SPLET mechanism. Considering, that EA^{2-} represents the dominant form only at higher pH values (pH > 10), it is reasonable to assume that SPLET mechanism cannot be responsible for the antioxidative action of EA$^-$ toward the studied selected free radicals [32,49]. On the other hand, the second step of the SPLET mechanism of EA deserves a careful inspection. Namely, electron transfer reaction is endergonic in the case of the highly reactive HO$^\bullet$, whereas it is isoergonic in the case of CCl$_3$OO$^\bullet$ and should, therefore, be further examined. The higher reactivity of CCl$_3$OO$^\bullet$ in comparison to HO$^\bullet$ during the electron transfer reaction can be explained by the strong negative inductive effect of the three chlorine atoms which increases the electron affinity of the radical. High ΔG_r values for the SET reactions between EA and both studied free radicals indicate that this mechanism does not occur, whereas the SET reaction pathway of EA$^-$ is identical to the second step of the SPLET mechanism of EA.

3.2. Kinetic Considerations

All exergonic and isoergonic reaction pathways were subjected to kinetic examination aimed at revealing the TSs and at calculating the corresponding activation free energies and reaction rate constants (Table 2).

Table 2. Activation energies $\Delta G_a^{\ddagger}$ (kJ mol^{-1}) and rate constants k (M^{-1} s^{-1}) for exergonic reaction pathways of the reactions of EA and EA$^-$ with HO$^{\bullet}$ and CCl$_3$OO$^{\bullet}$.

Mechanism	Position	HO$^{\bullet}$ EA $\Delta G_a^{\ddagger}$	k	HO$^{\bullet}$ EA$^-$ $\Delta G_a^{\ddagger}$	k	Cl$_3$COO$^{\bullet}$ EA $\Delta G_a^{\ddagger}$	k	Cl$_3$COO$^{\bullet}$ EA$^-$ $\Delta G_a^{\ddagger}$	k
HAT	1a	~0.0	1.91 × 10^9			64.9	7.74 × 10^3		
	2a	~0.0	1.91 × 10^9	~0.0	1.91 × 10^9	56.7	7.54 × 10^4	/	/
	1a'	~0.0	1.91 × 10^9	~0.0	1.91 × 10^9	64.9	7.74 × 10^3	/	/
	2a'	~0.0	1.91 × 10^9	~0.0	1.91 × 10^9	56.7	7.54 × 10^4	198.8	4.06 × 10^{-20}
RAF	1	36.9	6.17 × 10^7	17.0	5.30 × 10^7				
	2	40.8	1.33 × 10^7	~0.0	1.91 × 10^9				
	3	39.3	2.47 × 10^7	26.8	4.60 × 10^7				
	4	46.5	1.40 × 10^6	9.3	3.59 × 10^7				
	5	52.1	1.58 × 10^7	49.3	4.12 × 10^5				
	6	40.7	1.43 × 10^7	~0.0	1.91 × 10^9				
	1'	36.9	6.17 × 10^7	33.7	8.27 × 10^7				
	2'	40.8	1.33 × 10^7	37.4	4.69 × 10^7				
	3'	39.3	2.47 × 10^7	36.2	7.02 × 10^7				
	4'	46.5	1.40 × 10^6	44.3	3.12 × 10^6				
	5'	52.1	1.58 × 10^5	51.9	1.49 × 10^5				
	6'	40.7	1.43 × 10^7	38.4	3.14 × 10^7				
SPLET(I)	1a	/	/	/	/	~0.0	1.91 × 10^9	/	/
SPLET(II)		/	/	/	/	0.7	1.56 × 10^9	/	/
SET		/	/	/	/	/	/	/	/
$k_{overall}$			9.70 × 10^9				1.59 × 10^9		
$k_{overall}^{exp}$			8.9 × 10^9				0.84 × 10^9		

All our attempts to locate TSs for the HAT reactions of EA and EA$^-$ with HO$^{\bullet}$ were unsuccessful, so it was reasonable to assume that all these processes are barrierless. To confirm this assumption, each reactive position was further investigated in the following manner. HO$^{\bullet}$ radical was positioned in the vicinity of the corresponding H atom and then allowed to approach the reactive center up to the formation of the products. Dependence of the total energy on the corresponding scan coordinate (HO$^{\bullet}$–H distance) was analyzed. Based on the monotonous decrease of total energy with decreasing of HO$^{\bullet}$–H distance it was concluded that these reactions are indeed barrierless and therefore diffusion-controlled, with the corresponding reaction rate constant of 1.91×10^9 M^{-1} s^{-1}. Two representative total energy profiles (one for the neutral form EA and one for the monoanion EA$^-$) for HAT reactions are depicted in Figure 2.

A majority of TSs involved in the RAF mechanism of EA and EA$^-$ with HO$^{\bullet}$ were successfully allocated (Cartesian coordinates of all TSs are provided in the Supplementary Materials). Two exceptions represent the reaction pathways at positions 2 and 6 of EA$^-$, for which we were not able to locate TSs, despite numerous attempts. For this reason, the relaxed scan procedure applied for the HAT reaction pathways has also been employed in these two cases. The total energy of the system indeed monotonously decreases with decreasing HO$^{\bullet}$–C distance, so it can be concluded that these two processes are also diffusion-controlled (Figure S2). The increased affinity of C2 and C6 atoms toward HO$^{\bullet}$ in comparison to other positions is not surprising due to the strong mesomeric activating effect of O$^-$ at ortho and para positions. The rate constants for the reactions at other positions are correspondingly reduced mostly by two orders of magnitude. The mutual characteristics of TSs obtained for the studied RAF reactions include relatively strong interactions of hydroxyl radical with π electrons of the aromatic ring, as well as the preserved planarity of the molecule (Figure 3a). Slower rates are observed for the reactions at positions 4 = 4' of EA and 4' of EA$^-$, whereas the slowest reactions are those in positions 5 = 5′ of EA, as well as 5 and 5′ of EA⁻. In the first case, the π-interactions between the hydrogen of the hydroxyl radical and the aromatic ring is lost in TS (Figure 3b), whereas in the second, the reacting system becomes nonplanar and therefore less stable (Figure 3c). Additionally, the results of the IRC calculations for the representative TSs for the RAF mechanism with HO• are shown in Figure S3.

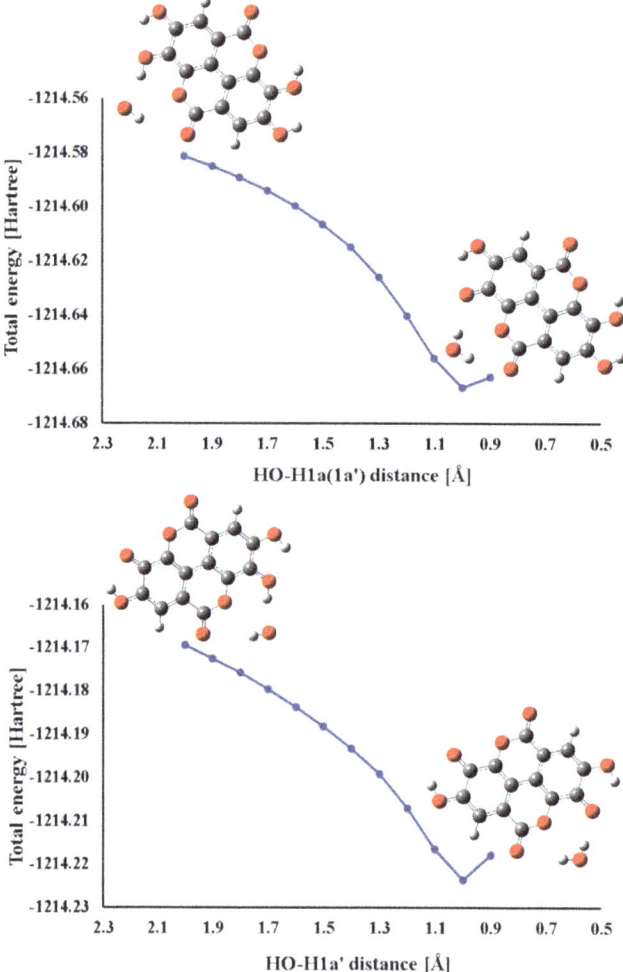

Figure 2. Dependence of total energy on the characteristic HO•–H distance during the hydrogen atom transfer between ellagic acid (top) or its monoanion (bottom) and HO•.

For the HAT reactions between EA and $CCl_3OO^\bullet$ both TSs were successfully located (Figure 4). The results of the IRC calculations are shown in Figure S4. In both TSs, the planarity of the system is preserved. As expected, the HAT reaction pathways with $CCl_3OO^\bullet$ are slower than the corresponding reactions with HO• (Table 2). On the other hand, we have encountered significant difficulties to locate TSs for the reactions of EA⁻ with $CCl_3OO^\bullet$. Only one approximation of TS was revealed, using a similar procedure described in detail in a previous study of Tošović and Marković [32]. Namely, the energy profile of the reaction in 2a′ position is characterized by an extremely steep decrease to the energy minimum (Figure S5). It is worth pointing out that the corresponding energy maximum is characterized by a single desired strong imaginary vibrational frequency (1339.94i cm^{-1}). Considering that the calculated $\Delta G_a^{\ddagger}$ value is extremely high (~200 kJ mol^{-1}) and the corresponding rate constant is tremendously small, the contribution of this reaction pathway to the overall antioxidative capacity of EA toward CCl$_3$OO$^{\bullet}$ remains negligible. It is reasonable to assume that similar results would be observed in the case of the two remaining HAT reaction paths (at positions 2a and 1a'), so they were not considered further.

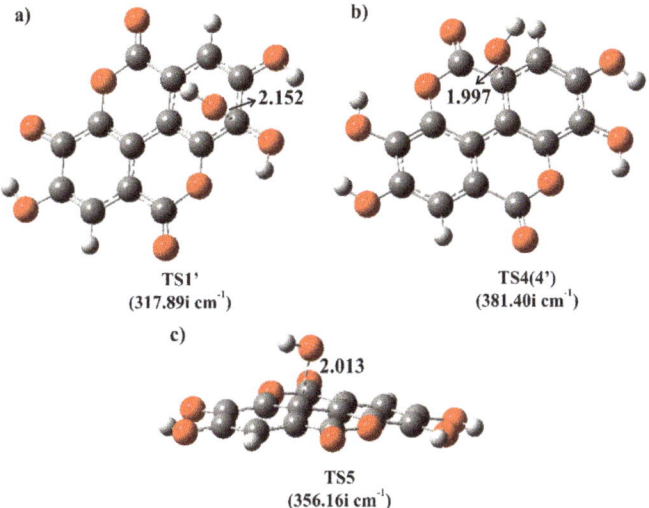

Figure 3. Representative examples of transition states obtained for the RAF reaction of EA and EA$^-$ with HO$^{\bullet}$ at positions: (a) 1' (EA$^-$), (b) 4=4' (EA) and (c) 5 (EA$^-$). All distances are reported in Å.

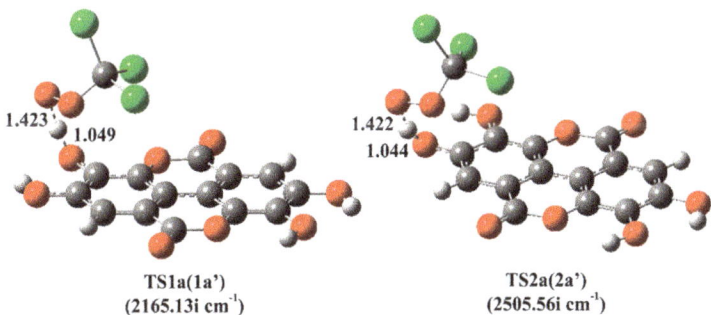

Figure 4. Optimized geometries of transition states for the hydrogen atom transfer (HAT) reaction pathways of ellagic acid with CCl$_3$OO$^{\bullet}$ at positions 1a=1a' and 2a=2a'. All distances are reported in Å.

Figure S6 demonstrates a barrierless formation of EA$^-$ in a proton loss reaction of the SPLET mechanism of EA, whereas the rate constant value of 1.56 × 10^9 M^{-1} s^{-1} for the second step of the SPLET mechanism, i.e., the electron transfer reaction, indicates that this reaction is also practically diffusion controlled.

The obtained $k_{overall}$ values amount to 9.70 × 10^9 and 3.71 × 10^8 M^{-1} s^{-1} for the reactions with HO$^{\bullet}$ and CCl$_3$OO$^{\bullet}$ (Table 2), respectively and it is very interesting to compare them with the existing experimental results. In the study of Priyadarsini et al. [18], the rate constants for these reactions were determined in aqueous solution at pH=7 using pulse radiolysis technique and amount to 8.9 × 10^9 and

1.4×10^8 M^{-1} s^{-1} for the HO$^\bullet$ and CCl$_3$OO$^\bullet$ radicals, respectively. Considering that the agreement between experimental and calculated reaction rate constants is very good, it can be concluded that the utilized computational approach successfully quantified reactivity of EA toward both studied free radicals.

To estimate the importance of each individual path to the overall antioxidative capacity of EA, the branching ratios were calculated (Table S1). The greatest Γ values in the case of HO$^\bullet$ belong to the diffusion-controlled reactions of monoanion, i.e., all HAT reaction pathways and two specific RAF reactions. On the other hand, the highest Γ values were obtained for the SPLET reaction paths between CCl$_3$OO$^\bullet$ and the neutral form of EA.

Galano et al. reported the overall rate constant values for the reactions of EA with HO$^\bullet$ and CCl$_3$OO$^\bullet$ radicals (among others) calculated solely based on the mechanisms in which the electron transfer reactions are involved, i.e., SPLET and SET, using a different theoretical model [17]. Our work suggests that in the case of CCl$_3$OO$^\bullet$ radical the electron transfer reaction is indeed the predominant antioxidative pathway and the comparison of our results with the study of Galano et al. for overall rate gives a good agreement. On the other hand, our results indicate that SPLET and SET mechanisms are not favorable for scavenging of HO$^\bullet$ and no meaningful comparison with the work of Galano et al. can be made.

3.3. Relative Antioxidative Activity

According to the QM-ORSA protocol, a thermodynamic and kinetic study needs to also be performed for the reference compound, Tx, to determine relative antioxidative value, r^T. The $k_{overall}$ value for the reaction of Tx with HO$^\bullet$, calculated using an identical methodology and theoretical model under equal conditions, has been recently reported and amounts to 1.94×10^9 M^{-1} s^{-1} [32]. On the other hand, to the best of our knowledge, the $k_{overall}$ value for the reaction of Tx with Cl$_3$COO$^\bullet$ is yet unknown. For this reason, all necessary calculations regarding this reaction had to be performed. The corresponding results and short discussion are provided in the Supplementary Materials. The obtained $k_{overall}$ value for Tx reacting with Cl$_3$COO$^\bullet$ is equal to 1.91×10^9 M^{-1} s^{-1}.

Based on the calculated $k_{overall}$ values for the reactions of EA and Tx with HO$^\bullet$ and CCl$_3$OO$^\bullet$ in aqueous solution the r^T values were determined. The obtained r^T values of 5.00 and 0.19 for the reactions with HO$^\bullet$ and CCl$_3$OO$^\bullet$, respectively, imply that EA is more reactive toward HO$^\bullet$, but less reactive toward CCl$_3$OO$^\bullet$ in comparison to Tx.

4. Conclusions

Antioxidants represent an important group of functional compounds that possess the ability to extend shelf life and maintain the quality of foods. More important, in biologic systems, antioxidants protect against oxidative stress and consequently help to prevent numerous diseases.

In this work, we investigated the antioxidative mechanisms of a dietary polyphenol EA by utilizing the QM-ORSA methodology. For this purpose, the reactions of EA with HO$^\bullet$ and CCl$_3$OO$^\bullet$ radicals were simulated.

Highly exergonic ΔG_r values indicate that EA and EA$^-$ can scavenge both investigated free radicals through HAT reaction pathways. The RAF reaction pathways are thermodynamically possible in the case of the reactions with HO$^\bullet$, whereas the SPLET reaction mechanism is thermodynamically feasible in the case of CCl$_3$OO$^\bullet$ radical. High ΔG_r values for the SET reactions between EA and both studied free radicals indicate that this mechanism does not play a vital role.

Based on the obtained kinetic results, EA can scavenge HO$^\bullet$ primarily through HAT and RAF mechanisms, whereas SPLET mechanism is responsible for scavenging of the CCl$_3$OO$^\bullet$ radical. Moreover, based on the calculated r^T values, EA is more reactive toward HO$^\bullet$, but less reactive toward CCl$_3$OO$^\bullet$ than Tx.

Last but not least, the calculated overall reaction rate constants, $k_{overall}$, for the reactions of EA with HO$^\bullet$ and CCl$_3$OO$^\bullet$, respectively, are in a very good agreement with the experimental values, indicating that the applied computational methodology successfully quantified the reactivity of EA toward both investigated free radicals. Considering that antioxidative mechanisms in aqueous environments are extremely complex, the consensus between the calculated and available experimental data strongly supports the reaction mechanisms proposed in this work.

Supplementary Materials: The supplementary materials are available online at http://www.mdpi.com/2076-3921/9/7/587/s1.

Author Contributions: Methodology, investigation, data analysis, visualization, writing—original draft preparation, J.T.; conceptualization, supervision, writing—review and editing, U.B. Both authors have read and agreed to the published version of the manuscript. All authors have read and agreed to the published version of the manuscript.

Funding: This research was funded by the Ministry of Education, Science and Sport of the Republic of Slovenia through Project Grant AB FREE as well as through Slovenian Research Agency grants J1-6736 and P2-0046.

Acknowledgments: The authors are grateful to Svetlana Marković for her useful suggestions regarding this work.

Conflicts of Interest: The authors declare no conflict of interest. The funders had no role in the design of the study; in the collection, analyses or interpretation of data; in the writing of the manuscript or in the decision to publish the results.

References

1. Craft, B.D.; Kerrihard, A.L.; Amarowicz, R.; Pegg, R.B. Phenol-Based Antioxidants and the In Vitro Methods Used for Their Assessment. *Compr. Rev. Food Sci. Food Saf.* **2012**, *11*, 148–173. [CrossRef]
2. Verotta, L.; Panzella, L.; Antenucci, S.; Calvenzani, V.; Tomay, F.; Petroni, K.; Caneva, E.; Napolitano, A. Fermented Pomegranate Wastes as Sustainable Source of Ellagic Acid: Antioxidant Properties, Anti-inflammatory Action, and Controlled Release Under Simulated Digestion Conditions. *Food Chem.* **2018**, *246*, 129–136. [CrossRef]
3. Bobinaitė, R.; Viškelis, P.; Venskutonis, P.R. Variation of Total Phenolics, Anthocyanins, Ellagic Acid and Radical Scavenging Capacity in Various Raspberry (Rubus spp.) Cultivars. *Food Chem.* **2012**, *132*, 1495–1501.
4. García-Estévez, I.; Escribano-Bailón, M.T.; Rivas-Gonzalo, J.C.; Alcalde-Eon, C. Validation of a Mass Spectrometry Method To Quantify Oak Ellagitannins in Wine Samples. *J. Agric. Food Chem.* **2012**, *60*, 1373–1379. [CrossRef]
5. González-Sarrías, A.; Miguel, V.; Merino, G.; Lucas, R.; Morales, J.C.; Tomás-Barberán, F.; Álvarez, A.I.; Espín, J.C. The Gut Microbiota Ellagic Acid-Derived Metabolite Urolithin A and Its Sulfate Conjugate Are Substrates for the Drug Efflux Transporter Breast Cancer Resistance Protein (ABCG2/BCRP). *J. Agric. Food Chem.* **2013**, *61*, 4352–4359. [CrossRef]
6. Rogerio, A.P.; Fontanari, C.; Borducchi, É.; Keller, A.C.; Russo, M.; Soares, E.G.; Albuquerque, D.A.; Faccioli, L.H. Anti-inflammatory Effects of Lafoensia pacari and Ellagic Acid in a Murine Model of Asthma. *Eur. J. Pharmacol.* **2008**, *580*, 262–270. [CrossRef]
7. Goodwin, E.C.; Atwood, W.J.; DiMaio, D. High-Throughput Cell-Based Screen for Chemicals That Inhibit Infection by Simian Virus 40 and Human Polyomaviruses. *J. Virol.* **2009**, *83*, 5630–5639. [CrossRef]
8. Nohynek, L.; Alakomi, H.-L.; Kähkönen, M.; Heinonen, M.; M Helander, I.; Oksman-Caldentey, K.-M.; Puupponen-Pimiä, R. Berry Phenolics: Antimicrobial Properties and Mechanisms of Action Against Severe Human Pathogens. *Nutr. Cancer* **2006**, *54*, 18–32. [CrossRef]
9. Lall, R.K.; Syed, D.N.; Adhami, V.M.; Khan, M.I.; Mukhtar, H. Dietary Polyphenols in Prevention and Treatment of Prostate Cancer. *Int. J. Mol. Sci.* **2015**, *16*, 3350–3376. [CrossRef]
10. Santos, I.S.; Ponte, B.M.; Boonme, P.; Silva, A.M.; Souto, E.B. Nanoencapsulation of Polyphenols for Protective Effect Against Colon–rectal Cancer. *Biotechnol. Adv.* **2013**, *31*, 514–523. [CrossRef]
11. Brglez Mojzer, E.; Knez Hrnčič, M.; Škerget, M.; Knez, Ž.; Bren, U. Polyphenols: Extraction Methods, Antioxidative Action, Bioavailability and Anticarcinogenic Effects. *Molecules* **2016**, *21*, 901. [CrossRef] [PubMed]
12. Stoner, G.D.; Mukhtar, H. Polyphenols as Cancer Chemopreventive Agents. *J. Cell. Biochem.* **1995**, *59*, 169–180. [CrossRef]
13. Hostnik, G.; Gladović, M.; Bren, U. Tannin Basic Building Blocks as Potential Scavengers of Chemical Carcinogens: A Computational Study. *J. Nat. Prod.* **2019**, *82*, 3279–3287. [CrossRef] [PubMed]
14. Larrosa, M.; García-Conesa, M.T.; Espín, J.C.; Tomás-Barberán, F.A. Ellagitannins, Ellagic Acid and Vascular Health. *Mol. Asp. Med.* **2010**, *31*, 513–539. [CrossRef]

15. Malik, A.; Afaq, S.; Shahid, M.; Akhtar, K.; Assiri, A. Influence of ellagic acid on prostate cancer cell proliferation: A caspase–dependent pathway. *Asian Pac. J. Trop. Med.* **2011**, *4*, 550–555. [CrossRef]
16. Alkayali, A. Ellagic Acid Food Supplement Prepared from Pomegranate Seed. U.S. Patent US 2006/0280819 A1, 14 December 2006.
17. Galano, A.; Francisco Marquez, M.; Pérez-González, A. Ellagic Acid: An Unusually Versatile Protector against Oxidative Stress. *Chem. Res. Toxicol.* **2014**, *27*, 904–918. [CrossRef] [PubMed]
18. Priyadarsini, K.I.; Khopde, S.M.; Kumar, S.S.; Mohan, H. Free Radical Studies of Ellagic Acid, a Natural Phenolic Antioxidant. *J. Agric. Food Chem.* **2002**, *50*, 2200–2206. [CrossRef]
19. Hassoun, E.A.; Walter, A.C.; Alsharif, N.Z.; Stohs, S.J. Modulation of TCDD-induced Fetotoxicity and Oxidative Stress in Embryonic and Placental Tissues of C57BL/6J Mice by Vitamin E Succinate and Ellagic Acid. *Toxicology* **1997**, *124*, 27–37. [CrossRef]
20. Marković, Z.; Milenković, D.; Đorović, J.; Dimitrić Marković, J.M.; Lučić, B.; Amić, D. A DFT and PM6 Study of Free Radical Scavenging Activity of Ellagic Acid. *Mon. Chemie-Chem. Mon.* **2013**, *144*, 803–812. [CrossRef]
21. Mazzone, G.; Toscano, M.; Russo, N. Density Functional Predictions of Antioxidant Activity and UV Spectral Features of Nasutin A, Isonasutin, Ellagic Acid, and One of Its Possible Derivatives. *J. Agric. Food Chem.* **2013**, *61*, 9650–9657. [CrossRef]
22. Tiwari, M.K.; Mishra, P.C. Modeling the Scavenging Activity of Ellagic Acid and its Methyl Derivatives Towards Hydroxyl, Methoxy, and Nitrogen Dioxide Radicals. *J. Mol. Model.* **2013**, *19*, 5445–5456. [CrossRef] [PubMed]
23. Galano, A.; Mazzone, G.; Alvarez-Diduk, R.; Marino, T.; Alvarez-Idaboy, J.R.; Russo, N. Food Antioxidants: Chemical Insights at the Molecular Level. *Annu. Rev. Food Sci. Technol.* **2016**, *7*, 335–352. [CrossRef]
24. Leopoldini, M.; Russo, N.; Toscano, M. The Molecular Basis of Working Mechanism of Natural Polyphenolic Antioxidants. *Food Chem.* **2011**, *125*, 288–306. [CrossRef]
25. Lee, C.Y.; Sharma, A.; Semenya, J.; Anamoah, C.; Chapman, K.N.; Barone, V. Computational Study of Ortho-Substituent Effects on Antioxidant Activities of Phenolic Dendritic Antioxidants. *Antioxidants* **2020**, *9*, 189. [CrossRef]
26. Cossi, M.; Rega, N.; Scalmani, G.; Barone, V. Energies, Structures, and Electronic Properties of Molecules in Solution with the C-PCM Solvation Model. *J. Comput. Chem.* **2003**, *24*, 669–681. [CrossRef] [PubMed]
27. Frisch, M.J.; Trucks, G.W.; Schlegel, H.B.; Scuseria, G.E.; Robb, M.A.; Cheeseman, J.R.; Scalmani, G.; Barone, V.; Mennucci, B.; Petersson, G.A.; et al. *Gaussian 09, Revision D.01*; Gaussian, Inc.: Wallingford, CT, USA, 2013.
28. Zhao, Y.; Truhlar, D.G. The M06 Suite of Density Functionals for Main Group Thermochemistry, Thermochemical Kinetics, Noncovalent Interactions, Excited States, and Transition Elements: Two New Functionals and Systematic Testing of Four M06-class Functionals and 12 Other Function. *Theor. Chem. Acc.* **2008**, *120*, 215–241. [CrossRef]
29. Zhao, Y.; Truhlar, D.G. Density Functionals with Broad Applicability in Chemistry. *Acc. Chem. Res.* **2008**, *41*, 157–167. [CrossRef]
30. Tošović, J.; Marković, S.; Dimitrić Marković, J.M.; Mojović, M.; Milenković, D. Antioxidative Mechanisms in Chlorogenic Acid. *Food Chem.* **2017**, *237*, 390–398. [CrossRef]
31. Tošović, J.; Marković, S. Reactivity of Chlorogenic Acid Toward Hydroxyl and Methyl Peroxy Radicals Relative to Trolox in Nonpolar Media. *Theor. Chem. Acc.* **2018**, *137*, 76. [CrossRef]
32. Tošović, J.; Marković, S. Antioxidative Activity of Chlorogenic Acid Relative to Trolox in Aqueous Solution—DFT Study. *Food Chem.* **2019**, *278*, 469–475. [CrossRef]
33. Marković, S.; Tošović, J. Comparative Study of the Antioxidative Activities of Caffeoylquinic and Caffeic Acids. *Food Chem.* **2016**, *210*, 585–592. [CrossRef] [PubMed]
34. Villuendas-Rey, Y.; Alvarez-Idaboy, J.R.; Galano, A. Assessing the Protective Activity of a Recently Discovered Phenolic Compound Against Oxidative Stress Using Computational Chemistry. *J. Chem. Inf. Model.* **2015**, *55*, 2552–2561. [CrossRef] [PubMed]
35. Glendening, E.D.; Reed, A.E.; Carpenter, J.E.; Weinhold, F. *NBO Version 3.1.*; ScienceOpen, Inc.: Burlington, MA, USA, 2001.
36. Galano, A.; Alvarez-Idaboy, J.R. A Computational Methodology for Accurate Predictions of Rate Constants in Solution: Application to the Assessment of Primary Antioxidant Activity. *J. Comput. Chem.* **2013**, *34*, 2430–2445. [CrossRef] [PubMed]

37. Cordova-Gomez, M.; Galano, A.; Alvarez-Idaboy, J.R. Piceatannol, a Better Peroxyl Radical Scavenger than Resveratrol. *RSC Adv.* **2013**, *3*, 20209–20218. [CrossRef]
38. Mazzone, G.; Russo, N.; Toscano, M. Antioxidant Properties Comparative Study of Natural Hydroxycinnamic Acids and Structurally Modified Derivatives: Computational Insights. *Comput. Theor. Chem.* **2016**, *1077*, 39–47. [CrossRef]
39. Marino, T.; Russo, N.; Galano, A. A Deeper Insight on the Radical Scavenger Activity of Two Simple Coumarins Toward OOH Radical. *Comput. Theor. Chem.* **2016**, *1077*, 133–138. [CrossRef]
40. Francisco-Marquez, M.; Galano, A. Detailed Investigation of the Outstanding Peroxyl Radical Scavenging Activity of Two Novel Amino-pyridinol-based Compounds. *J. Chem. Inf. Model.* **2019**, *59*, 3494–3505. [CrossRef]
41. Castañeda-Arriaga, R.; Alvarez-Idaboy, J.R. Lipoic Acid and Dihydrolipoic Acid. A Comprehensive Theoretical Study of Their Antioxidant Activity Supported by Available Experimental Kinetic Data. *J. Chem. Inf. Model.* **2014**, *54*, 1642–1652.
42. Ramis, R.; Ortega-Castro, J.; Caballero, C.; Casasnovas, R.; Cerrillo, A.; Vilanova, B.; Adrover, M.; Frau, J. How Does Pyridoxamine Inhibit the Formation of Advanced Glycation End Products? The Role of Its Primary Antioxidant Activity. *Antioxidants* **2019**, *8*, 344. [CrossRef]
43. Eckart, C. The Penetration of a Potential Barrier by Electrons. *Phys. Rev.* **1930**, *35*, 1303–1309. [CrossRef]
44. Duncan, W.T.; Bell, R.L.; Truong, T.N. TheRate: Program for Ab initio Direct Dynamics Calculations of Thermal and Vibrational-state-selected Rate Constants. *J. Comput. Chem.* **1998**, *19*, 1039–1052. [CrossRef]
45. Marcus, R.A. Electron Transfer Reactions in Chemistry. Theory and Experiment. *Rev. Mod. Phys.* **1993**, *65*, 599–610. [CrossRef]
46. Pan, J.X.; Wang, W.F.; Lin, W.Z.; Lu, C.Y.; Han, Z.H.; Yao, S.D.; Lin, N.Y. Interaction of Hydroxycinnamic Acid Derivatives with the Cl3COO Radical: A Pulse Radiolysis Study. *Free. Radic. Res.* **1999**, *30*, 241–245. [CrossRef]
47. Wang, A.; Lu, Y.; Du, X.; Shi, P.; Zhang, H. A Quantum Chemical Study on the Reactivity of Four Licorice Flavonoids Scavenging ·OOCl3C. *Struct. Chem.* **2019**, *30*, 1795–1803. [CrossRef]
48. Aruoma, O.I.; Murcia, A.; Butler, J.; Halliwell, B. Evaluation of the Antioxidant and Prooxidant Actions of Gallic Acid and Its Derivatives. *J. Agric. Food Chem.* **1993**, *41*, 1880–1885. [CrossRef]
49. Alberto, M.E.; Russo, N.; Grand, A.; Galano, A. A Physicochemical Examination of the Free Radical Scavenging Activity of Trolox: Mechanism, Kinetics and Influence of the Environment. *Phys. Chem. Chem. Phys.* **2013**, *15*, 4642. [CrossRef]

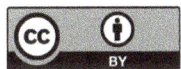

© 2020 by the authors. Licensee MDPI, Basel, Switzerland. This article is an open access article distributed under the terms and conditions of the Creative Commons Attribution (CC BY) license (http://creativecommons.org/licenses/by/4.0/).

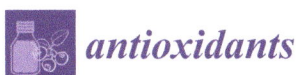

Article

Chemical Composition and Biological Activities of the Nord-West Romanian Wild Bilberry (*Vaccinium myrtillus* L.) and Lingonberry (*Vaccinium vitis-idaea* L.) Leaves

Bianca-Eugenia Ștefănescu [1,2], Lavinia Florina Călinoiu [2,*], Floricuța Ranga [3], Florinela Fetea [3], Andrei Mocan [1,4], Dan Cristian Vodnar [3,*] and Gianina Crișan [1]

[1] Department of Pharmaceutical Botany, "Iuliu Hațieganu" University of Medicine and Pharmacy, 23, Ghe. Marinescu Street, 400337 Cluj-Napoca, Romania; stefanescu.bianca@umfcluj.ro (B.-E.Ș.); mocan.andrei@umfcluj.ro (A.M.); gcrisan@umfcluj.ro (G.C.)
[2] Institute of Life Sciences, University of Agricultural Sciences and Veterinary Medicine Cluj-Napoca, Calea Mănăștur 3-5, 400372 Cluj-Napoca, Romania
[3] Faculty of Food Science and Technology, University of Agricultural Sciences and Veterinary Medicine Cluj-Napoca, Calea Mănăștur 3-5, 400372 Cluj-Napoca, Romania; florcutza_ro@yahoo.com (F.R.); florinelafetea@yahoo.com (F.F.)
[4] Laboratory of Chromatography, Institute of Advanced Horticulture Research of Transylvania, University of Agricultural Sciences and Veterinary Medicine, 400372 Cluj-Napoca, Romania
* Correspondence: lavinia.calinoiu@usamvcluj.ro (L.F.C.); dan.vodnar@usamvcluj.ro (D.C.V.)

Received: 4 April 2020; Accepted: 3 June 2020; Published: 5 June 2020

Abstract: This study was performed to evaluate and compare the in vitro antioxidant, antimicrobial, and antimutagenic activities, and the polyphenolic content of the Nord-West Romanian wild bilberry (*Vaccinium myrtillus* L.) and lingonberry (*Vaccinium vitis-idaea* L.) leaves from three different natural habitats (Smida, Turda, Borsa). In the case of both species, the flavanols level was higher in Smida habitat (altitude 1100 m), whereas quercetin derivates were more abundant in Borsa habitat (altitude 850 m). The bilberry leaf extracts contained in the highest amounts the feruloylquinic acid (59.65 ± 0.44 mg/g for Borsa habitat) and rutin (49.83 ± 0.63 mg/g for Borsa habitat), and showed relevant 2,2-diphenyl-1-picrylhydrazyl (DPPH) antioxidant activity (271.65 mM Trolox/100 g plant material for Borsa habitat, 262.77 mM Trolox/100 g plant material for Smida habitat, and 320.83 mM Trolox/100 g plant material for Turda habitat), for all the three extracts. Gallocatechin was the dominant flavanol in lingonberry species, with the highest amount being registered for Smida habitat (46.81 ± 0.3 mg/g), revealing a DPPH antioxidant activity of 251.49 mM Trolox/100 g plant material. The results obtained in the antimicrobial tests showed that the best inhibitory effect among bilberry species was attributed to the Turda (altitude 436 m) and Smida locations, against both Gram-positive and Gram-negative bacterial strains. For lingonberry, the differences in habitat did not influence the antibacterial effect, but the antifungal effect, only in the case of *Candida zeylanoides*. A strong antimutagenic effect was registered by the bilberry leaves toward *Salmonella typhimurium* TA100. Our study may be able to provide a better understanding of the correlation between natural habitat conditions and the accumulation of secondary metabolites and their related bioactivities in studied leaves.

Keywords: bilberry; lingonberry; polyphenols; antioxidant compounds; antimicrobial activity; antimutagenicity; altitude variations

1. Introduction

Most recent epidemiological studies have reported that certain medicinal plants can be responsible for preventing the development or evolution of several diseases [1–4]. The naturally-derived antioxidants are a topic of major interest considering their proven health effects on humans [2,5], but also to gradually replace the synthetic antioxidants that have been reported as endocrine disrupters or even carcinogenic compounds [6,7]. Dietary polyphenols have diverse therapeutic uses and several proven biological properties [1,8–11], being of important consideration to study their varieties in medicinal plants and natural foods [12].

The development of newly plant-derived functional products and nutraceuticals, known as edible sources with high antioxidant content, have been the intensively studied research topics in recent years [13]. Among them, *Vaccinium* species are constantly reported for their diversity in phenolic compounds [14–16], whereas cranberry (*Vaccinium macrocarpon* Ait.) and bilberry (*Vaccinium myrtillus* L.), being more debated than lingonberry (*Vaccinium vitis-idaea* L.), contributed to their high consumption rate under several forms: as fresh fruits, processed products, and dietary supplements. Recent literature reported that lingonberry occupies a significant position in the antioxidant and antimicrobial capacity ranking of *Vaccinium*-derived species [17,18].

Bilberry (*Vaccinium myrtillus* L.), also known as the European blueberry, and lingonberry (*Vaccinium vitis-idaea* L.), commonly known as cowberry or partridgeberry, are two small, spontaneous growing shrubs belonging to the genus *Vaccinium*, *Ericaceae* family. Their berries mature from July to September, while the ripeness time is highly affected by the site conditions, precisely altitude, and habitat type. Usually, higher altitudes generate later plant ripening when compared with lower elevations.

The bilberry and lingonberry leaves are the main by-products of berry harvesting and recent investigations [14,19] have reported a significantly higher content of phenolic compounds in the leaves and stems of *Vaccinium* species in contrast to the berries, in line with the strongest antioxidant activities registered by these aerial parts than fruits [20], indicating that they may be utilized as an alternative source of bioactive natural products for the development of food supplement, nutraceuticals, or functional food. Literature studies have shown that the leaves of bilberry and lingonberry contain fewer anthocyanins than fruits, but the content of phenolic compounds is higher in leaves than in fruits [16,21,22]. Several studies have reported the presence of hydroxycinnamic acids, flavonols, proanthocyanidins, cinchonains, and iridoids in the bilberry leaves [19,23–25]. Traditionally, bilberry leaves extracts are used for treating urinary tract affection and diabetes. Owing to the presence of various phenolic compounds, bilberry leaves also have antibacterial, anti-inflammatory, and antioxidant activities [26–28]. Chemical composition and biological properties of lingonberry leaves are similar to those of bilberry. Phenolic compounds found in lingonberry leaves are hydroxycinnamic acids, proanthocyanidins. flavonols, cinchonains, iridoids, and arbutin derivatives [14,23,27]. Extracts of lingonberry leaves have shown multiple beneficial diuretics and antiseptic properties for the urinary tract, anti-cough, phlegm removing, anti-inflammatory, neuroprotective, and antioxidant activity [21,29,30].

The genetic factor must be considered when referring to polyphenol biosynthesis in the different parts of the plant, including leaves. Moreover, the biotic and abiotic conditions may be responsible for certain variations (increases or decreases) in phenolic concentration, as reported in the recent literature for bilberry leaf and stem [19,24] and lingonberry leaf [25,31]. A multitude of environmental factors change with the altitude of the growing site, precisely precipitation, mean temperature, soil, wind speed, low- and high-temperature extremes, duration of snow cover, length of vegetation period, and intensity of radiation under clear sky conditions. Enhanced UV-B radiation and lower temperatures at high altitudes have been constantly debated as having an impact on plant secondary metabolism [32,33]. As a protective mechanism towards damage induced by excessive UV-B radiation, plants support and stimulate the biosynthesis of UV-B-absorbing phenolic compounds with an antioxidant capacity [32,34]. The stimulation of enzymes responsible for flavonoid biosynthesis in UV-enhanced radiation experiments was highly underlined [35,36].

The latitude-related factor was discussed in particular for *V. myrtillus* L., being reported for the high influence on the quality and quantity of phenolic compounds [24,37–40], suggesting that higher phenolic amounts may be supported by northern latitudes, altitude, and sunny weather. However, most studies have aimed to investigate an individual morphological part of the bilberry plant, with fruits as most debated, and leaves in a small percentage. In this context, this study aims to provide a better understanding of the correlation between natural habitats and the accumulation of phenolic compounds in the leaves of *Vaccinium myrtillus* L. and *Vaccinium vitis-idaea* L. and their related bioactivities: antioxidant, antimicrobial, and antimutagenic. Thus, the investigation on the differences, derived from natural habitats within the same region (Nord-West), on polyphenolic content of the Romanian wild bilberry and lingonberry leaf extracts could be useful to broaden the knowledge on this field.

Considering that the chemical composition of the Nord-West Romanian wild bilberry and lingonberry leaves has never been the subject of a scientific paper to best of our knowledge, this study aimed to determine the phenolic composition of bilberry and lingonberry leaves and to measure their antioxidant, antibacterial, antifungal, and antimutagenic activities, whereas the antimutagenic and antimicrobial activities of the leaves are of significant novelty. Furthermore, the differences between the three different natural habitats of Romanian bilberry and lingonberry leaves were also investigated.

2. Materials and Methods

2.1. Plant Samples and Growing Conditions

The leaves of bilberry (*Vaccinium myrtillus* L.) and lingonberry (*Vaccinium vitis-idaea* L.) were collected in the autumn (September) of 2017 from spontaneous species of three different locations in Romania, differing in altitude and habitat type: (1) Turda (46°32′00″ N, 23°52′00″ E), Cluj County; (2) Smida (46°38′33″ N, 22°52′49″ E), Cluj County; and (3) Borsa (47°39′19″ N, 24°39′47″ E), Maramures County. Leaves of both species were randomly sampled from ca. 10 shrubs in the same 20 m × 20 m area for each habitat. The plant material was dried at room temperature for 7–10 days and grounded to a fine powder and kept in the dark prior to analyses. The results were calculated based on the dried and grounded plant material/powder. The numbers of Plant Voucher Specimens are VM103 and VVI105.

2.2. Description of Habitats

Turda is a municipality in the county of Cluj, Transylvania, Romania, and it is located about 30 km southeast of Cluj-Napoca. Turda developed mainly on the left side of the Arieș river. The minimum altitude is 310 m in the eastern extremity, on the Arieș valley, and the maximum is in the northeast of the city, on Slăninii Hill (436 m), from where the leaves were collected. The karst relief is present and develops into soluble rocks (limestone, salt, gypsum), being characterized by mineral soils. The climate in September is quite dry with 44 mm of rainfall, and involves a maximum temperature of 23 °C and a minimum of 15 °C. The collection place had a moderate solar exposition considering the slope exposure [41].

Smida is located in the heart of the Apuseni Natural Park, a protected area that is among the last large areas of large, forested karst (spreading its wild beauty on approximately 76,000 hectares) throughout Europe. Smida village is at an altitude of 1100 m and benefits from a moderate continental climate, whereas in September, there is a maximum temperature of 23 °C and a minimum of 1 °C, with 6.5 mm of rainfall. The soil is characterized by acid brown soils with medium texture, and good aquatic drainage considering the winters rich in snow. It possesses large areas of natural forests and meadows, with a variety of fauna and flora. The relief is a karstic one, well developed, and made up of caves [42]. The collection place had partial sun exposure considering the open-spaced areas surrounded by forest.

The Borsa town is located in the south of Maramureș county, Transylvania, Romania at an altitude of 850 m in the Rodnei Mountains, on the Vișeu river valley. The relief of the area is mountainous, very rugged, and with steep slopes and high-level differences, being characterized by the moderate continental climate sector, with a maximum temperature of 13 °C and a minimum of 8 °C, and with the average annual rainfall of 1100 mm and permanent exposure to the advection of the western air masses of oceanic nature, whose characteristics are reflected in the evolution of all climatic elements. The collection place is characterized by acid brown soils and good solar exposition [43].

2.3. Chemicals and Reagents

Catechin, chlorogenic acid, quercetin, cyanidin chloride, and gallic acid used as standards for the HPLC-DAD-ESI-MS analysis were purchased from Sigma-Aldrich (Steinheim, Germany). Folin–Ciocalteu's phenol reagent, sodium carbonate (Na2CO3), sodium nitrate (NaNO2), hydrochloric acid (HCl), aluminum chloride (AlCl3), sodium hydroxide (NaOH), acetic acid, acetonitrile, methanol, ethanol, DPPH (2,2-diphenyl-1-picrylhydrazyl), and Trolox (6-hydroxy-2,5,7,8-tetramethylchroman-2-carboxylic acid) were purchased from Sigma-Aldrich (Steinheim, Germany). For antimicrobial assays, Mueller–Hinton agar, thioglycollate broth with resazurin, and Mueller–Hinton broth were purchased from BioMerieux (France), and Tween 80 and Broth Malt medium were purchased from Sigma-Aldrich (Steinheim, Germany).

2.4. Ultrasound-Assisted Extraction Procedure

The fine powder obtained from the leaves (0.25 g) was extracted with 7 mL 40% v/v ethanol in water for 30 min in an ultrasonic bath, at 20 °C. After centrifugation (5000 rpm for 10 min at 24 °C), the supernatant was filtered and stored (−18 °C) until analysis (total phenolic content, total flavonoid content, total anthocyanin content, antioxidant, antimutagenic and antimicrobial activities, and HPLC-DAD-MS analysis).

2.5. Analysis of Phenolic Compounds

2.5.1. HPLC-DAD-ESI-MS Analysis

Identification and quantification of phenolic compounds in the leave extract were performed on an HPLC-DAD-ESI-MS system consisting of an Agilent 1200 HPLC with DAD detector, coupled to an MS-detector single-quadrupole Agilent 6110. For phenolic compounds' separation, the Eclipse column, XDB C18 (4.6 × 150 mm, particle size 5 µm) (Agilent Technologies, USA), was used at 25 °C. The binary gradient was prepared from 0.1% acetic acid/acetonitrile (99:1) in distilled water (v/v) (solvent A) and 0.1% acetic acid in acetonitrile (v/v) (solvent B) with a flow rate of 0.5 mL/min, according to the elution program described by Dulf et al. [44]. For MS fragmentation, the ESI (+) module was used, with a scanning range between 100 and 1200 m/z, capillary voltage 3000 V, at 350 °C, and with a nitrogen flow of 8 l/min. The eluent was monitored by DAD, and the absorbance spectra (200–600 nm) were measured and collected during each run. For analyzing the data, Agilent ChemStation Software (Rev B.04.02 SP1, Palo Alto, CA, USA) was performed. The phenolic compounds from the extracts were identified by comparing the retention times, UV visible, and mass spectra of the peaks with four reference standards, as follows: the compounds of the flavanol subclass were quantified using the calibration curve performed with catechin standard on the concentration ranges of 10–200 µg/mL and expressed as equivalents of catechin (mg catechin/g plant material) ($r^2 = 0.9985$); for the hydroxycinnamic acid subclass, the compounds were quantified using the calibration curve performed with chlorogenic acid on the concentration range of 10–50 µg/mL, expressed as chlorogenic equivalents (mg chlorogenic acid/g plant material) ($r^2 = 0.9937$); flavonols were quantified using the calibration curve performed with quercetin on the concentration ranges of 10–200 µg/mL, expressed as quercetin equivalents (mg quercetin/g plant material) ($r^2 = 0.9951$); and anthocyanins were quantified using the calibration curve made with cyanidin on the concentration ranges of 10–100 µg/mL, expressed as cyaniding equivalents (mg cyanidin/g plant material) ($r^2 = 0.9951$).

2.5.2. Total Phenolic Content

The determination of total phenolic content (TPC) was performed by the Folin–Ciocalteu method [44,45]. Briefly, 25 µL of sample extract was combined with 125 µL of Folin–Ciocalteu reagent (0.2 N) and 100 µL of sodium carbonate solution (Na_2CO_3, 7.5% w/v). Afterward, the mixture was incubated for 2 h in the dark at room temperature (25 °C). The absorbance was recorded at 760 nm, using ethanol as blank. A standard curve was prepared using gallic acid (0.01–1 mg/mL), and the TPC in the extract was expressed as gallic acid equivalents (GAE) (mg GAE/100 g plant material).

2.5.3. Total Flavonoid Content

Total flavonoid content (TFC) was determined by a spectrophotometric method [46] based on the formation of a complex flavonoid—aluminum. Shortly, 1 mL of sample extract was mixed with 0.3 mL $NaNO_2$ (5%); after 5 min, 0.3 mL $AlCl_3$ (10%) was added; afterward, 2 mL NaOH (1M) and water to a total volume of 10 mL. The absorbance was measured immediately, at 510 nm. A standard curve was prepared using quercetin (0.117–1 mg/mL) and the TFC was expressed as quercetin equivalents (QE) (mg QE/ 100 g plant material).

2.5.4. Total Anthocyanin Content

The total anthocyanin content (TAC) was determined by UV/visible spectrophotometric method [47]. The extracts were diluted with 40% ethanol, and the absorption was measured at 530 nm using a Jasco UV-VIS Spectrophotometer (V-530 double beam, Tokyo, Japan). The anthocyanin content was estimated as cyanidin-3-glucoside at 530 nm using a molar absorptivity coefficient of 26,900 and was expressed as milligrams per 100 g of plant material [47].

2.6. DPPH Free-Radical-Scavenging-Assay

DPPH free-radical–scavenging activity was performed using the method described by Ebrahimabadi et al. [48] with slight modifications. First, 250 µL of each leaf hydroethanolic extract was mixed with 1750 µL of freshly prepared DPPH solution (0.1 mM in 40% ethanol). The absorbance was measured after 30 min of rest under dark conditions, at 517 nm, using the spectrophotometer Biotek and 40% ethanol as blank. In the DPPH assay, the antioxidant activity of the extracts was evaluated using the calibration curve performed with Trolox, and then the absorbance was recorded for all the tested extracts, to calculate the percentage inhibition (expressed as percentage inhibition of the DPPH radicals). The percentage inhibition (I%) was calculated as I% = $[(A_B - A_A)/A_B] \times 100$, where A_B = absorbance of blank and A_{A-} = absorbance of hydroethanolic extract.

2.7. Antimicrobial and Antifungal Capacity

2.7.1. Stains and Cultivation Conditions

To determine the antimicrobial activity for all extracts, six bacterial strains were used: three Gram-positive bacteria: *Staphylococcus aureus* (ATCC 49444), *Enterococcus faecalis* (ATCC 29212), *Rhodococcus equi* (ATCC 6939), and three Gram-negative bacteria: *Pseudomonas aeruginosa* (ATCC 27853), *Klebsiella pneumonia* (DSMZ 2026), *Escherichia coli enterotoxigen* (ATCC 25922). All tested microorganisms were obtained from the Food Biotechnology Laboratory, UASVM CN, Romania.

2.7.2. Microdilution Technique

Evaluation of the antimicrobial activity was done according to the guidelines of the Clinical Laboratory Standards Institute (CLSI) [49], using the standard broth microdilution technique for bacteria that grow aerobically, with slight modifications. Briefly, all the bacteria were cultured on Mueller–Hinton agar, followed by their storage at 4 °C and subculture once a month. Before antibacterial susceptibility testing, each strain was inoculated on Mueller–Hinton agar plates and incubated at 37 °C for 24 h. The medium used for susceptibility testing was Mueller–Hinton broth. Inoculums (density of 0.5 in McFarland scale) were prepared in a 0.9% NaCl sterile solution. Then, tested strains were suspended in Mueller–Hinton broth medium, to give a final density of 2×10^5 colony-forming units (CFU)/mL. The inoculum was stored at 4 °C for further use. Determinations of minimum inhibitory concentrations (MICs) were performed by a serial dilution technique using 96-well plates. The 100 µL Mueller–Hinton broth was placed into each of the 96 wells of the microplates. Aliquots of 100 µL of each extract (concentration of 0.1 g/mL) were added into the first rows of the microplates and twofold dilutions of the extracts were made by dispensing the solutions into the remaining wells. Then, 10 µL of the culture suspensions was inoculated into the wells. We used ethanol (40%) in water as a control. The microplates were incubated for 24–48 h at 37 °C. The MIC of the plant extracts was detected after the addition of 20 µL (0.2 mg/mL) of resazurin solution to each well, and the plates were incubated for 2 h at 37 °C. A change from blue to pink indicates the reduction of resazurin and, therefore, bacterial growth. The MIC was defined as the lowest concentration of the extract that inhibited the growth of the bacterial strain [50], which respectively prevented this color change. The minimum bactericidal concentrations (MBCs) were determined by serial subcultivation of 2 µL into 96-well plates containing 100 µL of Mueller–Hinton broth per well and further incubation for 48 h at 37 °C. The MBC was defined as the lowest concentration of the tested extract/compound/antibiotic killing the majority (99.9%) of bacterial inoculum, thus with no visible growth [50]. Streptomycin (Sigma P 7794, Santa Clara, CA, USA) (0.05–3 mg/mL) was used as a positive control for bacterial growth. Water was used as a negative control.

2.7.3. Antifungal Assay

Evaluation of the antifungal activity was done according to the guidelines of the CLSI [51], using the reference method for broth dilution antifungal susceptibility testing of yeasts, with slight modifications. To determine the minimum inhibitory concentration (MIC) and minimum fungicidal concentration (MFC) of the tested extracts, three fungi were used: *Candida albicans* (ATCC 10231), *Candida zeylanoides* (ATCC 20367), and *Candida parapsilosis* (ATCC 22019). All the tested fungal strains were obtained from the above-mentioned source. The cultures were stored on malt agar at 4 °C and subcultured monthly. Before antifungal susceptibility testing, each strain was inoculated on malt agar plates to ensure optical growth characteristics and purity. The medium used for susceptibility testing was broth malt. The initial density of *Candida* spp. was approximately 2×10^6 colony-forming units/mL (CFU/mL). Inoculums (density of 0.5 in McFarland scale) were prepared in a 0.9% NaCl sterile solution. Then, tested strains were suspended in broth malt medium, to give a final density of 1.5×10^5 CFU/mL. For the minimum inhibitory concentration test, the broth microdilution method was applied by preparing a serial of dilutions in 96-well plates. The 100 µL medium was placed into each of the 96 wells of the microplates. Aliquots of 100 µL of each extract diluted in 0.85% saline (concentration of 0.1 g/mL) were added into the first rows of the microplates, and twofold serial dilutions were made by dispensing the solutions into the remaining wells. Then, 10 µL of the inoculum was added to the wells. Plates were incubated at 28 °C for 72 h on a rotary shaker. Minimum inhibitory concentration (MIC) values were determined by adding resazurin (20 µL, 0.02%) followed by incubation for 2 h. The MIC was defined as the lowest concentration required to inhibit the growth of the fungal strain (observed through a binocular microscope). The MFCs were determined by serial subcultivation of 2 µL of tested extracts dissolved in medium and inoculated for 72 h into microtiter plates containing 100 µL of broth per well, followed by further incubation 72 h at 28 °C. The lowest concentration with no visible growth was defined as the MFC, indicating the death of 99.9% of the original inoculum. The positive control used was fungicide fluconazole (1–3500 µg/mL) (Sigma F 8929,

Santa Clara, CA, USA), while the negative control used was water. All the tests were done in duplicate and repeated thrice.

2.8. Mutagenic and Antimutagenic Assay

According to the plate incorporation method [52], described in more detail by Sarac and Sen [53], the plant extracts were tested for mutagenicity and antimutagenicity towards *S. typhimurium* TA98 and *S. typhimurium* TA100, whereas the positive controls used were 4-nitro-ophenylenediamine (4-NPD, 3 mg/plate) for TA98 and sodium azide (NaN3, 8 mg/plate) for TA100. The negative control was ethanol/water (1:1, *v/v*), and the concentration of plant extracts was established to 5 mg/plate. According to the equation described by Ong et al. [54], the antimutagenicity was calculated as follows: %Inhibition = [1 − T/M] × 100, where T is the number of revertants per plate in the presence of mutagen and the plant extract, and M is the number of revertants per plate without plant extract (positive control). The antimutagenicity of the reference mutagens in the absence of the plant extract was defined as 0% inhibition. For each of the two species, the testing was done in duplicate with three subsamples each, and in accordance, the data are reported as the mean ± standard deviation (SD). The following percentage ranges were used to express the antimutagenicity: strong: 40% or more inhibition; moderate: 25–40% inhibition; low/none: 25% or less inhibition [55].

2.9. Statistical Analysis

All of the analyses were done in triplicate, and the data were reported as the means ± standard deviation (SD). The statistical differences among the leave extracts of the three different locations for each type of species were performed using one-way analysis of variance (ANOVA) (Tukey multiple comparison tests) via GraphPad Prism Version 8.0.1 (Graph Pad Software Inc., San Diego, CA, USA). Differences between means at the 5% level were reported to be statistically significant.

3. Results and Discussion

3.1. Phenolic Profile of Wild Bilberry and Lingonberry Leaves

In this study, in the leaves of bilberry and lingonberry, 21 phenolic compounds were identified, originating from four phenolic groups: hydroxycinnamic acids, flavonols, flavanols, and anthocyanins, whereas 19 were found in bilberry leave extracts and 18 in lingonberry leave extracts (Table 1). In the case of bilberry leaves, the most abundant compounds for all three locations were represented by the flavonols class comprising only quercetin derivatives. The second most abundant class was flavanols. For lingonberry leaves, the most abundant class of compounds was flavanols, as reported in the literature [56], for all the three different altitude habitats, followed by hydroxycinnamic acids. In the case of lingonberry leaves, the flavonols class registered small levels for each compound, except rutin. Moreover, the anthocyanins group was not detected.

Table 1. The phenolic compounds content in the leaves of bilberry and lingonberry using HPLC-DAD-ESI-MS and expressed as mg/g.

	Phenolic Compounds	Retention Time R_t (min)	UV λ_{max} (nm)	$[M+H]^+$ (m/z)	VMT	VMS	VMB	VVIT	VVIS	VVIB
Flavanols	Gallocatechin	2.97	279	307, 290	7.59 ± 0.07 [b]	15.37 ± 0.14 [a]	4.84 ± 0.05 [c]	35.10 ± 0.24 [b]	46.81 ± 0.38 [a]	31.41 ± 0.21 [c]
	Epigallocatechin	4.24	279	307, 290	n.d	6.56 ± 0.06	n.d	25.24 ± 0.72 [b]	35.97 ± 0.23 [a]	23.35 ± 0.61 [c]
	Catechin	12.58	280	291	9.87 ± 0.07 [a]	4.79 ± 0.07 [c]	5.38 ± 0.09 [b]	18.51 ± 0.21 [b]	21.57 ± 0.2 [a]	17.43 ± 0.18 [b]
	Epicatechin	13.11	280	291	4.31 ± 0.03 [b]	9.66 ± 0.08 [a]	n.d	n.d	n.d	2.78 ± 0.03
	Procyanidin dimer I	11.33	280	579, 291	n.d	n.d	n.d	6.38 ± 0.05 [b]	8.36 ± 0.06 [a]	6.27 ± 0.03 [b]
	Procyanidin dimer II	19.74	280	579, 291	12.68 ± 0.11 [a]	12.13 ± 0.12 [a]	8.70 ± 0.07 [b]	2.20 ± 0.05 [b]	4.23 ± 0.04 [a]	4.61 ± 0.03 [a]
	Procyanidin trimer	13.89	280	865, 291	21.84 ± 0.21 [b]	24.30 ± 0.72 [a]	10.09 ± 0.12 [c]	12.92 ± 0.12 [c]	14.21 ± 0.16 [b]	18.84 ± 0.22 [a]
Hydroxycinnamic acids	Chlorogenic acid	12.01	281, 329	355, 163	3.34 ± 0.03 [c]	3.85 ± 0.02 [b]	5.94 ± 0.05 [a]	0.79 ± 0.01 [b]	n.d	1.16 ± 0.01 [a]
	Feruloylquinic acid	14.79	283, 330	369	55.37 ± 0.42 [b]	47.66 ± 0.39 [c]	59.65 ± 0.44 [a]	31.05 ± 0.18 [b]	24.61 ± 0.24 [c]	33.42 ± 0.37 [a]
	Caffeoylarbutin	17.20	288, 330	435	n.d	n.d	n.d	6.45 ± 0.04 [a]	3.42 ± 0.02 [c]	5.14 ± 0.05 [b]
	Dicaffeoylquinic acid	20.08	282, 329	517, 163	5.01 ± 0.05 [a]	4.05 ± 0.04 [b]	n.d	1.77 ± 0.02 [a]	0.93 ± 0.01 [b]	1.74 ± 0.01 [a]
Flavonols (quercetin derivatives)	Quercetin-rutinoside (Rutin)	15.35	263, 355	611, 303	44.91 ± 0.21 [b]	42.34 ± 0.19 [c]	49.83 ± 0.63 [a]	18.61 ± 0.19 [b]	11.45 ± 0.10 [c]	21.88 ± 0.19 [a]
	Quercetin-glucoside	16.20	263, 355	465, 303	1.42 ± 0.01 [b]	1.29 ± 0.01 [c]	2.37 ± 0.02 [a]	3.05 ± 0.03 [a]	2.23 ± 0.03 [b]	1.91 ± 0.02 [c]
	Quercetin-acetyl-rhamnoside	17.83	263, 356	493, 303	18.60 ± 0.16 [a]	12.67 ± 0.10 [c]	15.47 ± 0.14 [b]	6.10 ± 0.04 [b]	1.71 ± 0.01 [c]	8.01 ± 0.07 [a]
	Quercetin-arabinoside	18.69	262, 355	435, 303	1.55 ± 0.01 [a]	1.53 ± 0.01 [a]	1.39 ± 0.01 [b]	0.41 ± 0.01 [b]	0.07 ± 0.01 [c]	0.61 ± 0.01 [a]
	Quercetin-xyloside	18.98	262, 355	435, 303	1.47 ± 0.01 [b]	1.30 ± 0.01 [c]	1.53 ± 0.01 [a]	0.45 ± 0.01 [b]	0.05 ± 0.01 [c]	0.62 ± 0.01 [a]
	Quercetin-diglucoside	21.15	263, 355	628, 303	0.91 ± 0.01 [c]	1.42 ± 0.01 [a]	0.17 ± 0.01 [b]	3.11 ± 0.03 [b]	3.93 ± 0.05 [a]	1.12 ± 0.01 [c]
	Quercetin	21.88	261, 355	303	3.69 ± 0.03 [a]	3.26 ± 0.04 [b]	1.16 ± 0.06 [c]	4.78 ± 0.04 [a]	3.31 ± 0.02 [b]	2.61 ± 0.02 [c]
Anthocyanins	Cyanidin-glucoside	11.02	210, 517	449, 287	0.28 ± 0.01 [a]	0.29 ± 0.01 [a]	n.d	n.d	n.d	n.d
	Cyanidin-arabinoside	11.78	214, 517	419, 287	n.d	0.30 ± 0.01	n.d	n.d	n.d	n.d
	Cyanidin-acetyl-glucoside	14.28	218, 518	491, 287	0.33 ± 0.01 [a]	0.29 ± 0.01 [a]	n.d	n.d	n.d	n.d

Values (expressed as mean values ± SD, mg/g, $n = 3$) in the same row followed by different letters (a–c) indicate significant differences ($p < 0.05$) between the three different locations, individual for each type of species (one-way analysis of variance (ANOVA); multiple comparison test; Tukey multiple range test ($p = 0.05$); GraphPad Prism Version 8.0.1, Graph Pad Software, Inc., San Diego, CA, USA). VMT, *V. myrtillus* leaves from Turda; VMS, *V. myrtillus* leaves from Smida; VMB, *V. myrtillus* leaves from Borsa; VVIT, *V. vitis-idaea* leaves from Turda; VVIS, *V. vitis-idaea* leaves from Smida; VVIB, *V. vitis-idaea* leaves from Borsa; n.d, not detected.

The flavanols identified among the two studied species were catechin, epicatechin, gallocatechin, epigallocatechin, two procyanidin dimers, and procyanidin trimer. The procyanidin dimers and trimers are known as proanthocyanidins as well.

In the case of bilberry leaves, for almost all flavanols, the *V. myrtillus* leaves from Smida (VMS) reported the highest amounts. Exceptions were catechin and procyanidin dimers II, in which case *V. myrtillus* leaves from Turda (VMT) presented significantly higher values. The major flavanol identified was procyanidin trimer in all three natural habitats, whereas the VMS had the highest value (24.30 ± 0.72 mg/g plant material), closely followed by VMT, while *V. myrtillus* leaves from Borsa (VMB) registered a 2.5-fold lower value. In particular, gallocatechin was twofold more in VMS than VMT and threefold more when compared with VMB. Epigallocatechin presence only in VMS contributes to the range of differences found among the three different locations. Procyanidin dimer I was not detected in the bilberry leaves of any of the three habitats, whereas epicatechin was the minor compound identified. The VMB leaves had the lowest values among all the flavanols identified, whereas epigallocatechin, epicatechin, and procyanidin dimer I were not present. Compounds present in lower proportions were catechins, in line with the previous results on bilberry leaves from Northern Europe [24]. Significant differences in gallocatechin, epigallocatechin, epicatechin, and procyanidin trimer were detected among locations, and up to threefold higher levels (in the case of gallocatechin) were measured, which can be linked to specific growth conditions of the sites (soil, solar exposure, microclimatic conditions). The habitat can specifically influence the amounts of phenolics as follows: either by the influence of pedological or climatic factors and their interactions [57]. Likewise, Martz et al. [24] reported that high-light-intensity location, higher altitudes, and/or latitudes contributed to more than twofold higher levels of phenolics in the leaves in contrast to lower altitudes or low-light-intensity sites.

Exceptionally high levels of flavanols were quantified in lingonberry leaves, in agreement with the results of previous studies [14,16,56,58], whereas the most recent study of Tian et al. [59] found, as the two most common flavanols, (+)-catechin and (-)-epicatechin, at the highest level in lingonberry (*V. vitis-idaea*) leaf extract (118 mg/100 mL). In our study, gallocatechin was quantified in high amounts, whereas epigallocatechin was detected in significant levels ranging from 23.35 ± 0.61 to 35.97 ± 0.23 depending on the habitat. Their occurrence has never been reported in lingonberry so far, only in bilberry leaves [23] and bilberry stems [19]. However, Bujor et al. [14] reported only a trace amount in lingonberry leaves and quantified the gallocatechin in lingonberry stems. In our study, *V. vitis-idaea* leaves from Smida (VVIS) registered the highest values among almost all the flavanols identified, except for procyanidin trimer and procyanidin dimer II. Gallocatechin was the major flavanol identified in all the three locations, whereas VVIS had the highest amount (46.81 ± 0.38 mg/g plant material), while epigallocatechin and catechin were close behind. Epicatechin was the minor compound identified, and only in *V. vitis-idaea* leaves from Borsa (VVIB); moreover, VVIB registered the highest values for procyanidin dimer II and procyanidin trimer. Furthermore, recent literature reported rich contents of procyanidin dimers and trimers in the extracts of lingonberry leaf (85 mg/100 mL) [59]. All these results underline that rising concentrations of flavanols and especially gallocatechin, epigallocatechin, and catechin in lingonberry leaves, as well as procyanidin trimer in bilberry leaves, were observed in the habitats with higher altitude. This fact was explained in the previously reported results, whereas an increase of flavonoids level with elevation in herbal plants [60] and bilberry leaves [24] was registered. According to the literature, catechin dominated in the red berries, lingonberry, and cranberry, while epicatechin dominated in blue and blackberries [56], in agreement with our findings.

V. vitis-idaea L. yielded greater amounts of gallocatechin, epigallocatechin, catechin, and procyanidin dimer I with increasing altitude and its related climatic and soil conditions, except lower levels were found at the altitudes of 1100 when compared with 850 m in the case of procyanidin dimer II and procyanidin trimer (Table 1). The variation of the flavonoid fraction turned out to be closely related to the altitude-derived conditions, because we found the percentages of four out of six flavonoid compounds rising significantly at the highest altitude. It can be concluded that environmental factors at higher altitudes lead to elevated levels of flavanols, with gallocatechin and epigallocatechin above all, in dried and grounded lingonberry leaves.

Hydroxycinnamic acids are the most widespread phenolic acids in plants, which are described as cinnamic acid-derived compounds. Four derivates of hydroxycinnamic acid were identified: chlorogenic acid, feruloylquinic acid, dicaffeoylquinic acid, and caffeoylarbutin. In the case of bilberry species, VMB together with its environmental-derived conditions (good solar exposure, acid brown soil, low-temperature range) presented the highest levels among the four compounds, except for caffeoylarbutin and dicaffeoylquinic acid, which were not detected. The major compound reported was feruloylquinic acid (59.65 ± 0.44 mg/g plant material in VMB), followed by chlorogenic acid (5.94 ± 0.05 mg/g plant material in VMB) as 10-fold less than feruloylquinic acid. The study of Martz et al. [24] indicated that bilberry leaves from higher latitudes and higher altitudes (boreal forests in Finland, thus low solar exposure) had lower levels of chlorogenic acid derivatives. In the recent paper investigating the Finnish bilberry (*V. myrtillus* L.) leaf extract, hydroxycinnamic acid derivatives represented 82% of the total content of phenolics, mostly as 3-O-caffeoylquinic acid, whereas other hydroxycinnamic acids (coumaric acid, caffeic acid, and ferulic acid) were identified as esters of acids or hexoses [59].

Concerning the lingonberry species, a specific hydroxycinnamic acid was found, precisely the caffeoylarbutin (not detected in bilberry leaves), with an increase of three- to fourfold when compared with dicaffeoylquinic acid, depending on the location. Similarly, Liu et al. [25], Tian et al. [16], and Hokkanen et al. [23] found 2-caffeoylarbutin as the major caffeic acid derivative. The lowest levels of all hydroxycinnamic acids were reported for VVIS, whereas the highest levels were reported for VVIB (caffeoylarbutin). The major compound was again feruloylquinic acid (33.42 ± 0.37 mg/g plant material), as almost half the amount when compared with bilberry species.

Bidel et al. [61] found that the amount of hydroxycinnamic acid highly increased with a higher photosynthetic active radiation (PAR) level, while Li et al. [62] also reported a comparable pattern in apple peel. Hydroxycinnamic acids protect the fundamental tissues from adverse UV radiation; therefore, their expanded accumulation in intense light exposure is anticipated [36]. The high UV-B exposure at higher altitudes is the key determinant for the increased synthesis of phenolic acids in plants [63]. Moreover, lower temperatures at higher altitudes also sustain secondary metabolism [33,37], particularly the accumulation of hydroxycinnamic acids. Following all the above, the Borsa habitat, characterized by a good solar exposure, low-temperature range, and brown acid soils, may explain the highest levels of hydroxycinnamic acids when compared with a moderate/partial solar irradiation and higher temperature ranges (characterizing the other two habitats).

From the flavonols group, seven phenols were identified, all were quercetin derivatives: quercetin, quercetin-rutinoside (rutin), quercetin-glucoside, quercetin-acetyl-rhamnoside, quercetin-arabinoside, quercetin-xyloside, and quercetin-diglucoside. The major flavonol identified within both species was quercetin-rutinoside (rutin), being approximately 40 times higher than most of the flavonols compounds identified, and about 2 times higher than quercetin-acetyl-rhamnoside. Among studied bilberry leaves, VMB presented the highest level (49.83 ± 0.63 mg/g plant material), where all the extracts showed a level above 40 mg/g plant material. Concerning the lingonberry leaves, again, VVIB has shown the highest amount (21.88 ± 0.19 mg/g plant material), where VVIS was half of this level. The second major flavonol compound identified in both species was quercetin-acetyl-rhamnoside with VMT presenting the highest amount (18.60 ± 0.16 mg/g plant material) in the bilberry species, and VVIB in the lingonberry species (8.01 ± 0.01 mg/g plant material). In the case of almost all flavonol compounds, the Smida location (1100 m altitude) reported the lowest values. These results suggest that a Borsa habitat-type (altitude 850 m, good solar exposure, low-temperature range, brown acid soils) may be more beneficial for the biosynthesis of major flavonols compounds, whereas a good solar exposure (low forest environment) may positively contribute to flavonols level. The existing literature [19] on bilberry leaves reported, as major flavonols compound, the quercetin glycosides, namely, quercetin-3-O-galactoside, quercetin-3-O-glucoside, quercetin hexuronides, quercetin pentosides, and a quercetin rhamnoside.

Moreover, the specific quercetin-3-O-(400-(3-hydroxy-3-methyl glutaryl))-a-rhamnoside was identified in all of the morphological parts studied, being previously reported in leaves by Hokkanen et al. [23] and Ieri et al. [27]. In the study of Bujor et al. [14], investigating the lingonberry leaves, a range of 12–19% flavonols were found. There were 18 quercetin glycosides identified, whereas the quercetin-3-O-galactoside, quercetin-3-O-glucoside, quercetin rutinoside, quercetin pentosides, and quercetin-3-O-rhamnoside were in line with previous findings [16,23,25] and our study.

Concerning the anthocyanins class, the three anthocyanins identified were cyanidin-glucoside, cyanidin-arabinoside, and cyanidin-acetyl-glucoside. The anthocyanins group was present only in VMT and VMS leave extracts, but in a small amount (<0.35 mg/g). Our findings are in agreement with the study of Jaakola et al. [36], where elevated gene expression and, therefore, flavonoid biosynthesis including cyanidin glycosides owing to an increased UV exposure in bilberry leaves was described. Therefore, an assumption that anthocyanins from both bilberry leaves may have occurred in higher amounts with increased solar radiation can be made, if we consider the presence of cyanidin-arabinoside only in VMS. When compared with their related berries [64], anthocyanin synthesis is highly affected by light exposure and, as a consequence, bilberries from shaded sites [40] contained lower amounts of red pigments, as low light conditions limit photosynthetic activity. The mechanism involves firstly a decrease in carbohydrate synthesis, followed by a low level of substrate generated for secondary metabolism. Certain phenolic classes are then downregulated, with anthocyanin synthesis negatively influenced. Li et al. [62] also found that anthocyanin level as well as the flavonol content and activity of phenylalanine ammonia-lyase (PAL), and certain enzymes, were increased in the sun-exposed apple peel compared with the shaded peel, underlying the upregulation of the phenylpropanoid pathway generated by a favorable light condition. Rieger et al. [60] reported that the anthocyanins level in bilberries decreased with increasing altitude, while Roslon et al. [65] did not found a relationship between the content of anthocyanins in bilberry fruits and the position of habitats at different altitudes. In the same study, the leaves anthocyanins were not investigated as they were considered not specific for leaves.

3.2. Total Phenolics and Total Flavonoids

According to Figure 1A, the TPC among both species was very similar, whereas there were no statistical differences between the three types of lingonberry leaves. In the case of bilberry leaves, the highest level of TPC was registered by VMT with 13,588.95 ± 9.25 mg GAE/100 g plant material (135.8 ± 9.25 mg GAE/g plant material), being significantly different only from VMS, but not from VMB. In the study of Bujor et al. [19], on the same period of vegetation (September), for the bilberry leaf extracts, a TPC of 142.9 ± 19.2 (mg GAE/g dry extract) was reported, while in the most recent study on lingonberry of the same author [14], the lingonberry leaves extract shown a TPC of 158.9 ± 6.0 (mg GAE/g dry extract). These results are in the same range as our findings. Nevertheless, the *Vaccinium* plants have the same Romanian origin, but different habitats and environmental factors. In the study of Tian et al. [59], the lingonberry leaf ethanolic extracts showed a TPC of 859.5 ± 9.9 (GAE mg/100 mL), while for bilberry leaf ethanolic extracts, a TPC of 201.7 ± 18.2 (GAE mg/100 mL) was found. A possible explanation for the evident differences in contrast to our results may lie in the geographical location, Finnish versus Romanian. According to the same study [59], a higher value of Folin–Ciocalteau was found in the extracts from leaves than in the extract from berries and branches, and the leaf extracts showed higher antioxidative activities (3–20-fold in ORAC assay, 10–20 fold in TRAP) than the berry extracts, in association with the higher contents of phenolic compounds in the leaf extracts [59]. However, regarding our findings, it may be stated that the different habitats did not statistically influence the TPC of both bilberry and lingonberry leaves, considering the high fluctuation in amounts in the different phenolic sub-classes among the three different locations.

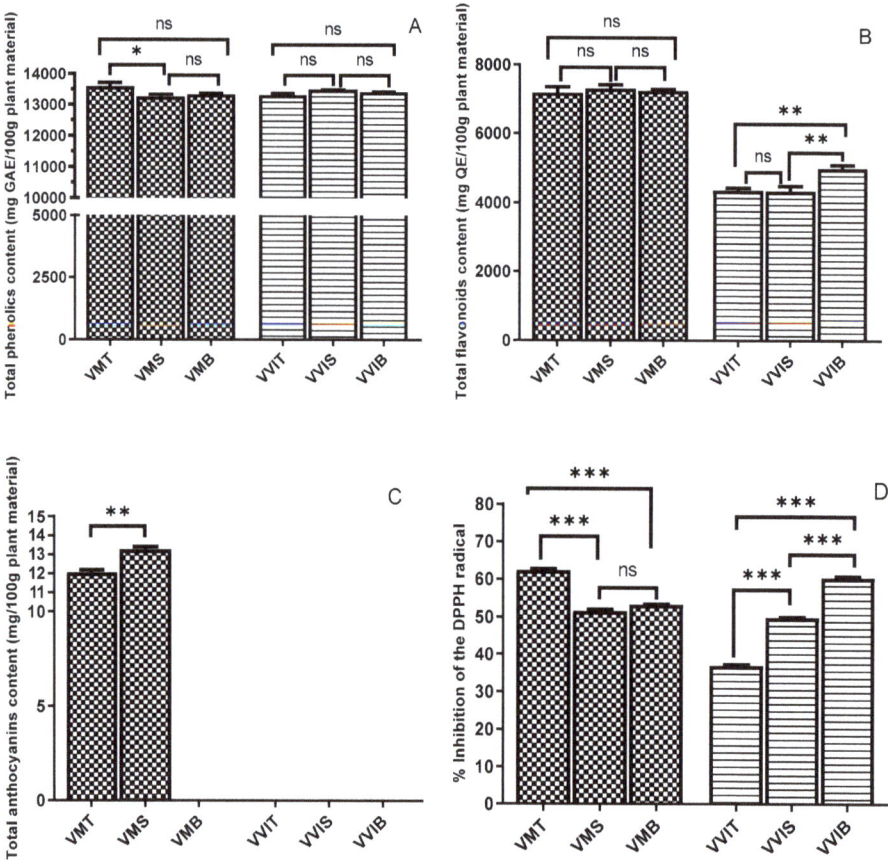

Figure 1. Total phenolic content (Folin–Ciocalteu method) (**A**), total flavonoids content (**B**), total anthocyanin content (**C**), and 2,2-diphenyl-1-picrylhydrazyl (DPPH) antioxidant activity (**D**) of the two species leave extracts, from all three locations. The total phenolic content of the extract is expressed as gallic acid equivalents (GAE) in mg/100 g plant material. Total flavonoid content is expressed as quercetin equivalents (QE) in mg/100 g plant material. The DPPH activity was expressed as percentage inhibition (I%). Values are reported as mean ± SD of triplicate determinations and different symbols (*, **, ***) indicate significant differences ($p < 0.05$) between the three different locations for each of the two species leave extracts, separately (one-way analysis of variance (ANOVA), multiple comparison tests, Tukey multiple range tests), while symbol (ns) indicate no significant difference. VMT, *V. myrtillus* leaves from Turda; VMS, *V. myrtillus* leaves from Smida; VMB, *V. myrtillus* leaves from Borsa; VVIT, *V. vitis-idaea* leaves from Turda; VVIS, *V. vitis-idaea* leaves from Smida; VVIB, *V. vitis-idaea* leaves from Borsa.

Figure 1B presents the TFC of the leaves extracts from both examined species. Among the studied bilberry leaves, there was no statistical difference with the habitat variation, with all three extracts having similar levels of approximately 7300 mg QE/100 plant material. The bilberry species had twofold higher TFC when compared with lingonberry. This may be explained by the fact that chromatographic profiles of flavonoids, but not only them, are different among bilberry, blueberry, lingonberry, and cranberry [66,67]. In the case of lingonberry extracts, the VVIB registered the highest value (4994.18 ± 8.03 mg QE/100 plant material), being statistically different from the other two habitats. Uleberg et al. [37] found that the amount of flavan-3-ols was higher in bilberries growing at lower temperatures, a fact that might explain why Borsa habitat, with lower temperatures (ranging between 13 °C and 8 °C), registered higher amounts. In the study of Mikulic-Petkovsek et al. [40], low levels of flavanols were found in fruits collected in shaded forests characterized by a low photosynthetic active radiation (PAR), and high flavanol amounts in bilberries from sun-exposed locations with high PAR. Jaakola et al. [36] reported that the levels of flavan-3-ols were significantly higher in bilberry leaves exposed to direct sunlight. Considering that Borsa collection place had a good solar exposure when compared with partial or moderate exposure in the other two habitats, these previous findings might explain our results.

Other articles [60,63] reported that increased solar exposure by higher altitudes contributes directly to increased flavonoids content in plants, which is partially true in our study considering that Borsa location (850 m altitude) had the highest level, and Smida location (1100 m) did not. Moreover, another study investigating the bilberry leaves concluded that leaves collected from open and forest areas showed that synthesis and accumulation of flavonoids were delayed in the forest compared with the high light open sites [24]. Several flavonoids and hydroxycinnamic acids act as characteristic UV shields and contribute to the plants' protective mechanism determined by high irradiation sites [60].

3.3. Total Anthocyanin Content

To our knowledge, this is the first study investigating the variation of the amounts of anthocyanins in wild-grown bilberries and lingonberries leaves in correlation to the geographical habitat. According to Figure 1C, only bilberry leaves via VMT and VMS extracts were found to have anthocyanin content. The anthocyanin profile contained small amounts of cyanidin glycosides, whereas VMS registered the highest level, precisely 13.29 ± 0.13 mg/100 g plant material. Our results matched well with the results of a previous comparison of eastern and southern European plants with those from Scandinavia [68], suggesting that a higher altitude may provide an increased sunlight exposure, and thus a higher anthocyanins content. The low levels of total anthocyanin content might be owing to a non-specificity in the leaves of berries when compared with the fruits.

3.4. DPPH Antioxidant Activity

The percentage inhibition of the DPPH radicals for tested leaf extracts is shown in Figure 1D. For bilberry leaves, VMT showed the best radical scavenging capacity based on the DPPH assay expressed as percentage inhibition of DPPH radicals (also as Trolox equivalents, precisely 310.74 mMT/100 g), while in the case of lingonberry leaves, the VVIB had the highest percentage inhibition of the DPPH radicals (and as Trolox equivalents, precisely 320.83 mMT/100 g). These results could be explained by the highest value registered for TPC, in the case of bilberry leaves, and considering the well-known correlation between increased phenolic content and strong antioxidant capacity, whereas for VVIB, the highest TFC value reported may be responsible for the scavenging capacity, as previously reported in the literature [69]. Previous articles have reported that more solar exposure at increased altitude contributed to elevated biosynthesis of ortho-dihydroxylated flavonoids [34,63], as well as a better radical scavenger capacity [70]. In the case of lingonberry leaves, flavanols, flavonols, and caffeic acid derivatives bring highly antioxidant 1,2-dihydroxyphenyl moieties, whereas coumaric acid derivatives display the less antioxidant monohydroxyphenyl moiety. For similar phenolic contents in the case of lingonberry leaves, the *V. vitis-idaea* leaves from Turda (VVIT) present significantly lower antioxidant capacity than both VVIS (−26%) and VVIB (−39%) (Figure 1D). Concerning the higher levels of flavanols, and precisely of procyanidin dimers and procyanidin trimer, compared with VVIT, as well as for VVIB, a significant contribution via feruloylquinic acid might explain the differences. Extension and terminal epicatechin units in flavanols were already proven to be similarly reactive in the quenching of the nitrogen-centered DPPH radical [71]. In the study of Tian et al. [59], the DPPH radical scavenging capacity of the berry leaf extracts varied among species and cultivars, whereas within 10 min, all the leaf extracts succeeded to capture around 80% of DPPH radicals.

The difference in reactivity of leaf extracts, from the three different habitats, in the DPPH test can be attributed to their varying contents in polyphenols containing dihydroxyphenyl moieties, molecular sizes, like for flavanols [14], or the presence of unidentified antioxidant substances. Soobrattee et al. [72] classified the antioxidant activity in the following order: procyanidin dimer > flavan-3-ols > flavonols > hydroxycinnamic acids > simple phenolic acids. Heim et al. [73] explained why the proanthocyanidins (procyanidin dimers and procyanidin trimer) as oligomers and polymers of flavan-3-ols exhibit stronger DPPH capacity, namely owing to more catechol groups, coupled with C3-OH and C4-C8 linkage.

3.5. Assessment of Antimicrobial Capacity

The studied leaves extract registered antibacterial and antifungal capacity towards bacteria and fungal strains. The results of MIC are described in Table 2, and those of MBC are provided in Table 3, for both bacteria and fungi strains. An important range of bacteriostatic effects of the bilberry and lingonberry leaves extracts was reported, depending on the tested strain.

Table 2. Minimum inhibitory concentration (MIC) of bilberry and lingonberry leaves expressed as mg/mL.

Type of Strains	Gram-Positive			Gram-Negative			Fungi		
Sample	S. aureus	E. fecalis	R. equi	E. coli enterotoxigen mg/mL	K. pneumonia	P. aeruginosa	Candida albicans	Candida zeylanoides	Candida parapsilosis
VMT	0.06	0.12	0.06	0.24	0.24	0.24	125	31.25	31.25
VMS	0.12	0.24	0.06	0.48	0.12	0.24	125	62.5	31.25
VMB	0.06	0.12	0.06	0.48	0.12	0.24	125	31.25	31.25
VVIT	0.12	0.12	0.06	0.48	0.12	0.96	125	62.5	31.25
VVIS	0.12	0.12	0.06	0.48	0.12	0.96	125	31.25	31.25
VVIB	0.12	0.12	0.06	0.48	0.12	0.96	125	62.5	31.25
Fluconazole µg/mL	-			-	-	-	15.62	7.81	15.62
Streptomicyn µg/mL	0.03	0.06	0.06	0.12	0.06	0.06			

Table 3. Minimum bactericidal/fungicidal concentration (MBC/MFC) of bilberry and lingonberry leaves expressed as mg/mL.

Type of Strains	Gram-Positive			Gram-Negative			Fungi		
Sample	S. aureus	E. fecalis	R. equi	E. coli enterotoxigen mg/mL	K. pneumonia	P. aeruginosa	Candida albicans	Candida zeylanoides	Candida parapsilosis
VMT	0.12	0.24	0.12	0.48	0.48	0.48	250	62.5	62.5
VMS	0.24	0.48	0.12	0.96	0.24	0.48	250	125	62.5
VMB	0.12	0.24	0.12	0.96	0.24	0.48	250	62.5	62.5
VVIT	0.24	0.24	0.12	0.96	0.24	1.92	250	125	62.5
VVIS	0.24	0.24	0.12	0.96	0.24	1.92	250	62.5	62.5
VVIB	0.24	0.24	0.12	0.96	0.24	1.92	250	125	62.5
Fluconazole µg/mL	-			-	-	-	31.24	15.62	31.24
Streptomicyn µg/mL	0.06	0.12	0.12	0.24	0.12	0.12			

In the case of bilberry leaves, towards *S. aureus*, the best antibacterial activity was registered for both VMT and VMB (MIC = 0.06 and MBC = 0.12 mg/mL). This result may be because of the increased TPC, considering that several studies underlined the fact that polyphenols may attack an important number of bacteria, and the antimicrobial capacity depends on interactions between polyphenols and bacterial cell surface [74,75]. *R. equi* was the most sensitive strain towards all the bilberry extracts, whereas *E. faecalis* Gram-positive strain was the most resistant one.

Towards the lingonberry extracts, S. aureus and E. faecalis exhibited a higher resistance in comparison with R. equi. Considering the Gram-negative strains, E. coli enterotoxigen was not as sensitive as K. pneumonia and P. aeruginosa towards extracts' antibacterial effects. In the case of lingonberry species, the same antibacterial pattern was registered as for Gram-positive ones.

The highest inhibitory activity among bilberry species against all the strains is attributed to the VMT and VMB, while for lingonberry, it seems that natural habitat conditions did not influence the antibacterial effect, but the antifungal effect, only in the case of Candida zeylanoides. It can be concluded that the Gram-positive strains were much more sensitive to all the tested extracts when compared with the Gram-negative ones.

There are only a few studies reporting the antibacterial capacity of bilberry and lingonberry species. In vitro antimicrobial effect of flavonol glycosides, anthocyanins, procyanidins, and flavan-3-ols groups derived from lingonberry juice were demonstrated towards S. mutans and F. nucleatum [76]. Moreover, the antibacterial capacity of fruits and leaves of bilberry in different types of solvents, like water, ethanol, and ethyl acetate, was tested on E. coli, E. faecalis, and P. vulgaris, and it was reported that all extracts had a higher effect towards E. faecalis and P. vulgaris [77]. The study of Tian et al. [59] demonstrated that the extracts of lingonberry leaves, hawthorn leaves, sea buckthorn leaves, Saskatoon leaves, and raspberry leaves registered high inhibitory effects towards S. aureus, L. monocytogenes, and B. cereus. The findings also suggested increased sensitivity of Gram-positive in contrast to Gram-negative bacteria to the phenolic extracts. Moreover, the same study found that the TPC and the content of non-flavonoid phenolics presented a stronger correlation with the inhibitory effects on S. aureus and Bacillus cereus when compared with TFC. Another study [78] established that lingonberry fruit extracts containing mainly type-A proanthocyanidins may be bactericidal against S. aureus or inhibit the hemagglutination of E. coli. Considering that both species had important amounts of proanthocyanidins (procyanidin dimer II, procyanidin trimer), this hypothesis could explain the antibacterial effects on S. aureus and E. coli. Several mechanisms of action in the growth inhibition of bacteria are involved, such as destabilization of the cytoplasmic membrane, permeabilization of the plasma membrane, inhibition of extracellular microbial enzymes, direct actions on microbial metabolism, and deprivation of the substrates required for microbial growth [79].

Regarding the antifungal capacity, both species, in the case of all three types of habitats, had the same effect towards Candida albicans, precisely none (MIC = 125 and MFC = 250 mg/mL) when compared with control Fluconazole (MIC = 15.62 and MFC = 31.25 mg/mL), with the highest antifungal effect towards Candida parapsilosis (MIC = 31.25 and MFC = 62.5). Against Candida zeylanoides, the highest inhibitory potential was registered by VMB and VMT (MIC = 31.25 and MFC = 62.5 mg/mL), as well as VVIS, respectively. A possible explanation of why Candida species were not sensitive to our berry leaf extracts could be explained by the lack of ellagitannins, reported previously as the main antimicrobial compounds against these microorganisms [80].

3.6. Assessment of Antimutagenic Effects of Bilberry and Lingonberry Leaves

The investigation and discovery of antimutagenic properties of plants are of great practical and therapeutic importance in pharmacology and medicine. Research over the past few years has revealed that mutation has a key role in carcinogenesis [81]. The wild bilberry and lingonberry leaf extracts were tested for their antimutagenic activity, considering our recent review study on their significant antioxidant capacity [1]. The influence of the habitat conditions, as well as the type of Vaccinium species, had an important influence on the number of revertants in S. typhimurium TA98 and TA100. The antimutagenicity potential of both species towards S. typhimurium TA98 and TA100 is reported in Table 4, whereas the tested direct-acting mutagens were 4-NPD for TA98 and sodium azide (NaN3) for TA 100.

Table 4. Antimutagenicity capacity towards *Salmonella typhimurium* TA98 and TA100 strains.

Samples	Number of Revertants			
	TA 98		TA100	
	Mean ± S.D	Inhibition %	Mean ± S.D	Inhibition %
Negative Control	9.25 ± 3.6 [a]		9.25 ± 2.4 [a]	
VMT	132 ± 3.2	31.95	198 ± 4.2	43.26
VMS	133 ± 4.4	31.44	201 ± 6.3	42.4
VMB	137 ± 3.6	29.38	202 ± 5.4	42.12
VVIT	144 ± 4.7	25.77	223 ± 2.6	36.1
VVIS	145 ± 2.1	25.25	245 ± 4.3	29.79
VVIB	144 ± 5.9	25.77	234 ± 7.9	32.95
4-NPD [b]	194 ± 3.3	-	-	-
NaN$_3$ [b]	-	-	349 ± 15.22	-

[a] Values expressed are means ± S.D of three replications. [b] 4-nitro-ophenylenediamine (4-NPD) and NaN$_3$ were used as positive controls for *Salmonella thyphimurium* TA98 and TA100 strains, respectively.

Concerning *S. typhimurium* TA98, the leaf extracts proved to significantly inhibit the number of revertants of strain TA98 induced by 4-NPD. Therefore, moderate antimutagenic activity was reported for both types of species, whereas the higher inhibition was registered by the bilberry leaves, precisely VMT (31.95%), closely followed by VMS (31.44%). A possible explanation for this could be the fact that the VMT sample had an increased scavenging capacity, as the literature constantly links the antioxidant potential with the antimutagenic capacity of different types of plant extracts [82,83]. Moderate inhibition of around 25% was registered by all the lingonberry types of leaves, a fact that might be explained by the lack of statistically significant levels of TPC among the three extracts.

Towards TA100, both types of species registered a higher antimutagenic activity, suggesting that *S. typhimurium* TA100 was much more sensitive to *Vaccinium*-type of leaf extracts. Following Table 4, all three types of bilberry leaves showed a strong inhibition capacity (>40%), whereas the best inhibition was exhibited by the VMT (43.26%) extract, closely followed by VMS and VMB. Regarding the lingonberry leaves, all of the extracts proved a moderate antimutagenic effect, whereas the VVIT extract inhibited the mutagenic effect of sodium azide of more than 36%, while the VVIS had the lowest inhibition percentage (29.79%). The best antimutagenic capacity was registered toward the strain *S. typhimurium* TA100 by all the leaf extracts.

In the case of both species, all the above-mentioned favorable effects are more likely to be associated with a high content of flavanols and flavonols, which significantly decrease the mutagenic activity of the standard mutagens examined. To the best of our knowledge, this is the first study evaluating the antimutagenic activity of Nord-West Romanian wild bilberry and lingonberry leaves, thus with significant novelty for the present paper. Moreover, the literature lacks in studies investigating this specific features of bilberry and lingonberry fruits or leaves. In the study of Smith et al. [84], the antimutagenic activity of different berry extracts was investigated. Among the tested berries were strawberry, raspberry, and blueberry of different fresh cultivars, and in several kinds of solvents (H_2O, ethanol, methanol). The antimutagenic inhibition range was between 23% and 53%. Another study [85] investigating the capacity to prevent mutation induced by two promutagenic dietary quinolines, namely MeIQ and 4-NQO of the *V. floribundum* and *V. myrtillus* berries extracts, reported being inactive at concentrations up to 1000 g/plate. In the recent review study on flavonoids' bioactivity [86], it was reported that plant flavonoids exhibit an important antimutagenic activity. Moreover, cranberry (*V. macrocarpon*), as a significant source of polyphenols, has been reported within vitro antimutagenic properties [2,87].

Therefore, regarding the existing data, we can state that the berries contain anthocyanins and procyanidins, constantly reported for their strong antioxidative activity, leading to both in vitro and in vivo antibacterial and antimutagenic activities [88]. In this study, the hydroethanolic extracts from leaves of *V. myrtillus* L. and *V. vitis-idaea* L. did inhibit the mutations on the Ames *Salmonella* test.

Besides, the present study has shown for the first time that hydroethanolic extracts from leaves of wild bilberry and lingonberry are a promising source for its antimutagenic compounds. These results indicate that it may be considered to be a safe and useful agent for the prevention of mutations.

4. Conclusions

The influence of natural habitats on the level of individual phenolic compounds and biological activities were examined, and considerable variations in phenolic profile and significant differences of bioactivities between bilberry and lingonberry leaves, collected from three different locations, were observed.

This study reports a qualitative analysis of bilberry and lingonberry leaves with structures proposed for 21 phenolic compounds. Quantitative analysis revealed that flavonoids class contribute more than half of the phenolic pool in leaves; whereas for bilberry species, rutin represents 50% of this subclass; and for lingonberry species, the flavanols comprise the majority via gallocatechin, epigallocatechin, catechin, and procyanidin trimer. Of significant novelty was the antimutagenic testing among these species, at different habitats, concluding that bilberry leaves have a stronger antimutagenic capacity, whereas better sun exposure may contribute to an increased flavonols synthesis, leading to better antioxidant and antimutagenic activities. Regarding the antimicrobial effects of the studies species, the Gram-positive bacteria were more susceptible to the activity of the extract, presenting high antibacterial effects, whereas the antifungal capacity was low.

Thus, the hypothesis that plants from higher altitudes contain higher amounts of radical scavenging compounds as a result of their exposure to more severe climatic conditions including enhanced solar radiation cannot be affirmed in general. On the basis of our results, distinct differences between the amounts of phenolic compounds due to habitat-derived conditions (altitude, solar exposure, temperature range, and so on) can be expected at least in the case of the flavanols, flavonols, hydroxycinnamic acids, and anthocyanins investigated in these species.

Author Contributions: Conceptualization, B.-E.Ș., and G.C.; methodology, B.-E.Ș.; software, L.F.C.; validation, G.C., A.M., and D.C.V.; investigation, B.-E.Ș., F.F., and F.R.; resources, D.C.V.; writing—original draft preparation, B.-E.Ș. and L.F.C.; writing—review and editing, G.C., A.M., and D.C.V.; supervision, G.C.; project administration, D.C.V.; funding acquisition, D.C.V. All authors have read and agreed to the published version of the manuscript.

Funding: This research was funded by MCI-UEFISCDI, grant number 2 PCCDI, Proiect PN-III-P1-1.2-PCCDI-2017-0056, and the publication was funded by 37 PFE.

Conflicts of Interest: The authors declare no conflict of interest.

References

1. Ștefănescu, B.E.; Szabo, K.; Mocan, A.; Crișan, G. Phenolic Compounds from Five Ericaceae Species Leaves and Their Related Bioavailability and Health Benefits. *Molecules* **2019**, *24*, 2046. [CrossRef] [PubMed]
2. Del Rio, D.; Rodriguez-Mateos, A.; Spencer, J.P.E.; Tognolini, M.; Borges, G.; Crozier, A. Dietary (Poly)phenolics in Human Health: Structures, Bioavailability, and Evidence of Protective Effects Against Chronic Diseases. *Antioxid. Redox Signal.* **2012**, *18*, 1818–1892. [CrossRef] [PubMed]
3. Shahidi, F.; Ambigaipalan, P. Phenolics and polyphenolics in foods, beverages and spices: Antioxidant activity and health effects—A review. *J. Funct. Foods* **2015**, *18*, 820–897. [CrossRef]
4. Shahidi, F.; Yeo, J.; Shahidi, F.; Yeo, J. Bioactivities of Phenolics by Focusing on Suppression of Chronic Diseases: A Review. *Int. J. Mol. Sci.* **2018**, *19*, 1573. [CrossRef] [PubMed]
5. Abbas, M.; Saeed, F.; Anjum, F.M.; Afzaal, M.; Tufail, T.; Bashir, M.S.; Ishtiaq, A.; Hussain, S.; Suleria, H.A.R. Natural polyphenols: An overview. *Int. J. Food Prop.* **2017**, *20*, 1689–1699. [CrossRef]
6. Popa, D.-S.; Bolfa, P.; Kiss, B.; Vlase, L.; Păltinean, R.; Pop, A.; Cătoi, C.; Crișan, G.; Loghin, F. Influence of Genista Tinctoria L or Methylparaben on Subchronic Toxicity of Bisphenol A in Rats. *Biomed. Environ. Sci.* **2014**, *27*, 85–96. [CrossRef]

7. Pop, A.; Berce, C.; Bolfa, P.F.; Cătoi, C.; Dumitrescu, I.-B.; Silaghi-Dumitrescu, L.; Loghin, F. Evaluation of the possible endocrine disruptive effect of butylated hydroxyanisole, butylated hydroxytoluene and propyl gallate in immature female rats. *Farmacia* **2013**, *61*, 202–211.
8. Dai, J.; Mumper, R.J. Plant phenolics: Extraction, analysis and their antioxidant and anticancer properties. *Mol. Basel Switz.* **2010**, *15*, 7313–7352. [CrossRef]
9. Călinoiu, L.F.; Vodnar, D.C. Whole Grains and Phenolic Acids: A Review on Bioactivity, Functionality, Health Benefits and Bioavailability. *Nutrients* **2018**, *10*, 1615. [CrossRef]
10. Calinoiu, L.-F.; Mitrea, L.; Precup, G.; Bindea, M.; Rusu, B.; Dulf, F.-V.; Stefanescu, B.-E.; Vodnar, D.-C. Characterization of Grape and Apple Peel Wastes' Bioactive Compounds and Their Increased Bioavailability After Exposure to Thermal Process. *Bull. Univ. Agric. Sci. Vet. Med. Cluj-Napoca-Food Sci. Technol.* **2017**, *74*, 80–89. [CrossRef]
11. Călinoiu, L.F.; Cătoi, A.-F.; Vodnar, D.C. Solid-State Yeast Fermented Wheat and Oat Bran as A Route for Delivery of Antioxidants. *Antioxidants* **2019**, *8*, 372. [CrossRef] [PubMed]
12. Martins, N.; Barros, L.; Ferreira, I.C.F.R. In vivo antioxidant activity of phenolic compounds: Facts and gaps. *Trends Food Sci. Technol.* **2016**, *48*, 1–12. [CrossRef]
13. Calinoiu, L.F.; Farcas, A.; Socaci, S.; Vodnar, D.C. *Innovative Sources*; Galanakis, C.M., Ed.; Academic Press Ltd-Elsevier Science Ltd.: London, UK, 2019; pp. 235–265. ISBN 978-0-12-817516-3.
14. Bujor, O.C.; Ginies, C.; Popa, V.I.; Dufour, C. Phenolic compounds and antioxidant activity of lingonberry (*Vaccinium vitis-idaea* L.) leaf, stem and fruit at different harvest periods. *Food Chem.* **2018**, *252*, 356–365. [CrossRef] [PubMed]
15. Ancillotti, C.; Ciofi, L.; Rossini, D.; Chiuminatto, U.; Stahl-Zeng, J.; Orlandini, S.; Furlanetto, S.; Del Bubba, M. Liquid chromatographic/electrospray ionization quadrupole/time of flight tandem mass spectrometric study of polyphenolic composition of different *Vaccinium* berry species and their comparative evaluation. *Anal. Bioanal. Chem.* **2017**, *409*, 1347–1368. [CrossRef] [PubMed]
16. Tian, Y.; Liimatainen, J.; Alanne, A.L.; Lindstedt, A.; Liu, P.; Sinkkonen, J.; Kallio, H.; Yang, B. Phenolic compounds extracted by acidic aqueous ethanol from berries and leaves of different berry plants. *Food Chem.* **2017**, *220*, 266–281. [CrossRef]
17. Grace, M.H.; Esposito, D.; Dunlap, K.L.; Lila, M.A. Comparative Analysis of Phenolic Content and Profile, Antioxidant Capacity, and Anti-inflammatory Bioactivity in Wild Alaskan and Commercial Vaccinium Berries. *J. Agric. Food Chem.* **2014**, *62*, 4007–4017. [CrossRef]
18. Ermis, E.; Hertel, C.; Schneider, C.; Carle, R.; Stintzing, F.; Schmidt, H. Characterization of in vitro antifungal activities of small and American cranberry (*Vaccinium oxycoccos* L. and *V. macrocarpon* Aiton) and lingonberry (*Vaccinium vitis*-idaea L.) concentrates in sugar reduced fruit spreads. *Int. J. Food Microbiol.* **2015**, *204*, 111–117. [CrossRef]
19. Bujor, O.C.; Le Bourvellec, C.; Volf, I.; Popa, V.I.; Dufour, C. Seasonal variations of the phenolic constituents in bilberry (*Vaccinium myrtillus* L.) leaves, stems and fruits, and their antioxidant activity. *Food Chem.* **2016**, *213*, 58–68. [CrossRef]
20. Bujor, O.-C.; Tanase, C.; Popa, M.E. Phenolic Antioxidants in Aerial Parts of Wild Vaccinium Species: Towards Pharmaceutical and Biological Properties. *Antioxid. Basel Switz.* **2019**, *8*, 649. [CrossRef]
21. Vyas, P.; Kalidindi, S.; Chibrikova, L.; Igamberdiev, A.U.; Weber, J.T. Chemical analysis and effect of blueberry and lingonberry fruits and leaves against glutamate-mediated excitotoxicity. *J. Agric. Food Chem.* **2013**, *61*, 7769–7776. [CrossRef]
22. Teleszko, M.; Wojdyło, A. Comparison of phenolic compounds and antioxidant potential between selected edible fruits and their leaves. *J. Funct. Foods* **2015**, *14*, 736–746. [CrossRef]
23. Hokkanen, J.; Mattila, S.; Jaakola, L.; Pirttila, A.M.; Tolonen, A. Identification of phenolic compounds from lingonberry (*Vaccinium vitis-idaea* L.), Bilberry (*Vaccinium myrtillus* L.) and Hybrid Bilberry (Vaccinium x intermedium Ruthe L.) Leaves. *J. Agric. Food Chem.* **2009**, *57*, 9437–9447. [CrossRef] [PubMed]
24. Martz, F.; Jaakola, L.; Julkunen-Tiitto, R.; Stark, S. Phenolic Composition and Antioxidant Capacity of Bilberry (*Vaccinium myrtillus*) Leaves in Northern Europe Following Foliar Development and Along Environmental Gradients. *J. Chem. Ecol.* **2010**, *36*, 1017–1028. [CrossRef] [PubMed]
25. Liu, P.; Lindstedt, A.; Markkinen, N.; Sinkkonen, J.; Suomela, J.-P.; Yang, B. Characterization of Metabolite Profiles of Leaves of Bilberry (*Vaccinium myrtillus* L.) and Lingonberry (*Vaccinium vitis-idaea* L.). *J. Agric. Food Chem.* **2014**, *62*, 12015–12026. [CrossRef]

26. Piterà, F. *Compedio di Gemmoterapia Clinica*; De Ferrari: Genova, Italy, 1994.
27. Ieri, F.; Martini, S.; Innocenti, M.; Mulinacci, N. Phenolic distribution in liquid preparations of *Vaccinium myrtillus* L. and *Vaccinium vitis idaea* L. *Phytochem. Anal.* **2013**, *24*, 467–475. [CrossRef]
28. Cignarella, A.; Nastasi, M.; Cavalli, E.; Puglisi, L. Novel lipid-lowering properties of *Vaccinium myrtillus* L. leaves, a traditional antidiabetic treatment, in several models of rat dyslipidaemia: A comparison with ciprofibrate. *Thromb. Res.* **1996**, *84*, 311–322. [CrossRef]
29. Wang, X.; Sun, H.; Fan, Y.; Li, L.; Makino, T.; Kano, Y. Analysis and bioactive evaluation of the compounds absorbed into blood after oral administration of the extracts of *Vaccinium vitis-idaea* in rat. *Biol. Pharm. Bull.* **2005**, *28*, 1106–1108. [CrossRef]
30. Raudone, L.; Vilkickyte, G.; Pitkauskaite, L.; Raudonis, R.; Vainoriene, R.; Motiekaityte, V. Antioxidant Activities of *Vaccinium vitis-idaea* L. Leaves within Cultivars and Their Phenolic Compounds. *Molecules* **2019**, *24*, 844. [CrossRef]
31. Alam, Z.; Morales, H.R.; Roncal, J. Environmental conditions affect phenolic content and antioxidant capacity of leaves and fruit in wild partridgeberry (*Vaccinium vitis-idaea*). *Botany* **2016**, *94*, 509–521. [CrossRef]
32. Körner, C. *Alpine Plant Life: Functional Plant Ecology of High Mountain Ecosystems; with 47 Tables*; Springer Science & Business Media: Berlin/Heidelberg, Germany, 2003; ISBN 978-3-540-00347-2.
33. Bilger, W.; Rolland, M.; Nybakken, L. UV screening in higher plants induced by low temperature in the absence of UV-B radiation. *Photochem. Photobiol. Sci.* **2007**, *6*, 190–195. [CrossRef]
34. Markham, K.R.; Tanner, G.J.; Caasi-Lit, M.; Whitecross, M.I.; Nayudu, M.; Mitchell, K.A. Possible protective role for 3′,4′-dihydroxyflavones induced by enhanced UV-B in a UV-tolerant rice cultivar. *Phytochemistry* **1998**, *49*, 1913–1919. [CrossRef]
35. Wellmann, E. UV dose-dependent induction of enzymes related to flavonoid biosynthesis in cell suspension cultures of parsley. *FEBS Lett.* **1975**, *51*, 105–107. [CrossRef]
36. Jaakola, L.; Määttä-Riihinen, K.; Kärenlampi, S.; Hohtola, A. Activation of flavonoid biosynthesis by solar radiation in bilberry (*Vaccinium myrtillus* L.) leaves. *Planta* **2004**, *218*, 721–728. [CrossRef] [PubMed]
37. Uleberg, E.; Rohloff, J.; Jaakola, L.; Trôst, K.; Junttila, O.; Häggman, H.; Martinussen, I. Effects of Temperature and Photoperiod on Yield and Chemical Composition of Northern and Southern Clones of Bilberry (*Vaccinium myrtillus* L.). *J. Agric. Food Chem.* **2012**, *60*, 10406–10414. [CrossRef]
38. Åkerström, A.; Jaakola, L.; Bång, U.; Jäderlund, A. Effects of Latitude-Related Factors and Geographical Origin on Anthocyanidin Concentrations in Fruits of *Vaccinium myrtillus* L. (Bilberries). *J. Agric. Food Chem.* **2010**, *58*, 11939–11945. [CrossRef]
39. Jovančević, M.; Balijagić, J.; Menković, N.R.; Scaron, K.; avikin; Zdunić, G.M.; Janković, T.; Dekić-Ivanković, M. Analysis of phenolic compounds in wild populations of bilberry (*Vaccinium myrtillus* L.) from Montenegro. *J. Med. Plant Res.* **2011**, *5*, 910–914.
40. Mikulic-Petkovsek, M.; Schmitzer, V.; Slatnar, A.; Stampar, F.; Veberic, R. A comparison of fruit quality parameters of wild bilberry (*Vaccinium myrtillus* L.) growing at different locations. *J. Sci. Food Agric.* **2015**, *95*, 776–785. [CrossRef]
41. Meteoblue. Available online: https://www.meteoblue.com/ro/vreme/historyclimate/weatherarchive/turda_rom%C3%A2nia_664460 (accessed on 4 June 2020).
42. Meteoromania. Available online: http://www.meteoromania.ro/servicii/date-meteorologice/arhiva-precipitatii/ (accessed on 4 June 2020).
43. Meteoblue. Available online: https://www.meteoblue.com/ro/vreme/historyclimate/weatherarchive/bor%c5%9fa_rom%c3%a2nia_684156 (accessed on 4 June 2020).
44. Dulf, F.V.; Vodnar, D.C.; Dulf, E.H.; Toşa, M.I. Total Phenolic Contents, Antioxidant Activities, and Lipid Fractions from Berry Pomaces Obtained by Solid-State Fermentation of Two Sambucus Species with *Aspergillus niger*. *J. Agric. Food Chem.* **2015**, *63*, 3489–3500. [CrossRef]
45. Dulf, F.V.; Vodnar, D.C.; Socaciu, C. Effects of solid-state fermentation with two filamentous fungi on the total phenolic contents, flavonoids, antioxidant activities and lipid fractions of plum fruit (*Prunus domestica* L.) by-products. *Food Chem.* **2016**, *209*, 27–36. [CrossRef]
46. Zhishen, J.; Mengcheng, T.; Jianming, W. The determination of flavonoid contents in mulberry and their scavenging effects on superoxide radicals. *Food Chem.* **1999**, *64*, 555–559. [CrossRef]
47. Giusti, M.M.; Wrolstad, R.E. Characterization and Measurement of Anthocyanins by UV-Visible Spectroscopy. *Curr. Protoc. Food Anal. Chem.* **2001**, F1.2.1–F1.2.13. [CrossRef]

48. Ebrahimabadi, A.H.; Mazoochi, A.; Kashi, F.J.; Djafari-Bidgoli, Z.; Batooli, H. Essential oil composition and antioxidant and antimicrobial properties of the aerial parts of *Salvia eremophila* Boiss. from Iran. *Food Chem. Toxicol. Int. J. Publ. Br. Ind. Biol. Res. Assoc.* **2010**, *48*, 1371–1376. [CrossRef] [PubMed]
49. Weinstein, M.P. *Methods for Dilution Antimicrobial Susceptibility Tests for Bacteria that Grow Aerobically*; Clinical and Laboratory Standards Institute (CLSI): Wayne, PA, USA, 2018; ISBN 978-1-56238-836-2.
50. Schwalbe, R.; Steele-Moore, L.; Goodwin, A.C. *Antimicrobial Susceptibility Testing Protocols*; CRC Press: Boca Raton, FL, USA, 2007; ISBN 978-1-4200-1449-5.
51. Alexander, B.D. *Reference Method for Broth Dilution Antifungal Susceptibility Testing of Yeasts*; Clinical and Laboratory Standards Institute: Wayne, PA, USA, 2017; ISBN 978-1-56238-826-3.
52. Maron, D.M.; Ames, B.N. Revised methods for the *Salmonella* mutagenicity test. *Mutat. Res. Mutagen. Relat. Subj.* **1983**, *113*, 173–215. [CrossRef]
53. Saraç, N.; Şen, B. Antioxidant, mutagenic, antimutagenic activities, and phenolic compounds of *Liquidambar orientalis* Mill. var. *orientalis*. *Ind. Crops Prod.* **2014**, *53*, 60–64. [CrossRef]
54. Ong, T.M.; Whong, W.Z.; Stewart, J.; Brockman, H.E. Chlorophyllin: A potent antimutagen against environmental and dietary complex mixtures. *Mutat. Res. Lett.* **1986**, *173*, 111–115. [CrossRef]
55. Evandri, M.G.; Battinelli, L.; Daniele, C.; Mastrangelo, S.; Bolle, P.; Mazzanti, G. The antimutagenic activity of *Lavandula angustifolia* (lavender) essential oil in the bacterial reverse mutation assay. *Food Chem. Toxicol.* **2005**, *43*, 1381–1387. [CrossRef]
56. Riihinen, K.; Jaakola, L.; Kärenlampi, S.; Hohtola, A. Organ-specific distribution of phenolic compounds in bilberry (*Vaccinium myrtillus*) and "northblue" blueberry (*Vaccinium corymbosum* x *V. angustifolium*). *Food Chem.* **2008**, *110*, 156–160. [CrossRef]
57. Dabbou, S.; Sifi, S.; Rjiba, I.; Esposto, S.; Taticchi, A.; Servili, M.; Montedoro, G.F.; Hammami, M. Effect of Pedoclimatic Conditions on the Chemical Composition of the Sigoise Olive Cultivar. *Chem. Biodivers.* **2010**, *7*, 898–908. [CrossRef]
58. Kähkönen, M.P.; Hopia, A.I.; Heinonen, M. Berry Phenolics and Their Antioxidant Activity. *J. Agric. Food Chem.* **2001**, *49*, 4076–4082. [CrossRef]
59. Tian, Y.; Puganen, A.; Alakomi, H.-L.; Uusitupa, A.; Saarela, M.; Yang, B. Antioxidative and antibacterial activities of aqueous ethanol extracts of berries, leaves, and branches of berry plants. *Food Res. Int.* **2018**, *106*, 291–303. [CrossRef]
60. Rieger, G.; Müller, M.; Guttenberger, H.; Bucar, F. Influence of Altitudinal Variation on the Content of Phenolic Compounds in Wild Populations of *Calluna vulgaris*, *Sambucus nigra*, and *Vaccinium myrtillus*. *J. Agric. Food Chem.* **2008**, *56*, 9080–9086. [CrossRef] [PubMed]
61. Bidel, L.P.R.; Meyer, S.; Goulas, Y.; Cadot, Y.; Cerovic, Z.G. Responses of epidermal phenolic compounds to light acclimation: *In vivo* qualitative and quantitative assessment using chlorophyll fluorescence excitation spectra in leaves of three woody species. *J. Photochem. Photobiol. B* **2007**, *88*, 163–179. [CrossRef] [PubMed]
62. Li, P.; Ma, F.; Cheng, L. Primary and secondary metabolism in the sun-exposed peel and the shaded peel of apple fruit. *Physiol. Plant.* **2013**, *148*, 9–24. [CrossRef] [PubMed]
63. Spitaler, R.; Winkler, A.; Lins, I.; Yanar, S.; Stuppner, H.; Zidorn, C. Altitudinal Variation of Phenolic Contents in Flowering Heads of *Arnica montana* cv. ARBO: A 3-Year Comparison. *J. Chem. Ecol.* **2008**, *34*, 369–375. [CrossRef] [PubMed]
64. Jakopic, J.; Stampar, F.; Veberic, R. The influence of exposure to light on the phenolic content of 'Fuji' apple. *Sci. Hortic.* **2009**, *123*, 234–239. [CrossRef]
65. Rosłon, W.; Osińska, E.; Pióro-Jabrucka, E.; Grabowska, A. Morphological and chemical variability of wild populations of bilberry (*Vaccinium myrtillus* L.). *Pol. J. Environ. Stud.* **2011**, *20*, 237–243.
66. Zheng, W.; Wang, S.Y. Oxygen Radical Absorbing Capacity of Phenolics in Blueberries, Cranberries, Chokeberries, and Lingonberries. *J. Agric. Food Chem.* **2003**, *51*, 502–509. [CrossRef]
67. Jaakola, L.; Määttä, K.; Pirttilä, A.M.; Törrönen, R.; Kärenlampi, S.; Hohtola, A. Expression of Genes Involved in Anthocyanin Biosynthesis in Relation to Anthocyanin, Proanthocyanidin, and Flavonol Levels during Bilberry Fruit Development. *Plant Physiol.* **2002**, *130*, 729–739. [CrossRef]
68. Määttä-Riihinen, K.R.; Kamal-Eldin, A.; Mattila, P.H.; González-Paramás, A.M.; Törrönen, A.R. Distribution and contents of phenolic compounds in eighteen Scandinavian berry species. *J. Agric. Food Chem.* **2004**, *52*, 4477–4486. [CrossRef]

69. Szakiel, A.; Pączkowski, C.; Koivuniemi, H.; Huttunen, S. Comparison of the triterpenoid content of berries and leaves of lingonberry *Vaccinium vitis-idaea* from Finland and Poland. *J. Agric. Food Chem.* **2012**, *60*, 4994–5002. [CrossRef]
70. Rice-Evans, C.A.; Miller, N.J.; Paganga, G. Structure-antioxidant activity relationships of flavonoids and phenolic acids. *Free Radic. Biol. Med.* **1996**, *20*, 933–956. [CrossRef]
71. Goupy, P.; Dufour, C.; Loonis, M.; Dangles, O. Quantitative Kinetic Analysis of Hydrogen Transfer Reactions from Dietary Polyphenols to the DPPH Radical. *J. Agric. Food Chem.* **2003**, *51*, 615–622. [CrossRef] [PubMed]
72. Soobrattee, M.A.; Neergheen, V.S.; Luximon-Ramma, A.; Aruoma, O.I.; Bahorun, T. Phenolics as potential antioxidant therapeutic agents: Mechanism and actions. *Mutat. Res.* **2005**, *579*, 200–213. [CrossRef] [PubMed]
73. Heim, K.E.; Tagliaferro, A.R.; Bobilya, D.J. Flavonoid antioxidants: Chemistry, metabolism and structure-activity relationships. *J. Nutr. Biochem.* **2002**, *13*, 572–584. [CrossRef]
74. Bouarab-Chibane, L.; Forquet, V.; Lantéri, P.; Clément, Y.; Léonard-Akkari, L.; Oulahal, N.; Degraeve, P.; Bordes, C. Antibacterial Properties of Polyphenols: Characterization and QSAR (Quantitative Structure–Activity Relationship) Models. *Front. Microbiol.* **2019**, *10*. [CrossRef] [PubMed]
75. Coppo, E.; Marchese, A. Antibacterial activity of polyphenols. *Curr. Pharm. Biotechnol.* **2014**, *15*, 380–390. [CrossRef]
76. Riihinen, K.R.; Ou, Z.M.; Gödecke, T.; Lankin, D.C.; Pauli, G.F.; Wu, C.D. The antibiofilm activity of lingonberry flavonoids against oral pathogens is a case connected to residual complexity. *Fitoterapia* **2014**, *97*, 78–86. [CrossRef]
77. Vučić, D.M.; Petković, M.R.; Rodić-Grabovac, B.B.; Stefanović, O.D.; Vasić, S.M.; Čomić, L.R. Antibacterial and antioxidant activities of bilberry (*Vaccinium myrtillus* L.) in vitro. *Afr. J. Microbiol. Res.* **2013**, *7*, 5130–5136.
78. Kylli, P.; Nohynek, L.; Puupponen-Pimiä, R.; Westerlund-Wikström, B.; Leppänen, T.; Welling, J.; Moilanen, E.; Heinonen, M. Lingonberry (*Vaccinium vitis-idaea*) and European Cranberry (*Vaccinium microcarpon*) Proanthocyanidins: Isolation, Identification, and Bioactivities. *J. Agric. Food Chem.* **2011**, *59*, 3373–3384. [CrossRef]
79. Puupponen-Pimiä, R.; Nohynek, L.; Alakomi, H.-L.; Oksman-Caldentey, K.-M. Bioactive berry compounds—Novel tools against human pathogens. *Appl. Microbiol. Biotechnol.* **2005**, *67*, 8–18. [CrossRef]
80. Nohynek, L.J.; Alakomi, H.-L.; Kähkönen, M.P.; Heinonen, M.; Helander, I.M.; Oksman-Caldentey, K.-M.; Puupponen-Pimiä, R.H. Berry Phenolics: Antimicrobial Properties and Mechanisms of Action Against Severe Human Pathogens. *Nutr. Cancer* **2006**, *54*, 18–32. [CrossRef] [PubMed]
81. Zahin, M.; Aqil, F.; Ahmad, I. Broad spectrum antimutagenic activity of antioxidant active fraction of punica granatum L. peel extracts. *Mutat. Res.* **2010**, *703*, 99–107. [CrossRef] [PubMed]
82. Brindzová, L.; Zalibera, M.; Jakubík, T.; Mikulášová, M.; Takácsová, M.; Mošovská, S.; Rapta, P. Antimutagenic and Radical Scavenging Activity of Wheat Bran. *Cereal Res. Commun.* **2009**, *37*, 45–55. [CrossRef]
83. Călinoiu, L.F.; Vodnar, D.C. Thermal Processing for the Release of Phenolic Compounds from Wheat and Oat Bran. *Biomolecules* **2020**, *10*, 21. [CrossRef]
84. Hope Smith, S.; Tate, P.L.; Huang, G.; Magee, J.B.; Meepagala, K.M.; Wedge, D.E.; Larcom, L.L. Antimutagenic activity of berry extracts. *J. Med. Food* **2004**, *7*, 450–455. [CrossRef]
85. Prencipe, F.P.; Bruni, R.; Guerrini, A.; Rossi, D.; Benvenuti, S.; Pellati, F. Metabolite profiling of polyphenols in *Vaccinium* berries and determination of their chemopreventive properties. *J. Pharm. Biomed. Anal.* **2014**, *89*, 257–267. [CrossRef]
86. Panche, A.N.; Diwan, A.D.; Chandra, S.R. Flavonoids: An overview. *J. Nutr. Sci.* **2016**, *5*, e47. [CrossRef]
87. Côté, J.; Caillet, S.; Doyon, G.; Sylvain, J.-F.; Lacroix, M. Bioactive Compounds in Cranberries and their Biological Properties. *Crit. Rev. Food Sci. Nutr.* **2010**, *50*, 666–679. [CrossRef]
88. Jurikova, T.; Mlcek, J.; Skrovankova, S.; Sumczynski, D.; Sochor, J.; Hlavacova, I.; Snopek, L.; Orsavova, J. Fruits of Black Chokeberry *Aronia melanocarpa* in the Prevention of Chronic Diseases. *Molecules* **2017**, *22*, 944. [CrossRef]

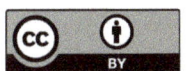

© 2020 by the authors. Licensee MDPI, Basel, Switzerland. This article is an open access article distributed under the terms and conditions of the Creative Commons Attribution (CC BY) license (http://creativecommons.org/licenses/by/4.0/).

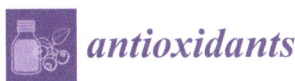

Article

(−)-Loliolide Isolated from *Sargassum horneri* Protects against Fine Dust-Induced Oxidative Stress in Human Keratinocytes

Mawalle Kankanamge Hasitha Madhawa Dias [1], Dissanayaka Mudiyanselage Dinesh Madusanka [1], Eui Jeong Han [1], Min Ju Kim [1], You-Jin Jeon [2,3], Hyun-Soo Kim [2,4], Ilekuttige Priyan Shanura Fernando [5,*] and Ginnae Ahn [1,5,*]

1. Department of Food Technology and Nutrition, Chonnam National University, Yeosu 59626, Korea; 198807@jnu.ac.kr (M.K.H.M.D.); 198793@jnu.ac.kr (D.M.D.M.); iosu5772@naver.com (E.J.H.); alswn1281@nate.com (M.J.K.)
2. Department of Marine Life Science, School of Marine Biomedical Sciences, Jeju National University, Jeju 63243, Korea; youjinj@jejunu.ac.kr (Y.-J.J.); gustn783@mabik.re.kr (H.-S.K.)
3. Marine Science Institute, Jeju National University, Jeju Self-Governing Province 63333, Korea
4. National Marine Biodiversity Institute of Korea, 75, Jangsan-ro 101-gil, Janghang-eup, Seocheon 33662, Korea
5. Department of Marine Bio-Food Sciences, Chonnam National University, Yeosu 59626, Korea
* Correspondence: shanura@chonnam.ac.kr (I.P.S.F.); gnahn@chonnam.ac.kr (G.A.); Tel.: +82-61-659-7213 (I.P.S.F. & G.A.)

Received: 11 April 2020; Accepted: 31 May 2020; Published: 2 June 2020

Abstract: The emergence of fine dust (FD) among air pollutants has taken a toll during the past few decades, and it has provided both controversy and a platform for open conversation amongst world powers for finding sustainable solutions and effective treatments for health issues. The present study emphasizes the protective effects of (−)-loliolide (HTT) isolated from *Sargassum horneri* against FD-induced oxidative stress in human HaCaT keratinocytes. The purification of (−)-loliolide was carried out by centrifugal partition chromatography. HTT did not show any cytotoxicity, and it further illustrated the potential to increase cell viability by reducing the reactive oxygen species (ROS) production in FD-stimulated keratinocytes. Furthermore, HTT suppressed FD-stimulated DNA damage and the formation of apoptotic bodies, and it reduced the population of cells in the sub-G_1 apoptosis phase. FD-induced apoptosis was advancing through the mitochondria-mediated apoptosis pathway. The cytoprotective effects of the HTT against FD-stimulated oxidative damage is mediated through squaring the nuclear factor E2-related factor 2 (Nrf2)-mediated heme oxygenase-1 (HO-1) pathway, dose-dependently increasing HO-1 and NAD(P)H dehydrogenase (quinone) 1 (NQO1) levels in the cytosol while concomitantly improving the nuclear translocation of Nrf2. Future studies could implement the protective functionality of HTT in producing pharmaceuticals that utilize natural products and benefit the diseased.

Keywords: *Sargassum horneri*; (−)-loliolide; fine dust; oxidative stress; HaCaT; apoptosis

1. Introduction

Recently, air pollution has become one of the most debated environmental issues throughout the globe. A real-time air quality index has been created to alert the public regarding levels of various air quality parameters, namely temperature, humidity, pressure, and pollutants such as nitric oxide ($NO_{2(g)}$), sulfur dioxide ($SO_{2(g)}$), and carbon monoxide ($CO_{(g)}$) with immediate updates. This system is operational in many cities around the globe. Fine dust (FD) is one of the principal contributors to air pollution that is prominently observed in highly industrialized East Asian countries, including China, Japan, and Korea [1,2]. Recent studies have predicted increasing global warming in the upcoming decades, fueled with various deleterious anthropogenic activities that can drastically catalyze the desertification process, which escalates the overall dust emissions from the desert areas and consequently affects environmental dynamics and ecosystems [3]. Strong winds from the northern and northwestern parts of the arid and semi-arid regions of Mongolia and China carry particulate matter as far as the North American continent that can be identified from the mineral signature of the aerosol composition [3,4]. The overexploited use of coal and petroleum for energy has become a major contributor to the emerging FD pollution with unburnt particles constantly being released into the atmosphere [2]. According to Raloff (2001), FD particles originating from industries may contain unburnt hydrocarbons, soot, $CO_{(g)}$, carcinogens (asbestos, pesticides, and silica), and heavy metals such as cadmium, mercury, led, chromium, arsenic, and copper [5]. The above environmental hazards can cause various detrimental effects on human health, triggering allergic reactions and oxidative stress. Chronic exposure would cause the development of conjunctivitis, asthma, rhinitis, and dermatitis [6,7]. In some instances, intercontinental FD clouds can also harbor pathogenic bacteria and viruses [5]. Though numerous studies have been carried out to understand the health impacts of FD, the available literature regarding the effects of FD-induced oxidative stress in human keratinocytes is insufficient.

The consumption of marine algae in East Asian countries has increased over the last few decades with the identification of a large number of bioactive natural products that benefit human health [8,9]. *Sargassum horneri* is an edible brown alga that is abundant along the coasts of China, South Korea, Japan, and the North American continent [10,11]. Due to its high biomass and nutritional value (as it is packed with vitamins, polysaccharides, amino acids, and dietary fibers), it is regarded as one of the delicacy dishes in Korea. Moreover, for centuries, *S. horneri* has been used as an ingredient in indigenous medicine [10]. Various studies have addressed the beneficial effects of bioactive compounds such as sargachromenol, phenolics, fucoxanthin, phlorotannins, proteoglycan, and sulfated polysaccharides isolated from *S. horneri* [7–10,12].

(−)-Loliolide ((6S,7aR)-6-hydroxy-4,4,7a-trimethyl-5,6,7,7a-tetrahydro-1-benzofuran-2(4H)-one) is a frequently available monoterpenoid lactone. First discovered in English Ryegrass (*Lolium perenne*) in 1964, (−)-loliolide (HTT) has since been found in many plants and animals in both terrestrial and marine ecosystems [13]. Various biological functions of HTT have been reported, including antioxidant, anti-fungal, antibacterial, and anti-cancer activities; in some instances, it has been used as an alternative medicine for depression and diabetes [13,14]. The major emphasis of the current study was to demonstrate that FD has the ability to induce keratinocytes to produce reactive oxygen species (ROS), inevitably resulting in oxidative stress that causes cell damage and apoptosis; another emphasis was the potential protective effects of HTT in developing future pharmaceuticals and cosmeceuticals.

2. Materials and Methods

2.1. Raw Materials, Chemicals, and Reagents

Urban aerosols (NIES CRM No. 28) were acquired from the National Institute for Environmental Studies (Tsukuba, Ibaraki, Japan). TrytonX-100, 3-(4-50dimethyl-2yl)-2-5-diphynyltetrasolium bromide (MTT), 2′,7′-dichlorofluorescin diacetate (DCFH-DA), dimethyl sulfoxide (DMSO) ethidium bromide, and low melting agarose were purchased from Sigma-Aldrich (ST. Louis, MO, USA). Human HaCaT keratinocytes were donated by the American Type Culture Collection (Manassas, VA, USA). Dulbecco's Modified Eagle Medium (DMEM) and antibiotics (streptomycin and penicillin) were purchased from GibcoBRL (Grand Island, NY, USA), and the fetal bovine serum (FBS) was obtained from Welgene (Gyeongsangbuk-do, South Korea). Relevant antibodies were purchased from Cell Signaling Technology Inc. (Beverly, MA, USA) and Santa Cruz Biotechnology Inc. (Dallas, TX, USA). All additional chemicals and reagents used were purchased from commercial sources with the highest quality.

2.2. Sample Preparation and Isolation of HTT

The collection of *S. horneri* samples was done during the spring season in 2015 along Jeju Island coasts in South Korea. Samples were washed with tap water to remove excess salts and other contaminants, and this process was followed by storage under refrigerated conditions. A detailed extraction and purification method of HTT was described in our previous publication [15]. Briefly, *S. horneri* dry powder was extracted with 80% methanol at 37 °C and concentrated using a rotary evaporator. The crude extract was sequentially fractioned into n-hexane, chloroform (CMSH), and ethyl acetate. CMSH was further purified by a high-performance centrifugal partition chromatography system (Sanki Engineering, Kyoto, Japan) using upper and lower phases of an equilibrated solvent system composed of n-hexane/ethyl acetate/methanol/water (5:5:5:5, v/v). The separation was monitored at 240 nm by an L-4000 UV detector (Hitachi, Japan). The eluant was collected into test tubes using a fraction collector (FC 203B, Gilson, South Korea). The further purification of the active fraction was carried out by a Prep HPLC system (Waters, Milford, MA, USA) using a semi-preparative C18 (YMC-Pack ODS-A, 5 µm, 10 × 250 mm) column. The gradient elution was carried out using acetonitrile: distilled water as; 0–60 min 5:95–100: 0 v/v; 60–70 min 100:0–100: 0 v/v at a flow rate of 3 mL min^{-1}, while the UV absorbance was observed at 230 and 254 nm by a Waters 2998 photodiode array detector (Waters, Milford, MA, USA).

2.3. In Vitro Analysis

2.3.1. Cell Culture and Maintenance

HaCaT (human keratinocyte) cells were cultured using DMEM media containing 10% (v/v) heat-inactivated FBS and 1% (v/v) streptomycin and penicillin (100 µg mL^{-1}). Cells were maintained inside a controlled environment with 5% CO_2 at 37 °C. Periodic subculturing was practiced, and cells with exponential growth were used for experiments that achieved a 95% confluency. HTT was initially dissolved in DMSO and diluted using DMEM for cell culture experiments. The final concentration of DMSO in treated samples was kept below 0.1%. DMEM was added to control cell groups to maintain a constant volume.

2.3.2. Cell Viability and ROS Production

The concentration of FD used, exposure time, and the method were based on previous observations and preliminary experiments [7]. Initially, FD was suspended in DMEM, followed by sonication for one minute to separate any clumps. FD suspended solvent was vortexed prior to each treatment. HaCaT cells were seeded at a concentration of 1×10^5 cells mL^{-1} in 96 well plates, with 2×10^4 cells in each well, which were incubated for 24 h. Different concentrations of HTT were used to treat the cells, and after one hour, cells were stimulated with FD (150 µg mL^{-1}) for one-hour. The FD-containing media were carefully removed and washed three times, followed by adding new media. MTT and DCFH-DA assays were conducted to measure the cell viability and intracellular ROS generation, respectively [16].

Simultaneously, the same concentration of cells was seeded in a 24 well plate and 6 cm culture dishes with 5×10^4 cells per well and 3×10^5 cells per dish for the respective detection of ROS levels by using fluorescence microscopy and flow cytometry under DCFH-DA staining. The side scatter vs. forward scatter (SSC vs. FSC) gating strategy was used in the flow cytometry to eliminate cell debris. Images of the fluorescence microscopy were obtained by using an Invitrogen™ EVOS™ Auto 2 fluorescence microscope (Thermo Fisher Scientific, Bothell, WA, USA), and flow cytometry analysis was conducted using a Beckman Coulter CytoFLEX system (Beckman Coulter, Brea, CA, USA).

2.3.3. Nuclear Morphological Analysis

Nuclear staining was carried out by using Hochest 33342 following the method described by Yang et al. (2011) with slight modifications [14]. HTT treatment and FD stimulation followed the same method mentioned in Section 2.3.2. After washing with phosphate-buffered saline (PBS), the Hoechst 33342 reagent was added, achieving a final concentration of 2 µg mL^{-1} per well, each of which were incubated for 20 min at 37 °C in the dark. The visualization of nuclear morphology was carried out using a fluorescence microscope.

2.3.4. Annexin V Assay

Early apoptosis detection was carried out by flow cytometry using an eBioscience™ Annexin V Apoptosis Detection Kit (Thermo Fisher Scientific, Carlsbad, CA, USA) according to the manufacture's guidelines. HTT-treated, FD-induced cells were incubated for six hours prior to harvesting for the assay.

2.3.5. Cell Cycle Analysis

Cell cycle analysis was conducted according to a pre-described method by Fernando et al. (2017) with slight alterations [17]. Briefly, HTT-treated and FD-induced cells, as described in Section 2.3.2, were used. Cell harvesting was carried out 24 h after the incubation, which was followed by fixing in 70% ethanol at 4 °C. Cells were washed using PBS, treated with 2 mM of ethylenediaminetetraacetic acid (EDTA), and resuspended in 300 µL of PBS–EDTA-containing RNase (0.2 µg mL^{-1}) and propidium iodide (50 µg mL^{-1}) for 30 min. The analysis was conducted using a flow cytometer.

2.3.6. Alkaline Comet Assay

The alkaline comet assay was carried out following the procedure by Fernando et al. (2017) with minor modifications [17]. The sample treated cells were incubated for 24 h and dispersed in 1% low melting agarose at 40 °C. The cell-agarose mixture was pipetted onto agarose pre-coated microscopic slides and rested for solidification. Then, the slides were lysed overnight by submerging in a 1% TrytonX-100-containing lysis buffer at 4 °C. Electrophoresis was conducted for 30 min at 30 V/300 mA, while the temperature was maintained at 4 °C. A neutralizing buffer was used to wash the slides three times, prior to staining with ethidium bromide (2 µg mL^{-1}) for five minutes. Pre-chilled water was used to wash away any excess dye, and the visualization was conducted using a fluorescence microscope.

2.3.7. Western Blot Analysis

As elucidated in Section 2.3.2, HTT-treated FD-induced cells were harvested and lysed using a NE-PER® nuclear and cytoplasmic extraction kit and radioimmunoprecipitation assay (RIPA) buffer (Thermo Scientific, Rockford, IL, USA). Isolated cytoplasmic and nuclear protein levels were determined by using Bio-Rad Protein Assay Dye (Bio-Rad Laboratories, Inc., Hercules, CA, USA), and a concentration gradient of bovine serum albumin was used as the reference standard. A normalized amount of protein was loaded into 10% polyacrylamide gels and electrophoresed. After transferring the protein bands to nitrocellulose membranes, blocking was carried out with 5% skim milk in tris buffered saline (TBS) containing Tween-20 for two hours. Primary antibodies were added to the membranes and incubated overnight at 4 °C with continuous agitation. Then, the membranes were incubated with their respective enzyme-linked secondary antibodies for two hours at room temperature and visualized using SuperSignal™ West Femto Maximum Sensitivity Substrate (Thermo Scientific Inc., Rockford, IL, USA) on a Core Bio DavinchChemi imager (Seoul, Korea).

2.4. Statistical Analysis

PASW Statistics 18 was used to conduct the statistical analysis, and data are expressed as mean ± standard error of the mean (SEM). The significant differences amongst data sets were determined by using the ANOVA with the Duncan's multiple range test. The significance of data was determined at $p < 0.05$.

3. Results

3.1. Effect of HTT on Cytotoxicity, Cell Viability and Intracellular ROS Production of FD-Induced HaCaT Cells

The extraction of *S. horneri* and further purification that led to the isolation of HTT is depicted in Figure 1A. Details of this isolation procedure were described in our previous publication [15]. According to Figure 1B, a non-significant increment of cell viability and ROS was observed, suggesting that the used concentrations of HTT had no cytotoxicity towards HaCaT cells. FD had induced the production of intracellular ROS compared to the control cell group while simultaneously reducing cell viability. However, treating cells with different concentrations of HTT significantly increased the cell viability compared to the cells that were exposed only to FD, concomitantly minimizing the production of intracellular ROS in a dose-dependent manner (Figure 1C). The highest concentration of HTT (200 µM) showed a similar cell viability activity to those of the positive control, indomethacin (IM). The protective effects of HTT against FD-induced ROS generation were confirmed by flow cytometry and fluorescence microscopic analysis (Figure 1D,E). FD-stimulated cells indicated a rightward shift of the cell population with a higher intensity of fluorescence compared to the control cells. The green fluorescence in Figure 1E was at its peak for the FD-stimulated cell group compared to the control. In both instances, treating with HTT dose-dependently reduced the fluorescence of DCFH-DA, confirming the protective effects of HTT against FD-induced oxidative stress.

3.2. HTT Inhibited Early Apoptosis and Apoptotic Body Formation in FD-Induced HaCaT Cells

Phosphatidylserine (PT) is an inner plasma membrane phospholipid that becomes translocated to the outer plasma membrane during the early stages of apoptosis. Annexin V is a phospholipid-binding protein that has a high affinity towards PT, and that can be utilized to detect early apoptotic cells [18]. The Hoechst 33342 nuclear staining is a unique fluorescent staining technique used to visualize apoptotic bodies and thereby determine the level of nuclear condensation and DNA damage [17]. According to the results of Figure 2A, HaCaT cells stimulated by FD indicated an apparent reduction of total cell density, with a notable increment of apoptotic bodies compared to the control; this indicated nuclear condensation. Cells that were pre-treated with HTT (200 µM) had the least amount of apoptotic bodies and the highest cell population compared to the rest of the treatment groups. Compared to the control, FD-induction increased the cell population in early apoptosis from 0.63% to 16.47%, as depicted in the lower right quadrants of the histograms in Figure 2B. The dose-dependent reduction of early apoptotic cell population further confirmed the protective effects of HTT against FD-induced apoptosis.

3.3. HTT Attenuates DNA Damage and Apoptotic Cells in the Sub-G_1 Phase

The alkaline comet assay—also known as single-cell gel electrophoresis—is a widely used method to detect DNA damage in cells. The comet tail length and tail DNA content are considered to be proportional to DNA damage [17]. As shown in Figure 3A, the tail DNA content drastically increased in the FD-treated cells compared to the control cell group, while the HTT pre-treatment reduced the tail DNA content in a dose-dependent manner suggesting the potential ability of HTT to reduce DNA damage induced by FD. Furthermore, as illustrated in Figure 3B, a significant proportion of FD-induced untreated cells were in the sub-G_1 phase (21.46%) compared to the control cell group (1.06%). However, the sub-G_1 cell population was dose-dependently reduced with HTT treatment. These results coincided with the results obtained for the Hoechst 33342 nuclear staining, further establishing the protective effect of HTT against FD-induced DNA damage in HaCaT cells.

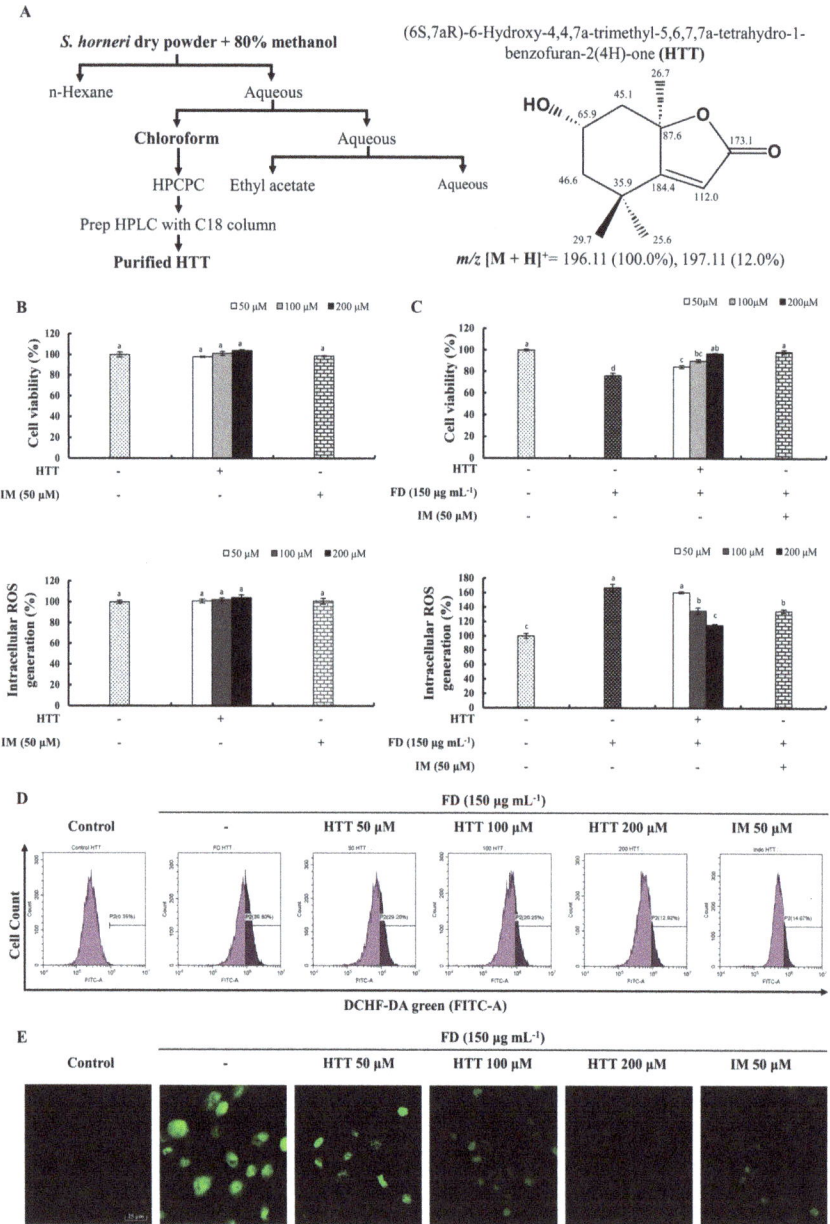

Figure 1. (**A**) Purification process and the chemical structure of (−)-loliolide (HTT) with ^{1}H NMR chemical shifts. The effects of HTT on cell viability and intracellular reactive oxygen species (ROS) production (**B**) in the absence of fine dust (FD) and (**C**) with FD-stimulated HaCaT cells. Analysis of ROS levels in 2′,7′-dichlorofluorescin diacetate (DCFH-DA)-stained HaCaT cells by (**D**) flow cytometry and (**E**) fluorescence microscopy. Seeded cells were pre-treated with different concentrations of HTT (50–200 µM) at one hour prior to stimulation with 150 µg mL^{-1} of FD. Indomethacin (IM) was used as the positive control. The experiments were conducted in three independent determinations ($n = 3$), and the values are given as means ± SEM. Error bars with different letters are significantly different ($p < 0.05$).

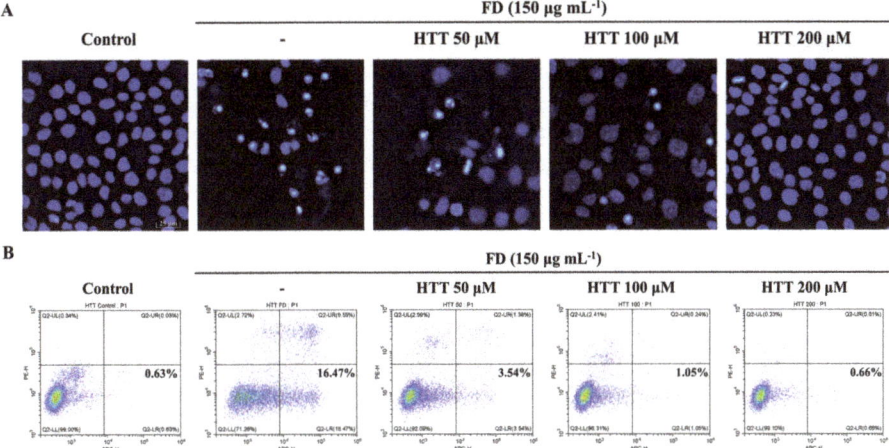

Figure 2. The effect of (−)-loliolide (HTT) on apoptotic body formation and early apoptosis in fine dust (FD)-induced HaCaT cells. Fluorescence microscopy of nuclear morphological analysis using (**A**) Hoechst 33342 dye and early apoptosis detection by (**B**) annexin V with flow cytometry. HTT pre-treated (50–200 μM) exposed to FD for one hour before replenishing with new media. The experiments were conducted in triplicates with three independent trials to confirm repeatability.

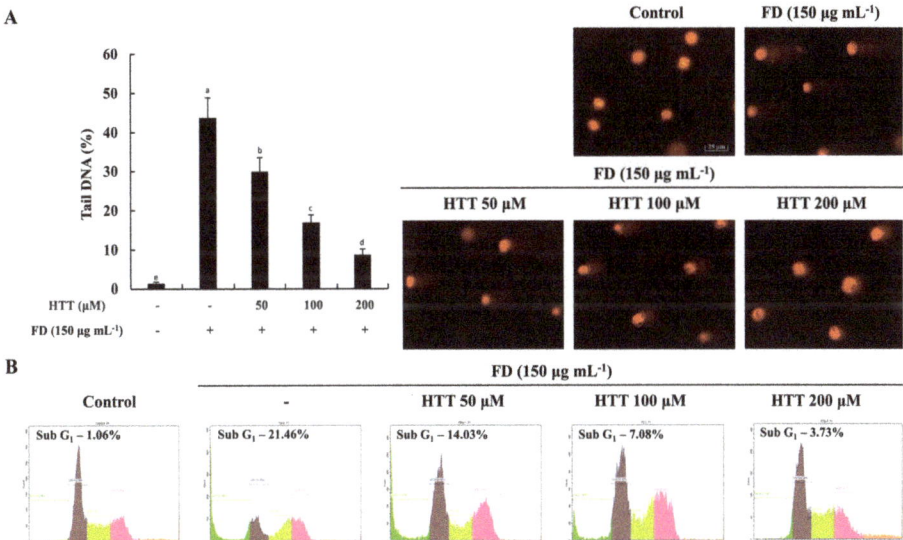

Figure 3. (−)-loliolide (HTT) inhibited DNA breakage and apoptosis in fine dust (FD)-stimulated HaCaT cells. (**A**) Comet tails and (**B**) sub-G_1 cell populations of FD-stimulated HaCaT cells treated with HTT. Cells were treated with different concentrations of HTT (50–200 μM) prior to stimulation with FD. Comet tail DNA percentages were analyzed using the OpenComet plugin of the ImageJ software. Results were analyzed as three independent determinations ($n = 3$) to confirm repeatability. Values are given as means ± SEM, and error bars representing different letters are significantly different ($p < 0.05$).

3.4. HTT Attenuates Apoptosis via the Mitochondrial Pathway

The effects of HTT on apoptosis-related proteins were analyzed using Western blotting. According to the results shown in Figure 4A, stimulating cells with FD increased the levels of pro-apoptotic proteins p53, B-cell lymphoma 2-associated X protein (Bax), cleaved caspase-9, cytochrome c, cleaved poly (ADP-ribose) polymerase (PARP), and caspase-3 while reducing the anti-apoptotic proteins B-cell lymphoma 2 (Bcl-2), PARP, and B-cell lymphoma extra-large (Bcl-xL) compared to the control cell group. Nonetheless, the HTT pre-treated cells showed increased levels of Bcl-2, Bcl-xL, and PARP while simultaneously suppressing the levels of Bax, cleaved PARP, cleaved caspase-9, caspase-3, cytochrome c, and p53 in a concentration-dependent manner that suggested the protective effect of HTT against FD-induced apoptosis in HaCaT cells. Furthermore, according to Figure 4B, treating cells with HTT (without FD stimulation) had no effect on apoptotic related protein levels (Bax, Bcl-2, and Bcl-xL) in HaCaT cells.

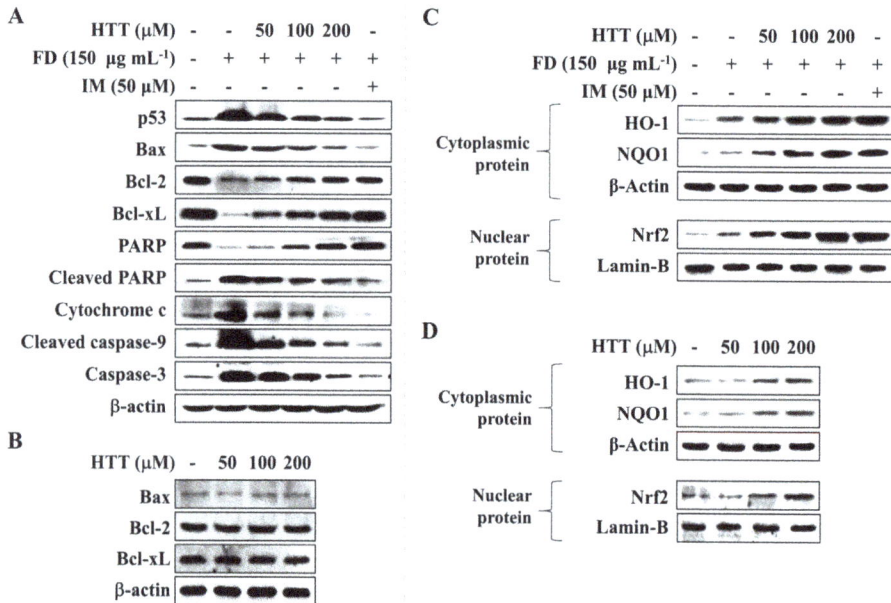

Figure 4. Effect of (−)-loliolide (HTT) on the levels of key apoptosis and antioxidant molecular mediators. Effect of HTT on key apoptotic mediators in (**A**) fine dust (FD)-induced and (**B**) non-induced cells. Effect of HTT on nuclear factor E2-related factor 2 (Nrf2)/heme oxygenase-1 (HO-1) signaling molecules in (**C**) FD-induced and (**D**) non-induced HaCaT cells. Seeded cells were treated with different concentrations of HTT one hour before stimulation. Indomethacin (IM) was used as the positive control. The experiment was done in three independent trials to confirm repeatability.

3.5. Effect of HTT on Upregulation of Nrf2/HO-1 Pathway Proteins

Figure 4C illustrates nuclear factor E2-related factor 2 (Nrf2) pathway-related protein level expressions. FD slightly increased the nuclear translocation of Nrf2. This was consistent with the increment of NAD(P)H dehydrogenase (quinone) 1 (NQO1) and heme oxygenase 1 (HO-1) protein levels in the cytosol compared to the control cells. However, the HTT pre-treated cells had gradually increased levels of NQO1, HO-1, and Nrf2 dose-dependently. Moreover, the levels of NQO1, HO-1, and Nrf2 had a slight dose-dependent increment without FD-stimulation, thus suggesting the potential of HTT to activate the Nrf2/HO-1 antioxidative pathway (Figure 4D). Indomethacin was used as a positive control in the experiment for the comparison of its effects with HTT.

4. Discussion

"Oxidative stress" and "ROS" are two frequently used terms that complement each other and play major roles in human health [19,20]. Weakened antioxidant defense mechanisms, coupled with excess production of ROS such as hydrogen peroxide (H_2O_2), superoxide anion radicals ($O_2^{\bullet-}$), hydroxyl radicals ($^{\bullet}OH$), hypochlorite (ClO^-), and nitric oxide radicals ($NO_x^{\bullet}$), is considered as primary causes of oxidative stress that damages major macromolecules of cells such as carbohydrates, proteins, lipids, and DNA, ultimately leading to cellular death. Moreover, the above incidents may trigger diseases such as diabetes, atherosclerosis, various neurodegenerative and cardiovascular disorders, and even cancer [19,21].

FD is one of the highly discussed issues in the modern world, as it affects countries all around the globe. Prolonged exposure to FD-polluted air containing various toxic substances, namely heavy metals and organic pollutants such as polycyclic aromatic hydrocarbons (PAHs) can synthesize ROS (e.g., the generation of $HO^{\bullet}$ via Fenton's reaction) inside the human body, subsequently leading to pulmonary and systemic oxidative stress [22–24]. According to Mori et al. (2008), the FD used in the current study mainly consisted of Si (14.9%), C (12%), Ca (6.69%), Al (5.04%), S (3.91%), Fe (2.92%), Mg (1.40%), K (1.37%), Cl (0.807%), Na (0.796%), N (0.79%), Ti (0.292%), P (0.145%), and Zn (0.114%), as well as minor amounts of other elements and substances including PAHs such as fluoranthene, benzo (b) fluoranthene, pyrene, indeno (1,3,3,-cd) pyrene, benzo (ghi) perylene, benz (a) anthracene, benzo (k) fluoranthene, and benzo (a) pyrene—all of which have the potential to induce oxidative stress in human keratinocytes [25]. Furthermore, FD reported from other heavily industrialized areas has shown similar general constituents (elements and PAHs) [26,27].

HTT is a crucial bio-active compound available in *S. horneri* that possesses potent medicinal properties and has been used as folk medicine in countries such as Japan, Mexico, Egypt, and the Philippines [13]. Therefore, the potential therapeutic use of HTT in attenuating FD-induced oxidative stress was investigated in the current study.

The HaCaT cell model is commonly used in dermatological studies to represent typical human keratinocytes. Located on the epithelium of the outer skin, these cells are prime candidates that have direct contact with FD and the potential to induce oxidative damage. This was further confirmed from the results shown in Figure 1C–E, where the concentration of the used FD increased the generation of ROS in HaCaT cells, thus increasing oxidative damage and inevitably reducing cell viability. However, the used concentrations of HTT increased the cell viability while minimizing the overall ROS production without any cytotoxicity, thus further illustrating the potential of HTT in attenuating the oxidative stress generated from exposure to FD. Further evidence was acquired from flow cytometry and fluorescence microscopy using DCFH-DA staining, which indicated the reduction of ROS levels upon HTT treatment. The flowcytometric analysis allows to omit the florescence incidents from dead cells and cell debris. The above results, together with fluorescence microscopy, confirmed the ability of HTT to attenuate oxidative stress caused by FD.

Apoptosis is considered to be the major outcome in cells and tissues that are regularly exposed to high levels of oxidative damage [19,21]. DNA fragmentation and nuclear condensation, along with the formation of apoptotic bodies, is a crucial identification criterion of controlled cell death [28]. Hoechst 33342 staining is a widely used staining technique that is implemented to visualize the formation of apoptotic bodies. The annexin V assay has the capability to identify different stages of apoptosis in particular cell lines and to provide the foundation to detect and differentiate between viable, early, and late apoptotic cells [18]. Based on the obtained results, HTT minimized the apoptotic body formation, an effect that was further confirmed by the results of the annexin V and alkaline comet assays. The cell cycle analysis histograms gave clear evidence of the ability of HTT on attenuating apoptosis from the reduction of sub-G_1 hypodiploid subpopulations in the cell cycle [29].

The mitochondrial-mediated apoptosis pathway is a highly complex cascade of reactions that regulates cell death. Bcl-2 family proteins, including pro-apoptotic proteins such as BH3 interacting-domain death agonist (Bid), Bcl-2-associated death promoter (Bad), Bcl-2 related ovarian killer (Bok), Bcl-2 homologous antagonist killer (Bak), Bcl-2-interacting killer (Bik), Bcl-2-modifying factor (Bmf), Bim, Nova, p53 upregulated modulator of apoptosis (Puma) and Bax; anti-apoptotic proteins (Bcl-xL, Bcl-2, and Mcl-1) coupled with caspases regulate the complex procedure [17,21]. The activation of the mitochondrial-mediated apoptosis pathway takes place with the activation of p53 and pro-apoptotic Bcl-2 family proteins in the cytosol, which leads to the inhibition of anti-apoptotic Bcl-2 family proteins localized on the mitochondria's outer membrane. This phenomenon increases the mitochondrial outer membrane permeabilization, which leads to the release of apoptosis-promoting proteins cytochrome c, endonuclease G, and the apoptosis-inducing factor to the cytosol. The combination of procaspase-9, apoptosis activating factor-1, and cytochrome c are known as the apoptosome. This complex is the prime candidate for activating caspase-9, which enables a cascade of reactions to take place activating caspases-3, -6, and -7 that further continue the apoptosis process [21]. Moreover, initiator caspases, namely caspase-2, -8, -9, and -10 are responsible for the apoptosis initiation and execution, while the effector caspases such as caspase-3, -6, and -7 are key intermediates that connect the cascade. This leads to the rise of morphological and biochemical modifications in key regulatory molecules such as PARP, which is a protein responsible for the repairing ability, transcription, and stability of DNA [17]. Results observed in the present study showed that HaCaT cells exposed to FD demonstrated apoptosis via the mitochondrial-mediated apoptosis pathway, and HTT dose-dependently minimized the pro-apoptotic molecule levels in cells. Furthermore, an in-depth analysis of mRNA expressions of key mediators related to the mitochondrial-mediated apoptosis pathway could be implemented in future studies and could be utilized to provide a thorough insight into the mechanism.

The activation of the Nrf2 pathway is considered to be one of the key regulatory processes that enable cells to exhibit resistance against redox imbalances and oxidative stress [30]. Inactive Nrf2 is localized in the cytosol bound with Kelch-like ECH-associated protein 1 (Keap1) that inhibits the activation of Nrf2 [31]. With the ongoing oxidative stress conditions in the cell, the Keap1 protein is inactivated by an upstream molecule known as p62 and promotes the nuclear translocation of activated Nrf2. This phenomenon is the key inducer of activating NQO1—a drug-metabolizing enzyme—and HO-1, which triggers protective effects by regulating redox imbalance. Nevertheless, the oxidative stress caused by the stimulant overwhelms the protective effects of antioxidative gene HO-1, limiting its potential ability to maintain redox imbalance [31]. However, based on the results, HTT potentially increased the Nrf2 levels in the nucleus, simultaneously increasing the HO-1 and NQO1 proteins in a concentration-dependent manner in the cytosol, suggesting that the cytoprotective effects of HTT against FD-induced oxidative damage was carried via the Nrf2/HO-1 signaling pathway.

5. Conclusions

Considering the results of the current study, HTT holds potent protective competence in attenuating FD-induced oxidative stress in human keratinocytes. Furthermore, new techniques and methods could be materialized to identify and increase the efficiency of extracting HTT like bio-active compounds from *S. horneri*. Future studies could be implemented on applications of HTT-based pharmaceutical and cosmetic products as a means of maintaining healthy skin.

Author Contributions: Conceptualization, M.K.H.M.D., I.P.S.F., and G.A.; methodology, H.-S.K., M.K.H.M.D., and D.M.D.M.; software, M.K.H.M.D. and D.M.D.M.; validation, E.J.H. and M.J.K.; formal analysis, M.K.H.M.D. and D.M.D.M.; investigation, M.K.H.M.D. and D.M.D.M.; resources, Y.-J.J. and G.A.; data curation, E.J.H. and M.J.K.; writing—original draft preparation, M.K.H.M.D.; writing—review and editing, I.P.S.F. and G.A.; visualization, M.K.H.M.D.; supervision, I.P.S.F. and G.A.; project administration, Y.-J.J. and G.A.; funding acquisition, G.A. All authors have read and agreed to the published version of the manuscript.

Funding: This research was supported by Basic Science Research Program through the National Research Foundation of Korea (NRF) funded by the Ministry of Education (2017R1D1A1B04035921).

Conflicts of Interest: The authors declare no conflict of interest.

References

1. Kang, D.; Kim, J.E. Fine, ultrafine, and yellow dust: Emerging health problems in Korea. *J. Korean Med. Sci.* **2014**, *29*, 621–622. [CrossRef]
2. Fernando, I.P.S.; Kim, H.S.; Sanjeewa, K.K.A.; Oh, J.Y.; Jeon, Y.J.; Lee, W.W. Inhibition of inflammatory responses elicited by urban fine dust particles in keratinocytes and macrophages by diphlorethohydroxycarmalol isolated from a brown alga Ishige okamurae. *Algae* **2017**, *32*, 261–273. [CrossRef]
3. Kim, H.S.; Kim, D.S.; Kim, H.; Yi, S.M. Relationship between mortality and fine particles during Asian dust, smog-Asian dust, and smog days in Korea. *Int. J. Environ. Health Res.* **2012**, *22*, 518–530. [CrossRef] [PubMed]
4. VanCuren, R.A.; Cahill, T.A. Asian aerosols in North America: Frequency and concentration of fine dust. *J. Geophys. Res. Atmos.* **2002**, *107*, 4804. [CrossRef]
5. Raloff, J. Ill winds Dust storms ferry toxic agents between countries and even continents. *Sci. News* **2001**, *160*, 218–220. [CrossRef]
6. Choi, H.; Shin, D.W.; Kim, W.; Doh, S.J.; Lee, S.H.; Noh, M. Asian dust storm particles induce a broad toxicological transcriptional program in human epidermal keratinocytes. *Toxicol. Lett.* **2011**, *200*, 92–99. [CrossRef]
7. Fernando, I.P.S.; Jayawardena, T.U.; Sanjeewa, K.K.A.; Wang, L.; Jeon, Y.J.; Lee, W.W. Anti-inflammatory potential of alginic acid from *Sargassum horneri* against urban aerosol-induced inflammatory responses in keratinocytes and macrophages. *Ecotox. Environ. Saf.* **2018**, *160*, 24–31. [CrossRef]
8. Yoshioka, H.; Ishida, M.; Nishi, K.; Oda, H.; Toyohara, H.; Sugahara, T. Studies on anti-allergic activity of *Sargassum horneri* extract. *J. Funct. Foods* **2014**, *10*, 154–160. [CrossRef]
9. Wen, Z.S.; Liu, L.J.; OuYang, X.K.; Qu, Y.L.; Chen, Y.; Ding, G.F. Protective effect of polysaccharides from *Sargassum horneri* against oxidative stress in RAW 264.7 cells. *Int. J. Biol. Macromol.* **2014**, *68*, 98–106. [CrossRef]
10. Kim, H.S.; Sanjeewa, K.K.A.; Fernando, I.P.S.; Ryu, B.; Yang, H.W.; Ahn, G.; Kang, M.C.; Heo, S.T.; Je, J.G.; Jeon, Y.J. A comparative study of *Sargassum horneri* Korea and China strains collected along the coast of Jeju Island South Korea: Its components and bioactive properties. *Algae* **2018**, *33*, 341–349. [CrossRef]
11. Marks, L.M.; Reed, D.C.; Holbrook, S.J. Life history traits of the invasive seaweed *Sargassum horneri* at Santa Catalina Island, California. *Aquat Invasions* **2018**, *13*, 339–350. [CrossRef]
12. Yende, S.R.; Harle, U.N.; Chaugule, B.B. Therapeutic potential and health benefits of *Sargassum* species. *Pharmacogn. Rev.* **2014**, *8*, 1–7. [CrossRef] [PubMed]
13. Grabarczyk, M.; Wińska, K.; Mączka, W.; Potaniec, B.; Anioł, M. Loliolide—The most ubiquitous lactone. *Folia Biol. Oecol.* **2015**, *11*, 1–8. [CrossRef]
14. Yang, X.; Kang, M.C.; Lee, K.W.; Kang, S.M.; Lee, W.W.; Jeon, Y.J. Antioxidant activity and cell protective effect of loliolide isolated from *Sargassum ringgoldianum* subsp. *coreanum*. *Algae* **2011**, *26*, 201–208. [CrossRef]
15. Jayawardena, T.U.; Kim, H.-S.; Sanjeewa, K.K.A.; Kim, S.-Y.; Rho, J.-R.; Jee, Y.; Ahn, G.; Jeon, Y.-J. *Sargassum horneri* and isolated 6-hydroxy-4,4,7a-trimethyl-5,6,7,7a-tetrahydrobenzofuran-2(4H)-one (HTT); LPS-induced inflammation attenuation via suppressing NF-κB, MAPK and oxidative stress through Nrf2/HO-1 pathways in RAW 264.7 macrophages. *Algal Res.* **2019**, *40*, 101513. [CrossRef]
16. Wang, L.; Ryu, B.; Kim, W.S.; Kim, G.H.; Jeon, Y.J. Protective effect of gallic acid derivatives from the freshwater green alga *Spirogyra* sp. against ultraviolet B-induced apoptosis through reactive oxygen species clearance in human keratinocytes and zebrafish. *Algae* **2017**, *32*, 379–388. [CrossRef]
17. Fernando, I.P.S.; Sanjeewa, K.K.A.; Kim, H.S.; Wang, L.; Lee, W.W.; Jeon, Y.J. Apoptotic and antiproliferative properties of 3β-hydroxy-Δ5-steroidal congeners from a partially purified column fraction of *Dendronephthya gigantea* against HL-60 and MCF-7 cancer cells. *J. Appl. Toxicol.* **2017**, *38*, 527–536. [CrossRef]
18. Chen, S.; Cheng, A.-C.; Wang, M.-S.; Peng, X. Detection of apoptosis induced by new type gosling viral enteritis virus in vitro through fluorescein annexin V-FITC/PI double labeling. *World J. Gastroenterol.* **2008**, *14*, 2174–2178. [CrossRef]
19. Lobo, V.; Patil, A.; Phatak, A.; Chandra, N. Free radicals, antioxidants and functional foods: Impact on human health. *Pharmacogn. Rev.* **2010**, *4*, 118–126. [CrossRef]

20. Haberzettl, P.; Bhatnagar, A.; Conklin, D.J. Particulate matter and oxidative stress—Pulmonary and cardiovascular targets and consequences. In *Systems Biology of Free Radicals and Antioxidants*; Laher, I., Ed.; Springer: Berlin/Heidelberg, Germany, 2014; pp. 1557–1586.
21. Redza-Dutordoir, M.; Averill-Bates, D.A. Activation of apoptosis signalling pathways by reactive oxygen species. *BBA Mol. Cell Res.* **2016**, *1863*, 2977–2992. [CrossRef]
22. Lakey, P.S.J.; Berkemeier, T.; Tong, H.J.; Arangio, A.M.; Lucas, K.; Poschl, U.; Shiraiwa, M. Chemical exposure-response relationship between air pollutants and reactive oxygen species in the human respiratory tract. *Sci. Rep. UK* **2016**, *6*. [CrossRef] [PubMed]
23. Lodovici, M.; Bigagli, E. Oxidative stress and air pollution exposure. *J. Toxicol.* **2011**. [CrossRef] [PubMed]
24. Wang, J.; Huang, J.A.; Wang, L.L.; Chen, C.C.; Yang, D.; Jin, M.L.; Bai, C.X.; Song, Y.L. Urban particulate matter triggers lung inflammation via the ROS-MAPK- NF-kappa B signaling pathway. *J. Thorac Dis.* **2017**, *9*, 4398–4412. [CrossRef] [PubMed]
25. Mori, I.; Sun, Z.; Ukachi, M.; Nagano, K.; McLeod, C.W.; Cox, A.G.; Nishikawa, M. Development and certification of the new NIES CRM 28: Urban aerosols for the determination of multielements. *Anal. Bioanal. Chem.* **2008**, *391*, 1997–2003. [CrossRef] [PubMed]
26. Piaścik, M.; Przyk, E.P.; Held, A. *The Certification of the Mass Fractions of Selected Polycyclic Aromatic Hydrocarbons (PAHs) in Fine Dust (PM10-Like Matrix) Certified Reference Material ERM®-CZ100*; Institute for Reference Materials and Measurements: Geel, Belgium; Publications Office of the European Union: Brussels, Belgium, 2010; pp. 1–50.
27. Mitkus, R.J.; Powell, J.L.; Zeisler, R.; Squibb, K.S. Comparative physicochemical and biological characterization of NIST Interim Reference Material PM2.5 and SRM 1648 in human A549 and mouse RAW264.7 cells. *Toxicol. In Vitro* **2013**, *27*, 2289–2298. [CrossRef]
28. Kijima, M.; Mizuta, R. Histone H1 quantity determines the efficiencies of apoptotic DNA fragmentation and chromatin condensation. *Biomed. Res. Tokyo* **2019**, *40*, 51–56. [CrossRef]
29. Kajstura, M.; Halicka, H.D.; Pryjma, J.; Darzynkiewicz, Z. Discontinuous fragmentation of nuclear DNA during apoptosis revealed by discrete "sub-G(1)" peaks on DNA content histograms. *Cytom. Part. A* **2007**, *71*, 125–131. [CrossRef]
30. Ma, Q. Role of Nrf2 in oxidative stress and toxicity. *Annu. Rev. Pharmacol.* **2013**, *53*, 401–426. [CrossRef]
31. Luo, J.F.; Shen, X.Y.; Lio, C.K.; Dai, Y.; Cheng, C.S.; Liu, J.X.; Yao, Y.D.; Yu, Y.; Xie, Y.; Luo, P.; et al. Activation of Nrf2/HO-1 Pathway by Nardochinoid C Inhibits Inflammation and Oxidative Stress in Lipopolysaccharide-Stimulated Macrophages. *Front. Pharmacol.* **2018**, *9*. [CrossRef]

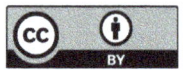
© 2020 by the authors. Licensee MDPI, Basel, Switzerland. This article is an open access article distributed under the terms and conditions of the Creative Commons Attribution (CC BY) license (http://creativecommons.org/licenses/by/4.0/).

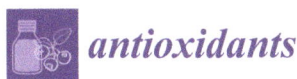

Article

Effect of *Quamoclit angulata* Extract Supplementation on Oxidative Stress and Inflammation on Hyperglycemia-Induced Renal Damage in Type 2 Diabetic Mice

Ji Eun Park [1], Heaji Lee [1], Hyunkyung Rho [1], Seong Min Hong [2], Sun Yeou Kim [2] and Yunsook Lim [1,*]

1. Department of Food and Nutrition, Kyung Hee Univerity, 26 Kyung Hee-Daero, Dongdamun-Gu, Seoul 02447, Korea; gh1003@khu.ac.kr (J.E.P.); ji3743@khu.ac.kr (H.L.); rho0408@khu.ac.kr (H.R.)
2. Department of Pharmacognosy, College of Pharmacy, Gachon University, Incheon 21936, Korea; hongsm0517@gmail.com (S.M.H.); sunnykim@gachon.ac.kr (S.Y.K.)
* Correspondence: ylim@khu.ac.kr; Tel.: +82-2-961-0262; Fax: +82-2-961-0260

Received: 19 May 2020; Accepted: 23 May 2020; Published: 27 May 2020

Abstract: Type 2 diabetes mellitus (T2DM) is caused by abnormalities of controlling blood glucose and insulin homeostasis. Especially, hyperglycemia causes hyper-inflammation through activation of NLRP3 inflammasome, which can lead to cell apoptosis, hypertrophy, and fibrosis. *Quamoclit angulata* (QA), one of the annual winders, has been shown ameliorative effects on diabetes. The current study investigated whether the QA extract (QAE) attenuated hyperglycemia-induced renal inflammation related to NLRP inflammasome and oxidative stress in high fat diet (HFD)-induced diabetic mice. After T2DM was induced, the mice were treated with QAE (5 or 10 mg/kg/day) by gavage for 12 weeks. The QAE supplementation reduced homeostasis model assessment insulin resistance (HOMA-IR), kidney malfunction, and glomerular hypertrophy in T2DM. Moreover, the QAE treatment significantly attenuated renal NLRP3 inflammasome dependent hyper-inflammation and consequential renal damage caused by oxidative stress, apoptosis, and fibrosis in T2DM. Furthermore, QAE normalized aberrant energy metabolism (downregulation of p-AMPK, sirtuin (SIRT)-1, and PPARγ-coactivator α (PGC-1 α)) in T2DM mice. Taken together, the results suggested that QAE as a natural product has ameliorative effects on renal damage by regulation of oxidative stress and inflammation in T2DM.

Keywords: *Quamoclit angulata*; type 2 diabetes; kidney damage; inflammation; oxidative stress; apoptosis; fibrosis

1. Introduction

Diabetes mellitus (DM) is considered as a metabolic disease that results in impaired glucose and insulin homeostasis [1]. Especially, insulin resistance caused by hyperglycemia, is the worldwide epidemic that is accompanied by various complications in type 2 DM (T2DM) [2]. The early stage of nephropathy (DN) is characterized by the structural changes of kidney such as damage of the glomerular basement membrane (GBM), enlargement of the mesangial cells, glomerulosclerosis, and fibrosis and renal function failure including microalbuminuria and reduced glomerular filtration rate (GFR) [3,4].

The main cause of renal damage is the hyperglycemic condition in T2DM. Hyperglycemia leads to overproduction of reactive oxygen species (ROS), which potentially causes oxidative stress and activates various cytokines, chemokines, and growth factors. Oxidative stress results from an imbalance between oxidants and antioxidants such as NAD(P)H quinone dehydrogenase-1 (NQO1), hemeoxygenase-1 (HO-1), catalase, superoxide dismutase (SOD), and glutathione peroxidase (GPx) [5–7]. The pathogenic changes caused by hyperglycemia-induced oxidative stress modify normal cell signaling and induce hyper-inflammation, apoptosis [8]. Moreover, formation of advanced glycation end products (AGEs) and activation of the AGE receptor due to hyperglycemia directly promote inflammatory states in the kidney by increasing oxidative stress [9].

Furthermore, oxidative stress activates the nucleotide-binding oligomerization domain (NOD)-like pyrin domain containing receptor 3 (NLRP3) inflammasome [10,11]. Activated NLRP3 recruits the apoptosis-associated speck-like protein containing a caspase recruitment domain (ASC) and pro-caspase-1, and contributes to the maturation of interleukin-1β (IL-1β) by activating caspase-1. NLRP3 inflammasome and mature IL-1β activate a transcription factor, nuclear factor-κB (NF-κB), and enhance multiple proinflammatory factors such as tumor necrosis factor-α (TNF-α), interleukin-6 (IL-6), and inducible nitric oxide synthase (iNOS) [12]. Hence, the activation of NLRP3 inflammasome contributes to chronic inflammatory response as well as insulin resistance in diabetes [13,14].

Moreover, chronic hyperglycemia-induced oxidative stress and hyper-inflammation accelerate renal apoptosis [5,13,15]. Cellular apoptosis is regulated by caspases through an extrinsic and intrinsic pathway. In ongoing-diabetes, hyperglycemia induces ROS-related apoptosis by increasing the Bax/Bcl-2 ratio, which is associated with progressive activation of pro-apoptotic caspase-3 [15,16]. ROS also increases protein kinase C (PKC), which activates transcription of transforming growth factor-β (TGF-β) [17]. In general, TGF-β leads to proliferation of fibroblasts and activates α-smooth muscle actin (α-SMA), which accommodates collagen formation and cellular hypertrophy. TGF-β also causes the proliferation of mesangial cells, consequentially leading to kidney fibrosis [18]. Therefore, suppression of renal cell apoptosis and pro-fibrotic change along with NLRP3 inflammasome related hyper-inflammation would be an effective target strategy on alleviating renal damage and the progress to DN [13].

Furthermore, abnormal energy metabolism in the kidney can cause renal damage. Sirtuin1 (SIRT1) mediates inflammatory signaling and apoptosis as a molecular response to glucotoxicity via deacetylation and inhibition of transcription factor NF-κB [19]. When the AMP/ATP ratio increases, 5′ adenosine monophosphate-activated protein kinase (AMPK) alleviates renal inflammation causing aberrant energy accumulation. The SIRT1/AMPK signaling pathway along with the peroxisome proliferator-activated receptor γ-coactivator α (PGC-1α) also suppresses renal hyper-inflammation and oxidative stress [20]. Hence, amelioration of SIRT1/AMPK signaling would be a possible therapeutic approach for diabetic renal damage.

In recent years, many medicinal plants have been reported as antidiabetic natural products including banaba, fenugreek, gymnema, yerba mate, etc. Among these plants, *Quamoclit angulata* (QA) is emerging as a source of therapeutic substance for diabetes and its complications. Although QA has not been fully investigated, a previously reported patent has shown that herbal agents of the *Quamoclit angulata* extract (QAE) decreased the fasting blood glucose (FBG) level and hemoglobin A1c (HbA1c) production by stimulating insulin secretion in pancreatic β cell. QAE also attenuated albuminuria, which is a major factor of DN in diabetic mice. Furthermore, QAE ameliorated angiogenesis by reducing the mRNA level of vascular endothelial growth factor (VEGF) in the ARPE 19 cell [21]. Nevertheless, little research has investigated the effects of QAE supplementation on renal damage in a hyperglycemic condition by molecular mechanisms. Hence, we examined if QAE supplementation has protective roles in renal damage via modulation of oxidative stress and inflammation in high fat diet-induced diabetic mice.

2. Materials and Methods

2.1. Quamoclit Angulata Extracts (QAE)

QA was obtained at Jeju, Korea. Aerial parts without the seed of QA (50 g) were extracted with 400 mL of water by incubation at 50 °C for 1 h. The sticky solid extract (50 g) was suspended in water, added to 1 kg of activated charcoal at room temperature for 1.5 h. After incubation, water, 20% ethanol fraction, and charcoal were removed through centrifugation and filtration (0.45 μm). Fractions were mixed, concentrated in vacuo, and frozen to dry. The yields of hot water extract and activated charcoal fractions were 25% and 11%, respectively.

2.2. Identification of Candidate Compounds of QAE

The standardization of QA was analyzed by using the HPLC system (Waters Corp., Milford, MA, USA) consisting of a separation module (e2695) and a photodiode array (PDA) detector. Twenty milligrams of dried QA were dissolved in 50% methanol/water. Protocatechuic acid, chlorogenic acid, syringic acid, myricetin, and quercetin were used as standard compounds and dissolved in methanol. For the analysis of each compound or sample, a Kromasil C^{18} column (150 × 4.6 mm, 5 μm) was used and a column temperature was set at 30 °C. The mobile phase consists of 3% acetic acid/water (solvent A) and methanol (solvent B) using a gradient program of 0–10% (B) in 0–10 min, 10–70% (B) in 10–44 min, 70–100% (B) in 44–50 min. The calibration was linear in a range of 0.1–1000 μg/mL for these five compounds. The flow rate was 0.9–1.0 mL/min and the PDA detector was set at 280 nm for acquiring chromatograms.

2.3. Animals Experiments

Male C57BL/6 mice at five weeks were housed in two or three per cages and maintained in a constant environment (temperature (22 ± 1 °C), humidity (50 ± 5%), and 12 h light/12 h dark cycle). After seven days of adaptation, the mice were randomly allocated into two groups. The first group was a non-diabetic control group (NC), which was fed an AIN-93G diet (10% kcal fat, Research Diets, New Brunswick, NJ, USA). The second was a diabetic group (DM), which was fed a high fat diet (40% kcal fat, Research Diets, New Brunswick, NJ, USA) for four weeks.

Then, the diabetic group received an intraperitoneal administration of 30 mg/kg body weight (BW) of streptozotocin (Sigma-Aldrich, St. Louis, MO, USA) in a citric acid buffer (pH 4.4). The NC mice received an equivalent amount of solvent. After five weeks from the last injection, fasting blood glucose (FBG) levels were measured once per week during the whole period of the animal experiment. Mice with FBG >140.4 mg/dL (7.8 mmol/L) more than two times were considered as the diabetic condition. The diabetes induction protocol was referred to the previous study by Zhang et al. [22].

Mice were separated in four groups; (1) CON: Non-diabetic normal mice were gavaged with distilled water, (2) DMC: Diabetic mice were gavaged with distilled water, (3) LQ: Diabetic mice were gavaged with a low dosage of QAE (5 mg/kg/day), (4) HQ: Diabetic mice were gavaged with a high dosage of QAE (10 mg/kg/day). QAE was dissolved in distilled water. Body weight, food intake, and fasting blood glucose level were weekly monitored during the animal experiment.

The animals were sacrificed after 12 weeks of oral supplementation. Blood was collected in a heparin (Sigma-Aldrich, St. Louis, MO, USA) coated syringe from the heart, centrifuged at 850 g at 4 °C for 10 min to obtain plasma. The kidney was removed from mice and stored at −80 °C before the experiment. All experiments with mice were approved by the Institutional Animal Care and Use Committee of Kyung Hee University (KHUASP(SE)-16-005 on 14 June, 2019).

2.4. Hemoglobin A1c (HbA1c) and Plasma Insulin Assay

HbA1c levels were measured using enzyme-linked immunosorbent assay (ELISA) commercial kits (Crystal Chem., Downers Grove, Elk Grove Village, IL, USA) according to directions of the manufacturer within two weeks from the sample collection.

The plasma insulin level was measured using ELISA kits (RayBiotech, Inc., Norcross, GA, USA). The homeostasis model assessment of insulin resistance (HOMA-IR) values were calculated as follows:

$$\text{HOMA-IR} = \text{fasting insulin (mmol/L)} \times \text{fasting glucose (μU/mL)}/22.5$$

2.5. Oral Glucose Tolerance Test (OGTT)

Fasted mice were administrated for 16 h with a 50% glucose solution (2 g/kg). The blood glucose level was detected at 0, 15, 30, 60, 90, and 120 min using a glucometer (OneTouch, LifeScan Inc., Malvern, PA, USA). The area under the curve (AUC) values of OGTT are calculated according to the trapezoidal rule as follows:

$$AUC = \sum (((\text{blood glucose})_i + (\text{blood glucose})_{i-1}) \times ((\text{time})_i - (\text{time})_{i-1})/2)$$
$$(i = \text{time sequence})$$

2.6. Renal Function Test

Urine samples were collected during three phases of the experiment (0–4 weeks; initial, 4–8 weeks; mid, and 8–12; late-points). Urinary albumin excretion was determined by the albumin assay kit (Bioassay, Hayward, CA, USA). The concentrations of urinary and plasma creatinine were calculated from interpolating the results of optical density at 515 nm into a standard curve. Concentrations of BUN were measured in accordance with the manufacturer's instructions using a commercial kit (Asan pharmaceutical, Seoul, South Korea).

2.7. Histological Observation of Kidney

Kidney tissues were fixed in 10% formaldehyde and then dehydrated through a series of alcohol. The tissues were cleared in xylene and embedded in paraffin. The sections were cut with a microtome into 5 μm, and stained with hematoxylin and eosin (H&E). Kidney morphology in stained tissue was observed using an optical microscope (Nikon ECLIPSE Ci, Nikon Instrument, Tokyo, Japan).

To calculate the glomerular area in H&E-staining, paraffin-embedded sections were measured by the Canvas 11 software (Deneba, Miami, FL, USA). The Glomerulus area was expressed as the mean of thirty glomeruli per each sample and a minimum of four samples from each group were examined. Area values are reported in $\mu m^2 \times 10^{-3}$.

2.8. Protein Extraction and Western Blot Analysis

The kidneys were ground and lysed on ice for 30 min. The lysate was centrifuged to remove tissue debris at 1945× g at 4 °C for 10 min. Each supernatant was centrifuged again at 9078× g at 4 °C for 30 min. Then, the final supernatant was collected for cytosolic extract. The pellet was re-crushed in a hypertonic lysis buffer for 1 h, and then the lysate was centrifuged at 9078× g at 4 °C for 20 min and the supernatant was used for nuclear extract. The protein concentration was quantified according to a BCA protein assay (ThermoFisher Scientific, Grand Island, NY, USA).

Thirty μg of each protein sample were loaded into an SDS-PAGE and transferred to poly-vinylidine fluoride (PVDF) membranes (Millipore, Marlborough, MA, USA). We used 8~12% SDS-PAGE gel according to the molecular weight (MW) of target protein(s). After the transfer, the membrane was blocked in 1~3% bovine serum albumin (BSA) in a phosphate buffed saline −0.1% Tween 20 (PBS-T), the membrane was incubated at 4 °C with each primary antibody. To detect primary antibodies, respective horseradish peroxide (HRP)-conjugated secondary antibodies were given to membranes. Protein bands were visualized using a chemiluminescent detector (Syngene, Cambridge, UK). Levels of targeted proteins were calculated using Syngene GeneSnap (Syngene, Cambridge, UK).

2.9. Statistical Analysis

Data were expressed as mean ± standard error of the mean (SEM). The significant differences between sample groups were determined using one-way ANOVA (significant level = 0.05).

3. Results

3.1. Identification of Major Natural Compounds in QAE

In this study, five compounds such as protocatechuic acid, chlorogenic acid, syringic acid, myricetin, and quercetin were analyzed by using the HPLC system. As shown in Table 1, the QA extract mainly involved protocatechuic acid (198.86 ± 2.26 µg/g). Meanwhile, chlorogenic acid (54.11 ± 1.81 µg/g), syringic acid (56.38 ± 0.57 µg/g), myricetin (12.42 ± 0.09 µg/g), and quercetin (13.41 ± 0.08 µg/g) were detected in QAE.

Table 1. Contents of protocatechuic acid, chlorogenic acid, syringic acid, myricetin, and quercetin compounds by HPLC analysis in the presence of *Quamoclit angulata* extract (QAE).

Samples	Content (µg/g)				
	Protocatechuic Acid	Chlorogenic Acid	Syringic Acid	Myricetin	Quercetin
QAE	198.86 ± 2.26	54.11 ± 1.81	56.38 ± 0.57	12.42 ± 0.09	13.41 ± 0.08

Data were expressed as means ± SEM ($n = 3$).

3.2. Effect of QAE Supplementation on Body Weight, Food Intake, and Kidney Weight in T2DM Mice

Body weight and food intake of all T2DM groups (the DMC group, the LQ group, and the HQ group) were significantly increased compared to the NC group. QAE supplementation for 12 weeks had no effect on body weight change in T2DM mice. With a slightly different result, kidney weight in the DMC group was significantly increased compared to the NC group, and there was no significant difference in the LQ group and the HQ group compared to the DMC group (Table 2).

Table 2. Effect of QAE on body weight, kidney weight, and food intake in type 2 diabetes mellitus (T2DM) mice.

Group	NC	DMC	LQ	HQ
Body Weight (g)				
before treatment	26.58 ± 0.45 [a]	32.04 ± 1.04 [b]	31.90 ± 1.25 [b]	30.80 ± 0.68 [b]
after treatment	30.42 ± 0.61 [a]	40.93 ± 1.57 [b]	40.20 ± 2.20 [b]	39.40 ± 1.89 [b]
Gain	3.85 ± 0.33 [a]	8.89 ± 0.70 [b]	8.31 ± 1.15 [b]	8.60 ± 1.33 [b]
Kidney Weight (mg)	151.00 ± 5.34 [a]	183.00 ± 14.37 [b]	175.00 ± 11.18 [a,b]	176.00 ± 4.30 [a,b]
Food Intake (g/day)	2.32 ± 0.21 [a]	3.48 ± 0.25 [b]	3.3 ± 0.12 [b]	3.76 ± 0.12 [b]

Data were expressed as means ± SEM. Mean values with the same superscript letter (a,b) are not significantly different ($p < 0.05$). NC: Normal mice; DMC: Type 2 diabetic mice; LQ: Type 2 diabetic mice supplemented with a low dose (5 mg/kg/day) of QAE; HQ: Type 2 diabetic mice supplemented with a high dose (10 mg/kg/day) of QAE.

3.3. Effect of QAE Supplementation on Fasting Blood Glucose and Plasma Insulin Levels, Homeostasis Model Assessment of Insulin Resistance (HOMA-IR), and Hemoglobin A1c (HbA1c) in T2DM Mice

Fasting blood glucose level, plasma insulin level, HOMA-IR, and HbA1c level were as follows (Table 3). At the end of the QAE treatment period, there was no difference in the fasting blood glucose level among all groups. The plasma insulin level in the HQ group was significantly lower than that in the DMC group. HOMA-IR was significantly reduced in both QAE treated diabetic groups. The HbA1c level was significantly decreased only in the HQ group compared with the DMC group (Table 3).

Table 3. Effect of QAE on plasma indices related to type 2 diabetes.

Plasma Indices	NC	DMC	LQ	HQ
FBG (mg/dL)	122 ± 7.51 [a]	173 ± 14.30 [b]	156 ± 9.94 [a,b]	150 ± 12.04 [a,b]
Insulin (uU/mL)	1.62 ± 0.30 [a]	2.62 ± 0.23 [b]	1.80 ± 0.38 [a,b]	1.61 ± 0.20 [a]
HOMA-IR	2.82 ± 0.58 [a]	8.45 ± 0.79 [b]	3.80 ± 1.01 [a]	4.19 ± 0.62 [a]
HbA1c (%)	6.61 ± 0.51 [a]	12.18 ± 2.82 [b]	8.64 ± 0.76 [a,b]	7.13 ± 0.39 [a]

Data were expressed as means ± SEM. Mean values with the same superscript letter (a,b) are not significantly different ($p < 0.05$). NC: Normal mice; DMC: Type 2 diabetic mice; LQ: Type 2 diabetic mice supplemented with a low dose (5 mg/kg/day) of QAE; HQ: Type 2 diabetic mice supplemented with a high dose (10 mg/kg/day) of QAE.

3.4. Effect of QAE Supplementation on Glucose Homeostasis in T2DM Mice

OGTT was performed to estimate insulin resistance and failure of glucose metabolism (Figure 1A), and glucose AUC was calculated as shown in Figure 1B. The figure showed that the DMC group had a high blood glucose level during 120 min after glucose administration compared to the NC group and there was no significant difference in the blood glucose level at 90 min after glucose administration among the DMC group and the QAE treatment groups. The blood glucose level of the LQ group at 120 min was remarkably reduced as compared to the DMC group and glucose AUC of the LQ group was significantly lower than that of the DMC group. On the other hand, the protein level of receptor for advanced glycation end products (RAGE) was remarkably increased in the DMC group compared to that of the NC group (Figure 1C). The HQ group showed a significant reduction of RAGE expression in comparison to the DMC group.

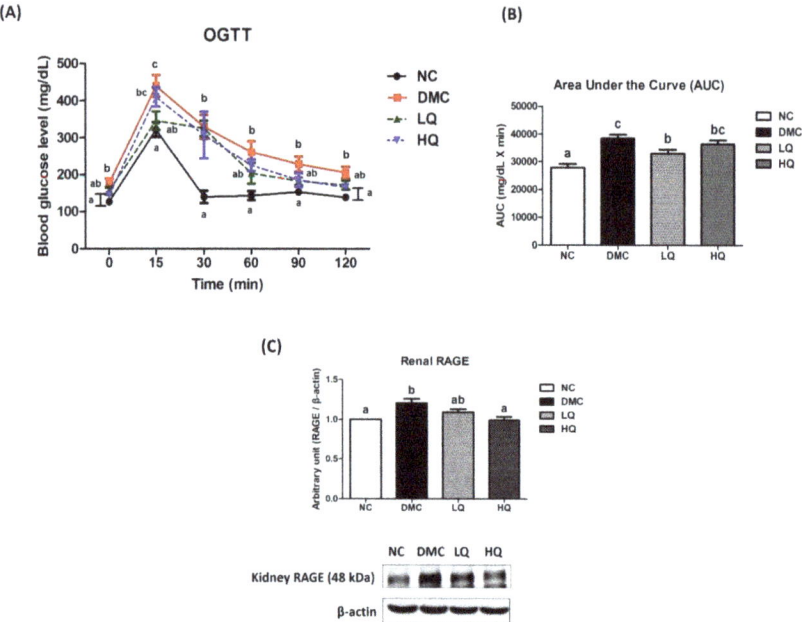

Figure 1. Effect of QAE on (**A**) glucose tolerance, (**B**) glucose area under the curve (AUC), and (**C**) renal receptor of AGE (RAGE) in T2DM mice. Data were expressed as means ± SEM. Mean values with the same superscript letter are not significantly different ($p < 0.05$). NC: Normal mice; DMC: Type 2 diabetic mice; LQ: Type 2 diabetic mice supplemented with a low dose (5 mg/kg/day) of QAE; HQ: Type 2 diabetic mice supplemented with a high dose (10 mg/kg/day) of QAE.

3.5. Effect of QAE Supplementation on Kidney Function in T2DM Mice

The ACRs of all T2DM groups were significantly higher than that in the NC group during the entire experimental period (Figure 2A). The ACRs of the QAE treatment groups decreased during the treatment period and showed a significant difference at the late stage of treatment in the diabetic mice. As shown in Figure 2B, the supplementation with a high dose of QAE significantly decreased the plasma creatinine and BUN compared with the DMC group. In representative H&E staining of the kidney (Figure 2C), the DMC group showed glomerular hypertrophy as compared to the NC group, while both the QAE treated groups ameliorated glomerular hypertrophy. The red arrow indicated mesangial expansion in the DMC group compared to the NC group. In the NC group, Bowman's space was observed as a thin white line. However, Bowman's space was broadened in the DMC group compared to that in the NC group, and was narrower in the QAE treatment groups than that in the DMC group. In addition, glomerular surface areas in histological sections of renal cortex were quantified to measure the degree of glomerular hypertrophy (Figure 2C). The glomerulus of the DMC group was significantly expanded compared with that of the NC group, while both QAE supplementation groups regardless of dose showed significantly reduced glomerular hypertrophy.

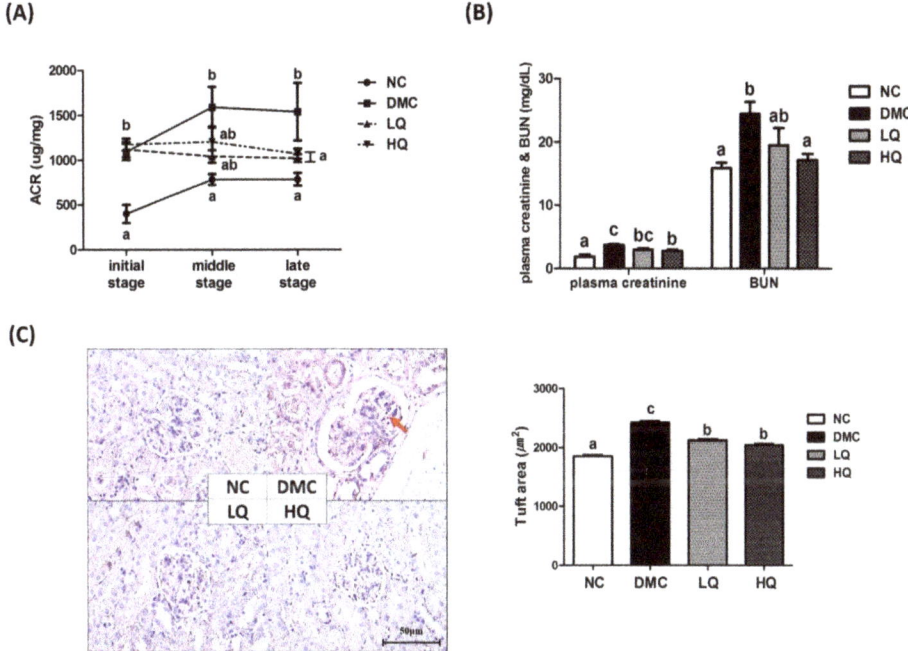

Figure 2. Effect of QAE on (**A**) urine albumin/creatinine ratio (ACR), (**B**) level of plasma creatinine and blood urea nitrogen (BUN), and (**C**) renal morphology and glomerular size in T2DM. Data were expressed as means ± SEM. Mean values with the same superscript letter (a,b and c) are not significantly different ($p < 0.05$). NC: Normal mice; DMC: Type 2 diabetic mice; LQ: Type 2 diabetic mice supplemented with a low dose (5 mg/kg/day) of QAE; HQ: Type 2 diabetic mice supplemented with a high dose (10 mg/kg/day) of QAE.

3.6. Effect of QAE Supplementation on Oxidative Stress in T2DM Mice

The renal 4-hydroxynonenal (4-HNE) level was examined for assessing lipid peroxidation and the level of renal protein carbonyls was used as a marker of protein oxidation caused by oxidative stress (Figure 3A). In the kidney, the 4-HNE protein level in the DMC group was significantly higher than that in the NC group. The HQ group presented a significant reduction of 4-HNE level compared to that of the DMC group. Renal levels of protein carbonyls in both QAE groups were significantly lower than that in the DMC group. In the DMC group, the protein levels of nuclear Nrf2 and its related markers such as HO-1, NQO1, catalase, MnSOD, and GPx were remarkably higher than those in the NC group. However, both QAE treatments significantly reduced the protein levels of nuclear Nrf2 and MnSOD. Moreover, a high dose of the QAE treatment significantly decreased the protein levels of HO-1, NQO1, and catalase in the diabetic mice. The protein levels of GPx and NOX4 were not significantly different among the DMC group and the QAE treatment groups (Figure 3B).

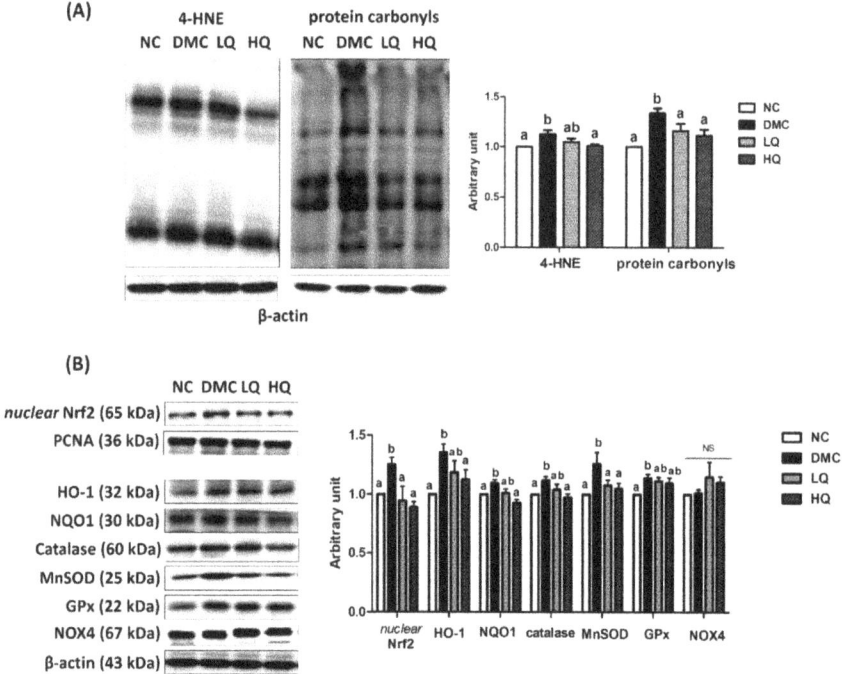

Figure 3. Effect of QAE on renal (**A**) 4-hydroxynonenal (4-HNE) and protein carbonyls and (**B**) antioxidant defense system in T2DM mice. Data were expressed as means ± SEM. Mean values with the same superscript letter (a,b) are not significantly different ($p < 0.05$). NC: Normal mice; DMC: Type 2 diabetic mice; LQ: Type 2 diabetic mice supplemented with a low dose (5 mg/kg/day) of QAE; HQ: Type 2 diabetic mice supplemented with a high dose (10 mg/kg/day) of QAE.

3.7. Effect of QAE Supplementation on Inflammation in T2DM Mice

The protein level of NLRP3 inflammasome was elevated in the DMC group compared to that of the NC group. However, the level of NLRP3 was significantly decreased in the QAE treatment groups compared to those in the DMC group. However, only a high dose of QAE treatment significantly lowered the protein levels of ASC, procaspase-1, caspase-1, and mature IL-1β in the diabetic mice. The protein levels of precursor IL-1β were not normalized in the QAE treatment groups compared to that in the DMC group (Figure 4A).

Furthermore, the DMC group demonstrated higher levels of inflammation related protein including monocyte chemoattractant protein (MCP)-1, CRP, nuclear NF-κB, TNF-α, IL-6, and iNOS than the NC group (Figure 4B). However, a high dose of QAE treatment in the diabetic mice reversed the protein levels of MCP-1 and nuclear NF-κB to the levels of the NC mice. In addition, the QAE treatment regardless of dose suppressed other inflammatory markers such as CRP, TNF-α, IL-6, and iNOS in the diabetic mice.

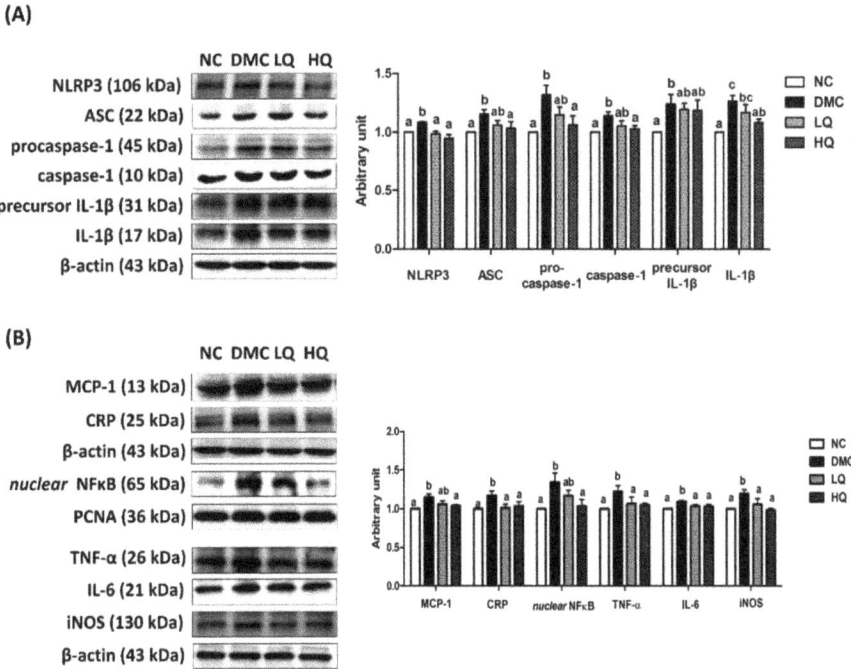

Figure 4. Effect of QAE on renal NLRP3 Inflammasome related hyper-inflammation in T2DM mice. Protein levels of (**A**) nucleotide-binding oligomerization domain-like pyrin domain containing receptor 3 (NLRP3) inflammasome: nucleotide-binding oligomerization domain-like pyrin domain containing receptor 3 (NLRP-3); apoptosis-associated speck-like proteins including caspase recruitment domain (ASC), caspase-1, and interleukin (IL)-1β; and (**B**) markers of pro-inflammatory response: monocyte chemoattractant protein-1 (MCP-1), C-reactive protein (CRP); and nuclear factor kappa B (NF-κB)-related inflammatory response: nuclear factor kappa B (NF-κB), tumor necrosis factor-α (TNF-α), interleukin (IL)-6, and inducible nitric oxide synthase (iNOS). Data were expressed as means ± SEM. Mean values with the same superscript letter (a,b and c) are not significantly different ($p < 0.05$). NC: Normal mice; DMC: Type 2 diabetic mice; LQ: Type 2 diabetic mice supplemented with a low dose (5 mg/kg/day) of QAE; HQ: Type 2 diabetic mice supplemented with a high dose (10 mg/kg/day) of QAE.

3.8. Effect of QAE Supplementation on Energy Metabolism in T2DM Mice

The protein levels of AMPK were not significantly different among the groups. The protein level of phosphorylated AMPK in the DMC group was significantly declined compared to that of the NC group, but those in the QAE treatment groups were increased compared to the DMC group. In addition, the QAE treatment elevated the pAMPK/AMPK ratio as much as the level of the NC group (Figure 5A). Furthermore, the protein levels of SIRT1 and PGC-1α were significantly declined in the DMC group compared to those in the NC group, but were increased in the QAE treatment groups regardless of dosage (Figure 5B).

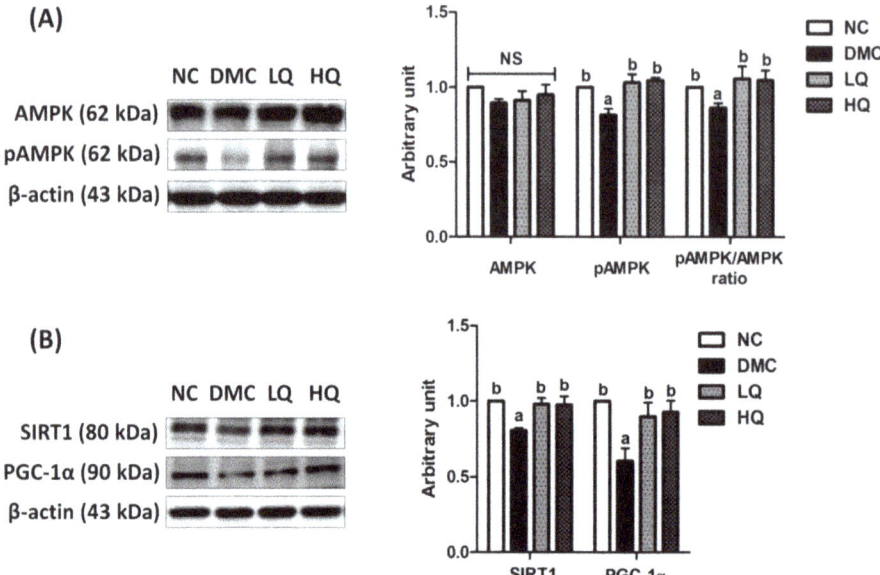

Figure 5. Effect of QAE on renal AMPK/SIRT1 signaling in T2DM mice. (**A**) Phosphorylation of AMPK and (**B**) SIRT-1 and PGC-1α. Data were expressed as means ± SEM. Mean values with the same superscript letter (a,b) are not significantly different ($p < 0.05$). NC: Normal mice; DMC: Type 2 diabetic mice; LQ: Type 2 diabetic mice supplemented with a low dose (5 mg/kg/day) of QAE; HQ: Type 2 diabetic mice supplemented with a high dose (10 mg/kg/day) of QAE.

3.9. Effect of QAE Supplementation on Apoptosis and Fibrosis in T2DM Mice

The protein levels of caspase-8, caspase-3, and nuclear p53 in the DMC group were significantly higher than those in the NC group, but the high dose of QAE supplementation decreased the protein levels of caspase-8 and p53 than those in the DMC group. Furthermore, the QAE treatment regardless of dose reduced caspase-3 compared to the DMC group (Figure 6A). The protein levels of Bax in the QAE treatment groups were significantly decreased in comparison to that of the DMC group. The QAE treatment regardless of dose remarkably lowered the protein level of Bax/Bcl-2 ratio in the diabetic mice (Figure 6A). In addition, the QAE treatments reduced the protein level of ERK compared to that of the DMC group. At the same time, the protein levels of phosphorylated ERK in the QAE treatment groups were reduced compared to that in the DMC group. Moreover, the pERK/ERK ratio, an index of ERK phosphorylation, in the QAE treatment groups was also decreased compared to that in the DMC group (Figure 6A).

To examine the effect of the QAE supplementation on renal fibrosis, the protein levels of PKC-βII, TGF-β, α-SMA, and COL1A were measured (Figure 6B). The renal protein levels of PKC, TGF-β, α-SMA, and COL1A in the DMC group were significantly higher than those in the NC group. However, the QAE treatments decreased the protein levels of PKC, TGF-β, and α-SMA in comparison to the DMC group, and, in particular, a high dose of the QAE treatment declined the protein level of COL1A in the diabetic mice.

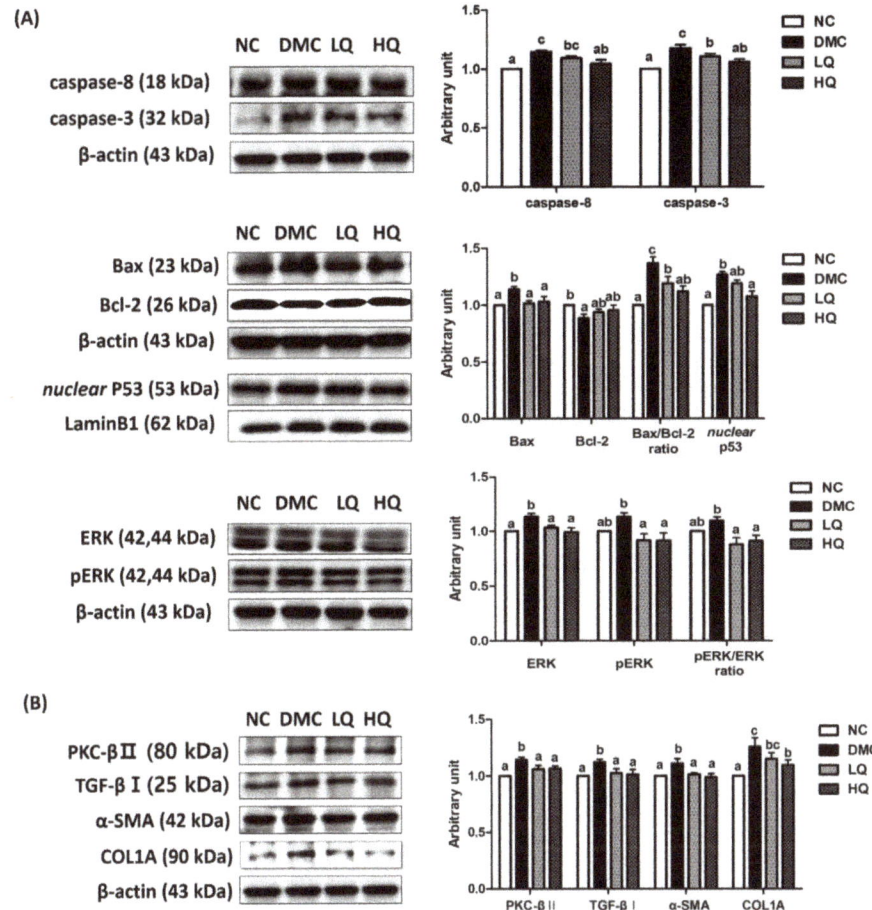

Figure 6. Effect of QAE on renal (**A**) apoptosis and (**B**) fibrosis in T2DM mice. Data were expressed as means ± SEM. Mean values with the same superscript letter (a,b and c) are not significantly different ($p < 0.05$). NC: Normal mice; DMC: Type 2 diabetic mice; LQ: Type 2 diabetic mice supplemented with a low dose (5 mg/kg/day) of QAE; HQ: Type 2 diabetic mice supplemented with a high dose (10 mg/kg/day) of QAE.

4. Discussion

Various studies noticed that many medicinal plants and natural products have potential biological activities. Among these plants, QA is a species of ipomoea morning glory and cultivated as an ornamental plant throughout the tropics. In this study, we aimed to investigate that dietary QAE supplementation could have beneficial effects on NLRP3 inflammasome dependent hyper-inflammation and consequential renal damage by stimulation of AMPK-SIRT1 signaling in type 2 diabetes.

The current study suggested a hypoglycemic effect of QAE presented by decreased plasma insulin, HOMA-IR, and HbA1c. HbA1c is considered as an index of average blood glucose control level, because the HbA1c level tends to increase with the averaged blood glucose levels over preceding three months. A previous study also showed a strong correlation between HbA1c and 6-h fasting glucose levels than overnight FBG levels in diabetic mice [23]. In this study, the QA supplementation ameliorated plasma insulin level, HOMA-IR, and HbA1c compared to the DMC group, although did not significantly decrease the FBG level. In glucose tolerance test, AUC was declined in the LQ group compared to the DMC group. As shown in Table 1, QA contained five compounds such as protocatechuic acid (PCA), chlorogenic acid, syringic acid, myricetin, and quercetin. A recent study showed similar tendency that PCA significantly reduced blood glucose and plasma insulin level in the hyperglycemic condition [24]. In addition, it is known that activated ligation of AGEs to renal RAGE activated production of ROS subsequently causing oxidative stress [25]. Furthermore, chlorogenic acid (CGA) and quercetin have been shown to decrease blood glucose level by stimulating glucose uptake through the activation of AMPK in diabetic mice [26,27]. CGA has been also reported as an inhibitor of carbonic anhydrase V which has an impact on gluconeogenesis [28]. The current results showed that a high dose of QAE treatment decreased RAGE expression compared to T2DM mice. These data suggest that the QAE treatment has ameliorative effects on a hyperglycemic condition due to synergistic or additive effects of PCA, chlorogenic acid, and quercetin these active ingredients.

Moreover, there are well-known renal malfunction indicators including albuminuria, plasma creatinine, BUN, and urinary ACR level in DN. Our data showed that the QAE treatment significantly decreased urinary ACR, plasma creatinine, and BUN in diabetic mice. From these changes, it could be inferred that the QAE treatment improved renal function in a diabetic condition.

In terms of molecules, major mechanisms of hyperglycemia-induced tissue damage are as follows—the increase of intracellular AGEs formation and its receptor expression, and activation of PKC. As indicated above, the current study demonstrated that QAE supplementation reduced the protein level of RAGE in the diabetic mice. In addition, elevated protein levels of 4-HNE were decreased in the HQ group and both doses of QAE supplementation lowered protein carbonyls in the DMC group. Previous studies showed that the increased level of Nrf2 as well as 4-HNE and protein carbonyls activated Nrf2 related antioxidant defense systems [12,29]. Our results particularly demonstrated that the protein level of Nrf2 and its related antioxidant defense enzymes including NQO1, HO-1, and catalase were increased in the DMC mice but these markers were reduced in the HQ group. Especially, PCA is known to attenuate oxidative stress by decreasing the levels of ROS and malondialdehyde (MDA) in a diabetic condition [30]. Hence, it can be concluded that QAE containing PCA and CGA supplementation could alleviate cellular oxidative stress as well as activations of RAGE in diabetes.

Oxidative stress also can contribute to inflammatory response via the activation of NF-κB and downstream factors such as TNF-α, IL-6, and iNOS in DN [31]. Furthermore, oxidative stress would potentially activate NLRP3 inflammasome by initial recognition as cellular danger [32,33]. In this study, the renal protein levels of NLRP3 inflammasome, nuclear NF-κB, and subsequent inflammatory factors were higher in the DMC group compared with the NC group. A previous study demonstrated that the PCA treatment significantly reduced the secretion of pro-inflammatory cytokines in T2DM rats [34]. Furthermore, syringic acid is known to reduce oxidative stress and inflammation in diabetes [35]. Simultaneously, QAE supplementation selectively reduced the renal inflammatory factors via suppression of NLRP3 inflammasome. Therefore, the current study suggested that QAE supplementation alleviated the activation of NLRP3 inflammasome and consequential hyper-inflammation under a diabetic condition.

In consistent hyperglycemia, chronic hyper-inflammation in the kidney results in renal apoptosis via activation of caspases, proapoptotic protein Bax, p53, and mitogen activated protein kinase (MAPK) signaling [36–39]. PCA is known to reduce the protein expression levels of type IV collagen, laminin, and fibronectin in high glucose-stimulated human mesangial cells (MCs) [40]. Our results showed that pro-fibrosis related markers including PKC-βII, TGF-βI, and α-SMA as well as apoptosis related markers such as caspase-8, caspase-3, Bax/Bcl-2 ratio, and pERK/ERK ratio were declined in the QAE treated group, regardless of dose, compared with the DMC group. The present study suggested that PCA and chlorogenic acid in QAE might play major roles in the protection of renal apoptosis and fibrosis in T2DM.

How could the QAE treatment ameliorate the renal damage through suppression of oxidative stress, NLRP3 inflammasome-dependent hyper-inflammation, cell apoptosis, and pro-fibrosis in a hyperglycemic condition? There are cumulative evidences that AMPK influences intracellular signaling pathway, especially amelioration of oxidative stress via activation of antioxidant defense enzymes [41]. Metformin, which is a well-known diabetic drug, shows therapeutic mechanisms related to AMPK, which suppresses the NF-κB through activation of SIRT1 and PGC-1α [21,42,43]. PCA also increased the phosphorylation of AMPK and then activated the expression of p-Nrf2 and HO-1 in oxidative damage in HUVECs [44]. Moreover, a recent study reported that the syringic acid improved energy metabolism by regulation of mitochondrial biogenesis in diabetic rats [33]. On the other hand, SIRT1, an intracellular energy sensor, beneficially affected glucose homeostasis, cellular immunity to oxidative stress, inflammation, apoptosis, and fibrosis in the kidney [45]. In DN, one of the earliest characteristics is the loss of podocyte, which plays a crucial role in albumin processing, but SIRT1 is known to attenuate podocyte depletion and albuminuria by downregulation of claudin-1 in podocytes [46,47]. Resveratrol, a natural plant polyphenol, respectively stimulates SIRT1 and AMPK, and has a protective effect on oxidative stress and inflammatory response in the kidney [20]. A previous study showed that SIRT1 suppressed NLRP3 inflammasome activation as well as the NF-κB associated inflammatory response [48,49]. PGC-1α also regulates oxidative stress via participation in cellular signaling to mitochondrial oxidative stress and independently inhibits the NF-κB related inflammatory response [50,51]. The current studies demonstrated that the treatment of QAE containing PCA and syringic acid elevated the protein levels of SIRT1 and PGC-1α and downregulated NLRP3 inflammasome dependent inflammatory mediators in the diabetic mice. In particular, both doses of QAE supplementation has an effect on the stimulation of AMPK/SIRT pathway and a high dose of QAE supplementation decreased NLRP3 inflammation accompanied by nuclear NF-κB activation in our study. Therefore, it can be inferred that the QAE treatment has a protective effect on renal oxidative stress and hyper-inflammation under a hyperglycemic condition by involving this antagonism of SIRT1/NF-κB/NLRP3 inflammasome.

The previous study reported by our group found that the *Lespedeza bicolor* extract (LBE) containing polyphenolic compounds such as quercetin, genistein, daidzein, and naringenin has shown to exert antioxidant and anti-inflammatory effects accompanied by upregulation of the AMPK-SIRT1 pathway in the same diabetic model [52]. The current findings supported that QAE at much lower concentrations compared to LBE and other plant extracts has shown antidiabetic effects through regulation of the AMPK-SIRT related mechanism as shown in LBE treated diabetic mice [52]. Moreover, QAE supplementation attenuated pro-fibrosis as well as apoptosis in the diabetic group, which was not shown in LBE treatment groups. Therefore, it can be concluded that QAE is more effective than LBE on renal fibrosis and apoptosis in diabetes.

5. Conclusions

Taken together, we reported that QAE supplementation at a high dose had ameliorative effects on renal NLRP3 inflammasome associated hyper-inflammation and consequent renal cell apoptosis and pro-fibrosis in the HFD/STZ-induced T2DM mice. In addition, QAE supplementation regardless of the dose stimulated AMPK/SIRT1 signaling and ameliorated oxidative stress, although some molecular markers were selectively regulated at different treatment doses of QAE in diabetic renal damage. In conclusion, the current study suggested that QAE could be a potential therapeutic for improving renal damage in T2DM.

Author Contributions: Conceptualization, Y.L.; Data curation, J.E.P. and H.L.; Formal analysis, Y.L. and J.E.P.; Investigation, Y.L. and S.Y.K.; Funding acquisition, Y.L.; HPLC analysis, S.M.H.; Methodology, Y.L., J.E.P., H.L., and H.R.; Supervision, Y.L.; Writing—Review and editing, J.E.P., H.L., H.R., and Y.L. All authors have read and agreed to the published version of the manuscript.

Funding: This research was supported by iPET [115045-03] (Korea Institute of Planning and Evaluation for Technology in Food, Agriculture, Forestry and Fisheries), Ministry of Agriculture, Food and Rural Affairs.

Conflicts of Interest: The authors declare no conflict of interest.

Abbreviations

ACR	Albumin/Creatinine ratio
AGEs	Advanced glycation end products
AMPK	5′ adenosine monophosphate-activated protein kinase
ASC	Apoptosis-associated speck-like protein containing a caspase recruitment domain
AUC	Area under the curve
BUN	Blood urea nitrogen
DM	Diabetes mellitus
DN	Diabetic nephropathy
FBG	Fasting blood glucose
GPx	Glutathione peroxidase
4-HNE	4-hydroxynonenal
HO-1	Hemeoxygenase-1
IL-1β	Interleukin-1β
IL-6	Interleukin-6
iNOS	Inducible nitric oxide synthase
NC	Normal control
NF-κB	Nuclear factor-κB
NLRP3	NOD-like pyrin domain containing receptor 3
NQO1	NAD(P)H quinone dehydrogenase-1
PKC	Protein kinase C
RAGE	Receptor for advanced glycation end products
ROS	Reactive oxygen species
SIRT1	Sirtuin1
SMA	Smooth muscle actin
SOD	Superoxide dismutase
T2DM	Type 2 diabetes mellitus
TGF-β	Transforming growth factor-β
TNF-α	Tumor necrosis factor-α
QA	*Quamoclit angulata*
QAE	*Quamoclit angulata* extract

References

1. Rains, J.L.; Jain, S.K. Oxidative stress, insulin signaling, and diabetes. *Free Radic. Biol. Med.* **2011**, *50*, 567–575. [CrossRef] [PubMed]
2. Wright, E., Jr.; Scism-Bacon, J.L.; Glass, L.C. Oxidative stress in type 2 diabetes: The role of fasting and postprandial glycaemia. *Int. J. Clin. Pract.* **2006**, *60*, 308–314. [CrossRef] [PubMed]
3. Tesch, G.H.; Allen, T.J. Rodent models of streptozotocin-induced diabetic nephropathy. *Nephrology* **2007**, *12*, 261–266. [CrossRef] [PubMed]
4. Ritz, E. Diabetic nephropathy. *Saudi J. Kidney Dis. Transpl.* **2006**, *17*, 481–490.
5. Turkmen, K. Inflammation, oxidative stress, apoptosis, and autophagy in diabetes mellitus and diabetic kidney disease: The Four Horsemen of the Apocalypse. *Int. Urol. Nephrol.* **2017**, *49*, 837–844. [CrossRef]
6. Eo, H.; Lee, H.J.; Lim, Y. Ameliorative effect of dietary genistein on diabetes induced hyper-inflammation and oxidative stress during early stage of wound healing in alloxan induced diabetic mice. *Biochem. Biophys. Res. Commun.* **2016**, *478*, 1021–1027. [CrossRef]
7. Newsholme, P. Molecular mechanisms of ROS production and oxidative stress in diabetes. *Biochem. J.* **2016**, *473*, 4527–4550. [CrossRef]
8. Habib, S.L. Diabetes and renal tubular cell apoptosis. *World J. Diabetes* **2013**, *4*, 27–30. [CrossRef]
9. Noh, H.; Ha, H. Reactive oxygen species and oxidative stress. *Contrib. Nephro.* **2011**, *170*, 102–112.
10. Lu, M. Curcumin Ameliorates Diabetic Nephropathy by Suppressing NLRP3 Inflammasome Signaling. *Biomed. Res. Int.* **2017**, *2017*, 1516985. [CrossRef]

11. He, Y.; Hara, H.; Nunez, G. Mechanism and Regulation of NLRP3 Inflammasome Activation. *Trends Biochem. Sci.* **2016**, *41*, 1012–1021. [CrossRef] [PubMed]
12. Eo, H.; Park, J.E.; Jeon, Y.J.; Lim, Y. Ameliorative Effect of Ecklonia cava Polyphenol Extract on Renal Inflammation Associated with Aberrant Energy Metabolism and Oxidative Stress in High Fat Diet-Induced Obese Mice. *J. Agric. Food Chem.* **2017**, *65*, 3811–3818. [CrossRef] [PubMed]
13. Shen, J.; Wang, L.; Jiang, N.; Mou, S.; Zhang, M.; Gu, L.; Shao, X.; Wang, Q.; Qi, C.; Li, S.; et al. NLRP3 inflammasome mediates contrast media-induced acute kidney injury by regulating cell apoptosis. *Sci. Rep.* **2016**, *6*, 34682. [CrossRef]
14. Klen, J.; Goricar, K.; Janez, A.; Dolzan, V. NLRP3 Inflammasome Polymorphism and Macrovascular Complications in Type 2 Diabetes Patients. *J. Diabetes Res.* **2015**, *2015*, 616747. [CrossRef] [PubMed]
15. Wagener, F.A.; Dekker, D.; Berden, J.H.; Scharstuhl, A.; van der Vlag, J. The role of reactive oxygen species in apoptosis of the diabetic kidney. *Apoptosis* **2009**, *14*, 1451–1458. [CrossRef] [PubMed]
16. Balasescu, E.; Ion, D.A.; Cioplea, M.; Zurac, S. Caspases, Cell Death and Diabetic Nephropathy. *Rom. J. Intern. Med.* **2015**, *53*, 296–303.
17. Dakshinamurty, K.V. Pathophysiology and pathology of Diabetic Nephropathy. In *Diabetic Kidney Disease—ECAB*; Elsevier Health Sciences: Amsterdam, The Netherlands, 2013; p. 223.
18. Chen, S.; Hong, S.W.; Iglesias-de la Cruz, M.C.; Isono, M.; Casaretto, A.; Ziyadeh, F.N. The key role of the transforming growth factor-beta system in the pathogenesis of diabetic nephropathy. *Ren. Fail.* **2001**, *23*, 471–481. [CrossRef]
19. Kitada, M.; Koya, D. SIRT1 in Type 2 Diabetes: Mechanisms and Therapeutic Potential. *Diabetes Metab. J.* **2013**, *37*, 315–325. [CrossRef]
20. Kim, Y.; Park, C.W. Adenosine monophosphate-activated protein kinase in diabetic nephropathy. *Kidney Res. Clin. Pract.* **2016**, *35*, 69–77. [CrossRef]
21. Chun, B.H. Pharmaceutical Composition for Treating Diabetes Containing Quamoclit Angulate Extracts. U.S. Patent Application 13/579,743, 3 January 2011.
22. Zhang, M.; Lv, X.Y.; Li, J.; Xu, Z.G.; Chen, L. The characterization of high-fat diet and multiple low-dose streptozotocin induced type 2 diabetes rat model. *Exp. Diabetes Res.* **2008**, *2008*, 704045. [CrossRef]
23. Han, B.G.; Hao, C.M.; Tchekneva, E.E.; Wang, Y.Y.; Lee, C.A.; Ebrahim, B.; Harris, R.C.; Kern, T.S.; Wasserman, D.H.; Breyer, M.D.; et al. Markers of glycemic control in the mouse: Comparisons of 6-h- and overnight-fasted blood glucoses to Hb A1c. *Am. J. Physiol. Endocrinol. Metab.* **2008**, *295*, E981–E986. [CrossRef] [PubMed]
24. Semaming, Y.; Kukongviriyapan, U.; Kongyingyoes, B.; Thukhammee, W.; Pannangpetch, P. Protocatechuic Acid Restores Vascular Responses in Rats With Chronic Diabetes Induced by Streptozotocin. *Phytother. Res.* **2016**, *30*, 227–233. [CrossRef] [PubMed]
25. Sourris, K.C.; Morley, A.L.; Koitka, A.; Samuel, P.; Coughlan, M.T.; Penfold, S.A.; Thomas, M.C.; Bierhaus, A.; Nawroth, P.P.; Yamamoto, H.; et al. Receptor for AGEs (RAGE) blockade may exert its renoprotective effects in patients with diabetic nephropathy via induction of the angiotensin II type 2 (AT2) receptor. *Diabetologia* **2010**, *53*, 2442–2451. [CrossRef] [PubMed]
26. Ong, K.W.; Hsu, A.; Tan, B.K. Chlorogenic acid stimulates glucose transport in skeletal muscle via AMPK activation: A contributor to the beneficial effects of coffee on diabetes. *PLoS ONE* **2012**, *7*, e32718. [CrossRef]
27. Dhanya, R.; Arya, A.D.; Nisha, P.; Jayamurthy, P. Quercetin, a Lead Compound against Type 2 Diabetes Ameliorates Glucose Uptake via AMPK Pathway in Skeletal Muscle Cell Line. *Front. Pharmacol.* **2017**, *8*, 336. [CrossRef]
28. Mollica, A.; Locatelli, M.; Macedonio, G.; Carradori, S.; Sobolev, A.P.; De Salvador, R.F.; Monti, S.M.; Buonanno, M.; Zengin, G.; Angeli, A.; et al. Microwave-assisted extraction, HPLC analysis, and inhibitory effects on carbonic anhydrase I, II, VA, and VII isoforms of 14 blueberry Italian cultivars. *J. Enzyme Inhib. Med. Chem.* **2016**, *31* (Suppl. S4), 1–6. [CrossRef] [PubMed]
29. Izumi, Y.; Yamamoto, N.; Matsushima, S.; Yamamoto, T.; Takada-Takatori, Y.; Akaike, A.; Kume, T. Compensatory role of the Nrf2-ARE pathway against paraquat toxicity: Relevance of 26S proteasome activity. *J. Pharmacol. Sci.* **2015**, *129*, 150–159. [CrossRef] [PubMed]
30. Adedara, I.A.; Fasina, O.B.; Ayeni, M.F.; Ajayi, O.M.; Farombi, E.O. Protocatechuic acid ameliorates neurobehavioral deficits via suppression of oxidative damage, inflammation, caspase-3 and acetylcholinesterase activities in diabetic rats. *Food Chem. Toxicol.* **2019**, *125*, 170–181. [CrossRef] [PubMed]

31. Salminen, A.; Hyttinen, J.M.; Kaarniranta, K. AMP-activated protein kinase inhibits NF-kappaB signaling and inflammation: Impact on healthspan and lifespan. *J. Mol. Med.* **2011**, *89*, 667–676. [CrossRef]
32. Harijith, A.; Ebenezer, D.L.; Natarajan, V. Reactive oxygen species at the crossroads of inflammasome and inflammation. *Front. Physiol.* **2014**, *5*, 352. [CrossRef]
33. Salminen, A.; Kaarniranta, K.; Kauppinen, A. Crosstalk between Oxidative Stress and SIRT1: Impact on the Aging Process. *Int. J. Mol. Sci.* **2013**, *14*, 3834–3859. [CrossRef] [PubMed]
34. Bhattacharjee, N.; Dua, T.K.; Khanra, R. Protocatechuic Acid, a Phenolic from Sansevieria roxburghiana Leaves, Suppresses Diabetic Cardiomyopathy via Stimulating Glucose Metabolism, Ameliorating Oxidative Stress, and Inhibiting Inflammation. *Front. Pharmacol.* **2017**, *8*, 251. [CrossRef] [PubMed]
35. Shariati, H.; Hassanpour, M.; Sharifzadeh, G.; Zarban, A.; Samarghandian, S.; Saeedi, F. Evaluation of diuretic and antioxidant properties in aqueous bark and fruit extracts of pine. *Curr. Drug Discov. Technol.* **2020**. [CrossRef] [PubMed]
36. Elmore, S. Apoptosis: A review of programmed cell death. *Toxicol. Pathol.* **2007**, *35*, 495–516. [CrossRef]
37. Towns, R.; Pietropaolo, M.; Wiley, J.W. Stimulation of autophagy by autoantibody-mediated activation of death receptor cascades. *Autophagy* **2008**, *4*, 715–716. [CrossRef] [PubMed]
38. Giacco, F.; Brownlee, M. Oxidative stress and diabetic complications. *Circ. Res.* **2010**, *107*, 1058–1070. [CrossRef]
39. Fu, J.; Lee, K.; Chuang, P.Y.; Liu, Z.; He, J.C. Glomerular endothelial cell injury and cross talk in diabetic kidney disease. *Am. J. Physiol. Renal Physiol.* **2015**, *308*, F287–F297. [CrossRef]
40. Ma, Y.; Chen, F.; Yang, S.; Chen, B.; Shi, J. Protocatechuic acid ameliorates high glucose-induced extracellular matrix accumulation in diabetic nephropathy. *Biomed. Pharmacother.* **2018**, *98*, 18–22. [CrossRef]
41. Wang, K.; Tang, Z.; Wang, J.; Cao, P.; Li, Q.; Shui, W.; Wang, H.; Zheng, Z.; Zhang, Y. RETRACTED: Polysaccharide from Angelica sinensis ameliorates high-fat diet and STZ-induced hepatic oxidative stress and inflammation in diabetic mice by activating the Sirt1-AMPK pathway. *J. Nutr. Biochem.* **2017**, *43*, 88–97. [CrossRef]
42. Yacoub, R.; Lee, K.; He, J.C. The Role of SIRT1 in Diabetic Kidney Disease. *Front. Endocrinol.* **2014**, *5*, 166. [CrossRef]
43. Wan, X.; Wen, J.J.; Koo, S.J.; Liang, L.Y.; Garg, N.J. SIRT1-PGC1alpha-NFkappaB Pathway of Oxidative and Inflammatory Stress during Trypanosoma cruzi Infection: Benefits of SIRT1-Targeted Therapy in Improving Heart Function in Chagas Disease. *PLoS Pathog.* **2016**, *12*, e1005954. [CrossRef] [PubMed]
44. Han, L.; Yang, Q.; Ma, W.; Li, J.; Qu, L.; Wang, M. Protocatechuic Acid Ameliorated Palmitic-Acid-Induced Oxidative Damage in Endothelial Cells through Activating Endogenous Antioxidant Enzymes via an Adenosine-Monophosphate-Activated-Protein-Kinase-Dependent Pathway. *J. Agric. Food Chem.* **2018**, *66*, 10400–10409. [CrossRef] [PubMed]
45. Guclu, A.; Erdur, F.M.; Turkmen, K. The Emerging Role of Sirtuin 1 in Cellular Metabolism, Diabetes Mellitus, Diabetic Kidney Disease and Hypertension. *Exp. Clin. Endocrinol. Diabetes* **2016**, *124*, 131–139. [CrossRef] [PubMed]
46. Hasegawa, K.; Wakino, S.; Simic, P.; Sakamaki, Y.; Minakuchi, H.; Fujimura, K.; Hosoya, K.; Komatsu, M.; Kaneko, Y.; Kanda, T.; et al. Renal tubular Sirt1 attenuates diabetic albuminuria by epigenetically suppressing Claudin-1 overexpression in podocytes. *Nat. Med.* **2013**, *19*, 1496–1504. [CrossRef]
47. Kong, L.; Wu, H.; Zhou, W.; Luo, M.; Tan, Y.; Miao, L.; Cai, L. Sirtuin 1: A Target for Kidney Diseases. *Mol. Med.* **2015**, *21*, 87–97. [CrossRef]
48. Lee, H.J.; Hong, Y.S.; Yang, S.J. Interaction between NLRP3 Inflammasome and Sirt1/6: Metabolomics Approach. *FASEB J.* **2015**, *29*, 913.12.
49. Li, Y.; Yang, X.; He, Y.; Wang, W.; Zhang, J.; Zhang, W.; Jing, T.; Wang, B.; Lin, R. Negative regulation of NLRP3 inflammasome by SIRT1 in vascular endothelial cells. *Immunobiology* **2017**, *222*, 552–561. [CrossRef]
50. Guo, K.; Lu, J.; Huang, Y.; Wu, M.; Zhang, L.; Yu, H.; Zhang, M.; Bao, Y.; He, J.C.; Chen, H.; et al. Protective role of PGC-1alpha in diabetic nephropathy is associated with the inhibition of ROS through mitochondrial dynamic remodeling. *PLoS ONE* **2015**, *10*, e0125176.

51. Liang, H.; Ward, W.F. PGC-1alpha: A key regulator of energy metabolism. *Adv. Physiol. Educ.* **2006**, *30*, 145–151. [CrossRef]
52. Park, J.E.; Lee, H.; Kim, S.Y.; Lim, Y. *Lespedeza bicolor* Extract Ameliorated Renal Inflammation by Regulation of NLRP3 Inflammasome-Associated Hyperinflammation in Type 2 Diabetic Mice. *Antioxidants* **2020**, *9*, 148. [CrossRef]

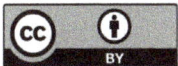

© 2020 by the authors. Licensee MDPI, Basel, Switzerland. This article is an open access article distributed under the terms and conditions of the Creative Commons Attribution (CC BY) license (http://creativecommons.org/licenses/by/4.0/).

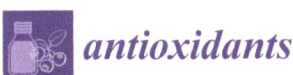

Article

Protective Effects of Myricetin on Benzo[a]pyrene-Induced 8-Hydroxy-2′-Deoxyguanosine and BPDE-DNA Adduct

Seung-Cheol Jee [1], Min Kim [1], Kyeong Seok Kim [2], Hyung-Sik Kim [2] and Jung-Suk Sung [1,*]

[1] Department of Life Science, Dongguk University-Seoul, Biomedi Campus, 32 Dongguk-ro, Ilsandong-gu, Goyang-si, Gyeonggi-do 10326, Korea; markjee@naver.com (S.-C.J.); pipikimmin@naver.com (M.K.)
[2] Department of Division of Toxicology, School of Pharmacy, Sungkyunkwan University-Suwon, Gyeonggi-do 16419, Korea; caion123@nate.com (K.S.K.); hkims@skku.edu (H.-S.K.)
* Correspondence: sungjs@dongguk.edu; Tel.: +82-31-961-5132; Fax: +82-31-961-5108

Received: 30 April 2020; Accepted: 19 May 2020; Published: 21 May 2020

Abstract: Benzo[a]pyrene (B[a]P), a group 1 carcinogen, induces mutagenic DNA adducts. Myricetin is present in many natural foods with diverse biological activities, such as anti-oxidative and anti-cancer activities. The aim of this study was to investigate the protective effects of myricetin against B[a]P-induced toxicity. Treatment of B[a]P induced cytotoxicity on HepG2 cells, whereas co-treatment of myricetin with B[a]P reduced the formation of the B[a]P-7,8-dihydrodiol-9,10-epoxide (BPDE)-DNA adduct, which recovered cell viability. Furthermore, we found a protective effect of myricetin against B[a]P-induced genotoxicity in rats, via myricetin-induced inhibition of 8-hydroxy-2′-deoxyguanosine (8-OHdG) and BPDE-DNA adduct formation in the liver, kidney, colon, and stomach tissue. This inhibition was more prominent in the liver than in other tissues. Correspondingly, myricetin regulated the phase I and II enzymes that inhibit B[a]P metabolism and B[a]P metabolites conjugated with DNA by reducing and inducing CYP1A1 and glutathione S-transferase (GST) expression, respectively. Taken together, this showed that myricetin attenuated B[a]P-induced genotoxicity via regulation of phase I and II enzymes. Our results suggest that myricetin is anti-genotoxic, and prevents oxidative DNA damage and BPDE-DNA adduct formation via regulation of phase I and II enzymes.

Keywords: Benzo[a]pyrene; myricetin; oxidative stress; BPDE-DNA adduct; phase detoxifying enzyme

1. Introduction

Polycyclic aromatic hydrocarbons (PAHs) are ubiquitous environmental chemical carcinogens that lead to genetic damage and possess highly bioaccumulation characteristic [1]. Benzo[a]pyrene (B[a]P) is a well-known PAH (Figure 1A), which is listed as group 1 carcinogens by the International Agency for Research on Cancer (IARC). B[a]P is toxic and its exposure is primarily due to the food chain [2] Previous studies have shown that the average amount of people's exposure to B[a]P is 8.09–9.20 ng/day [3]. This means that humans are exposed to a low dose of B[a]P over a lifetime. The long-term exposure of B[a]P can cause angiogenesis and metastasis in the skin, lungs, liver, colorectal and stomach [4]. Other studies support that long-term exposure of low-dose B[a]P induces cell angiogenesis and metastasis [5], and a low dose of B[a]P toxicity is enhanced by interaction with PM2.5 air pollutants [6]. B[a]P is converted to B[a]P-7,8-diol-9,10-epoxide (BPDE) which is ultimate metabolite of B[a]P (Figure 1B), and it leads to genetic toxicity via covalent binding with DNA [7].

In addition, B[a]P is linked to reactive oxygen species (ROS) formation, which induces genotoxicity via the formation of 8-hydroxy-2-deoxyguanosine (8-oxo-dG) [8].

B[a]P is metabolized by phase I enzymes, such as cytochrome P450 (CYP). Furthermore, CYP1A1 is associated with the B[a]P metabolism process [9]. Previous studies have shown that B[a]P is oxidized by CYP enzymes that induce a variety of B[a]P metabolite transitions that form DNA adducts [10,11]. After formation of DNA adducts, this leads to several diseases and cancers. The xenobiotic chemicals are generally converted into water-soluble metabolites by phase II enzymes in the cells, and are easily removed by phase III enzymes [12]. Uridine 5′-diphospho (UDP)-glucuronosyltransferases (UGTs), sulfotransferases (SULTs), glutathione S-transferases (GSTs), NAD(P)H: quinine oxidoreductase type 1 (NQO1), heme oxygenase-1 (HO-1), and N-acetyltransferase (NAT) are known as major phase II enzymes [13]. GST is a major enzyme of phase II detoxifying enzymes. It is activated when conjugated with BPDE and reduces DNA damage by counteracting B[a]P metabolites via inhibition of BPDE-DNA adduct formation [14,15]. In addition, GSH conjugates with B[a]P-7,8-dione, which attenuates the B[a]P-induced genotoxicity [16]. Following GSH–conjugation with B[a]P metabolites via phase II detoxifying enzymes, it is excreted by transporter genes, such as ABCC1 and ABCC2 [17]. Previous studies have showed that ABCC transporters are required to detoxify B[a]P [18]. The knockdown of ABCC2 increases the concentration of B[a]P metabolites in a variety of organs [19]. ABCC2 is required for the elimination of BPDE-DNA adducts in organs by B[a]P metabolite excretion.

B[a]P is produced during food processes such as broiling, frying, and roasting. These processes increase the concentration of B[a]P, which increases the risk of disease and cancer; therefore, it is important to prevent B[a]P-induced toxicity from the natural synthesis of B[a]P [20]. Natural compounds are widely used to reduce B[a]P-induced toxicity and in cancer therapy [21,22]. Myricetin (Figure 1C), which is found in vegetables, herbs, and fresh fruits, is used as a treatment against different cancers [23]. Previously, studies have showed that myricetin has potentially therapeutic properties, such as anti-oxidant, cytoprotective, and anti-cancer properties [24]. Additionally, another study has shown that myricetin is protective after B[a]P-induced DNA damage by regulating DNA strand breaks [25]. However, cancer-causing DNA mutations occur if the BPDE-DNA adducts and ROS-induced DNA damage are not repaired by base excision repair (BER) and nucleotide excision repair (NER). Therefore, it is important to prevent DNA damage by inhibiting DNA conjugation with B[a]P metabolites. In this study, we investigated the protective effect of myricetin against B[a]P-induced genotoxicity via the inhibition of DNA adduct formation by regulating phase I and II enzymes.

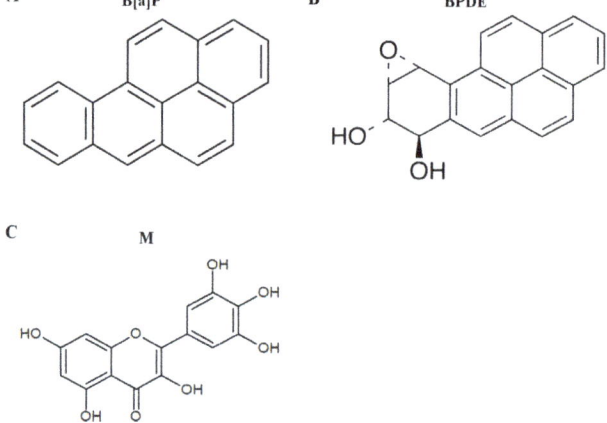

Figure 1. The structure of chemicals. (**A**) Benzo[a]pyrene (B[a]P), (**B**) B[a]P-7,8-dihydrodiol-9,10-epoxide (BPDE), and (**C**) myricetin.

2. Materials and Methods

2.1. Chemicals and Reagents

Benzo[a]pyrene (B[a]P), myricetin, dimethyl sulfoxide (DMSO), ammonium persulfate, nuclease P1, N,N,N'N'-Tetramethyl ethylenediamine (TEMED), protease inhibitor cocktail, phosphatase inhibitor cocktail II, phosphatase inhibitor cocktail III, glycine, sodium dodecyl sulfate (SDS), tris base, sodium chloride, tween 20, and 2-mercaptoethanol were obtained from Sigma-Aldrich Chemical (St. Louis, MO, USA). Sodium pyruvate, penicillin-streptomycin, and trypsin-ethylenediaminetetraacetic acid (EDTA) were obtained from Welgene (Daegu, Korea). Alkaline phosphatase (AP) was purchased from Takara Bio Inc (Shiga, Japan). Phosphate-buffered saline (PBS) was purchased from Biosesang (Seongnam, Korea). A total of 30% acrylamide/bis solution was purchased from Bio-Rad (Hercules, CA, USA). Antibodies, such as CYP1A1, CYP1B1, GST, ABCC2, β-actin, and HRP-conjugated anti-rabbit immunoglobulin G (IgG), were purchased from Santa Cruz Biotechnology (Santa Cruz, CA, USA).

2.2. Cell Culture

Human-derived liver cancer cells (HepG2) were purchased from the American Type Culture Collection (Manassas, VA, USA). HepG2 cells were grown with Eagle's minimum essential medium (MEM, Welgene, Daegu, Korea) containing 10% fetal bovine serum (FBS, Welgene), 100 μg/mL streptomycin, 100 U/mL penicillin, and 1 mM sodium pyruvate in 100 mm^2 cell culture dishes. The old media were replaced with a new medium every two days. The HepG2 cells were incubated at 37 °C in 5% CO_2 under a humidified atmosphere. The cells were used for further research when the confluency reached 80%.

2.3. Animals and Housing

Sprague-Dawley male rats (5-weeks-old; weight, 140–150 g) were purchased from Orient Bio (Seongnam-si, Korea) and were housed at a 23 ± 2 °C of temperature and 55 ± 1% of humidity. The room condition was maintained at specific pathogen free (SPF) with a 12 h light/12 h darkness cycle. Rodent chow and water were supplied ad libitum. The rats were randomly divided into three groups in each group (n = 6): (1) Control group, administration of corn oil (oral); (2) B[a]P-treated group, administration of B[a]P (2 mg/kg; daily, oral) dissolved in corn oil; (3) B[a]P co-treated with myricetin group, administration of myricetin (15 mg/kg) with B[a]P (2 mg/kg; daily, oral) dissolved in corn oil for 55 days. The concentration and period of B[a]P exposure were following other studies. To determine the B[a]P and myricetin concentration, we considered following reasons: (1) people are normally exposed to low-dose of B[a]P. Previous studies showed that people were exposed to 14 and 59.2 μg/kg/day of PAHs [26,27]. The average amount of people's exposure to B[a]P is 8.09–9.20 ng/day [3]. Additionally, previous studies showed that short-term treatment of B[a]P for in vivo used the dose of B[a]P at 25 to 200 mg/kg in rats [28]. Moreover, another study suggested that low-dose of B[a]P concentration was defined under 12 mg/kg/day [29]. On the other hand, the animals were treated with doses of 50, 100, and 200 mg/kg of myricetin to rats for a long time [30]. (2) People are unavoidably exposed to B[a]P through foods and polluted air for a lifetime. Therefore, we consider the results and determine the long-term effects of a low dose of B[a]P and myricetin. Treatments were administered at the same time daily. Behavioral tests were performed in the morning. The animal experiment protocol was approved by Sungkyunkwan University Laboratory Animal Care Service (SKKU-2013-000105, 23 March 2013) in accordance with the Ministry of Food and Drug Safety (MFDS) Animal Protection of Korea (Oh-Song, Korea).

2.4. Cell Viability Assay

To evaluate the cytotoxicity of B[a]P and myricetin on HepG2 cells, a cell viability assay was performed. A density of 1×10^4 cells/well of HepG2 cells were seeded in 96-well plates. A variety of concentrations of B[a]P (0, 1, 2.5, 5, and 10 μM) and myricetin (5, 10, 20, and 40 μM) were incubated in the wells for 48 h at 37 °C. After 48 h incubation, to evaluate the cell viability, 10 μL of EZ-CYTOX reagent (DOGEN, Daejeon, Korea) were treated with 100 μL MEM to each well and incubated for 2 h at 37 °C. Relative absorbance of each well was read at 450 nm to measure the amount of cell viability using a microplate reader (Molecular Devices, San Jose, CA, USA).

2.5. BPDE-DNA Adduct Formation Analysis

DNA extraction was performed using a QIAamp DNA Mini Kit (Qiagen, Valencia, CA, USA), according to the manufacturer's instructions. DNA was isolated and the level of BPDE-DNA adduct formation was assessed using BPDE-DNA adduct ELISA kit (Cell Biolabs, San Diego, CA, USA) and following manufacturer's instructions. Briefly, DNA samples of 2 μg/mL concentration are prepared. An amount of 100 μL of each sample is treated in 96 well plates for 2 h at 37 °C and rinsed two times. After washing, 100 μL of anti-BPDE antibody is treated in each well and incubated for 2 h at room temperature. Each well is rinsed 5 times using washing buffer, and then secondary antibody is added in each well for 1 h at room temperature. Each well is rinsed 3 times using washing buffer. All wells are reacted with 3,3′,5,5′-Tetramethylbenzidine (TMB) buffer at room temperature for 20 min. Finally, the reaction is stopped by adding stop solution. The BPDE-DNA adducts formation level was evaluated by measuring the relative absorbance using a microplate reader at 450 nm.

2.6. Quantification of DNA Damage via 8-Hydroxydeoxyguanosine

We evaluated the concentration of 8-hydroxydeoxyguanosine (8-OHdG) using an 8-OHdG DNA damage ELISA kit (Cell Biolabs, San Diego, CA, USA), according to manufacturer's instructions. Briefly, isolated DNA was denatured at 95 °C for 5 min and immediately transferred to ice. A total of 10 units of nuclease P1 and 20 mM sodium acetate (pH 5.2) were added to total DNA, and digested DNA to nucleosides for 2 h at 37 °C. Next, alkaline phosphatase (Takara, Japan) added for 15 min at 37 °C, followed by incubation for 15 min at 50 °C in 100 mM Tris buffer (pH 7.5). The reaction mixtures were centrifuged for 5 min at $6000 \times g$ and the supernatants were extracted for assay analysis. Briefly, 50 μL of each sample is treated in wells and incubated for 10 min at room temperature. An amount of 50 μL of anti-8-OHdG antibody is treated in each well and incubated for 1 h at room temperature on orbital shaker. Each well is rinsed 3 times, 100 μL secondary antibody is added in each well and incubated for 1 h at room temperature. After incubation, 100 μl of substrate solution buffer is added in each well for 20 min at room temperature and then the reaction is stopped by adding stop solution. The absorbance of 8-OHdG was measured using a microplate reader at 450 nm (VERSA max™, Molecular Devices, San Jose, CA, USA).

2.7. Western Blot Analysis

The protein in the liver was extracted using PRO-PREP™ protein extraction solution (iNtRON, Seongnam, Korea). The protein in cells was extracted in RIPA buffer (150 mM NaCl, 1% Nonidet P-40, 50 mM Tris-HCl, and 0.25% sodium deoxycholate) (Biosolution, Seoul, Korea) containing protease inhibitor cocktail, phosphatase inhibitor cocktail II and III. Each protein concentration was quantified using the Bio-Rad protein assay (Hercules, CA, USA). After protein quantification, it was denatured at 95 °C for 5 min in buffer. Next, samples (50 μg) were ran on 10% SDS-polyacrylamide gel electrophoresis (SDS-PAGE) at 50 V for 60 min in running buffer. The proteins were transferred to polyvinylidene difluoride (PVDF) membranes (BioRad, Hercules, CA, USA) at 100 V for 90 min in a transfer buffer. Membranes blocked with TNT buffer containing 5% skim milk for 1 h, followed by incubation with CYP1A1, CYP1B1, and β-actin antibodies overnight at 4 °C. After washing for 15 min at 4 times with TNT buffer, the membrane was incubated for 45 min with secondary antibodies, and then washed for 15 min at 4 times with TNT buffer. Immunoreactivity was visualized using chemiluminescence (ECL) Plus Western Blotting reagents (Amersham Bioscience, Buckinghamshire, UK). The protein level was quantified using Quantity One Image Software (Bio-Rad, Hercules, CA, USA).

2.8. Statistical Analysis

Experimental data were evaluated in triplicates and experiments were repeated at least three times. All data were expressed as mean ± standard error of the mean (SEM). The One-way analysis of variance (ANOVA) and Tukey's multiple comparison analysis were performed to determine the significant differences between groups using GraphPad Prism 5.0 (GraphPad Software, San Diego, CA, USA). Differences were considered statistically significant when $p < 0.05$.

3. Results

3.1. Protective Effect of Myricetin against B[a]P-Induced Toxicity

HepG2 cells were treated with different concentrations of B[a]P and myricetin to evaluate their toxicity. B[a]P treatment for 48 h induced cytotoxicity in a dose-dependent manner compared with the control group (Figure 2A). The 40% inhibitory concentration of B[a]P was calculated at 10 µM for 48 h and used in subsequent experiments. Treatment of myricetin at 5, 10, 20, and 40 µM for 48 h revealed no toxicity up to 10 µM; however, cytotoxicity was shown for treatments > 20 µM when compared with the control group (Figure 2B). Then, to confirm the protective effect of myricetin on B[a]P cytotoxicity, HepG2 cells were co-treated with or without B[a]P in the presence of myricetin and the amount of the viable cells continuously analyzed compared with non-treated group. We found that myricetin co-treatment with B[a]P recovered up to 85% cell viability (Figure 2C). These results suggest that myricetin has protective effect against B[a]P-induced cytotoxicity. Based on the cell viability data, 10 µM of myricetin was used for all further in vitro experiments.

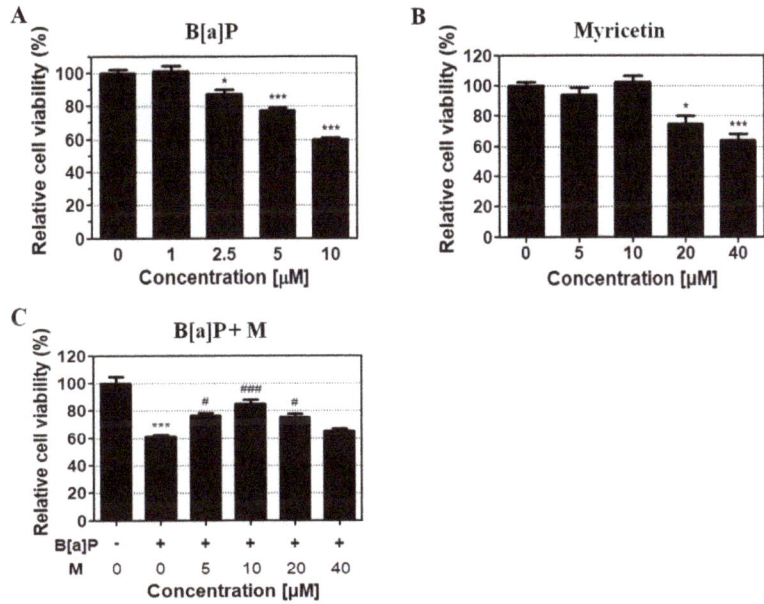

Figure 2. B[a]P and myricetin cytotoxicity in HepG2 cells. (**A,B**) HepG2 cells were treated with B[a]P (0, 1, 2.5, 5, and 10 µM) or myricetin (0, 5, 10, 20, and 40 µM) at different concentrations for 48 h. (**C**) The protective effect of myricetin against B[a]P-induced cytotoxicity was measured with B[a]P (10 µM) co-treatment with various concentrations of myricetin for 48 h. All treatment group values are significantly different when compared with controls (* $p < 0.05$, *** $p < 0.001$) and B[a]P (# $p < 0.05$, ### $p < 0.001$). Tukey's multiple comparison test. M: myricetin.

3.2. Protective Effects of Myricetin against B[a]P-Induced Oxidative DNA Damage

To confirm the B[a]P-induced oxidative DNA damage, we calculated the concentration of 8-OHdG in the liver, kidney, colon, and stomach tissue of rats following treatment with 2 mg/kg of B[a]P and 15 mg/kg of myricetin for 55 days. B[a]P significantly increased the concentration of 8-OHdG in the liver, stomach, colon, and kidney when compared with the control group but B[a]P co-treatment with myricetin significantly reduced the 8-OHdG in the liver, stomach, and kidney respectively (Figure 3A–D). These results confirmed that myricetin protects DNA from further oxidation that contributes to cell death prevention.

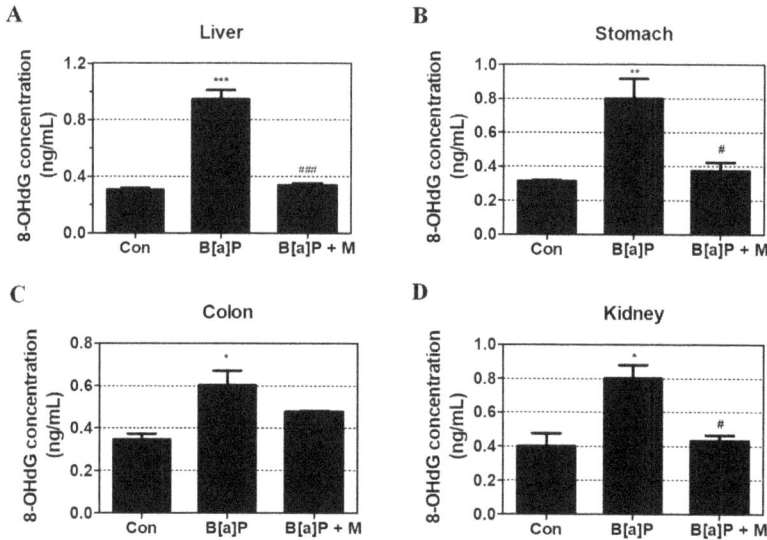

Figure 3. Oxidative DNA damage following B[a]P (2 mg/kg) and myricetin (10 mg/kg) co-treatment. Oxidative DNA damage was measured by the concentration of 8-OHdG in liver, stomach, colon, and kidney tissues. (**A–D**) Myricetin was protective against B[a]P-induced 8-OHdG formation following B[a]P treatment in all tissue when compared with controls (* $p < 0.05$, ** $p < 0.01$, *** $p < 0.001$) and B[a]P (# $p < 0.05$, ### $p < 0.001$). Tukey's multiple comparison test. M: myricetin.

3.3. Inhibition Effect of Myricetin against BPDE-DNA Adduct Formation

To evaluate the protective effect of myricetin against B[a]P-induced genotoxicity, the concentration of BPDE-DNA adducts was measured in HepG2 cells and the liver, stomach, colon, and kidney tissue of rats using BPDE-DNA Adduct ELISA Kit. Treatment with B[a]P, myricetin, and B[a]P + myricetin showed that B[a]P induced BPDE-DNA adduct formation when compared with the non-treatment group. However, B[a]P co-treatment with myricetin clearly decreased BPDE-DNA adduct formation when compared with B[a]P treatment alone (Figure 4A). Furthermore, B[a]P induced BPDE-DNA adduct formation in the liver, kidney, colon, and stomach of treated rats when compared with the control group. B[a]P co-treatment with myricetin inhibited the BPDE-DNA adduct formation in all rat tissue (Figure 4B–E). These results showed that the genotoxicity of B[a]P was attenuated by myricetin via inhibition of the formation of BPDE-DNA adduct.

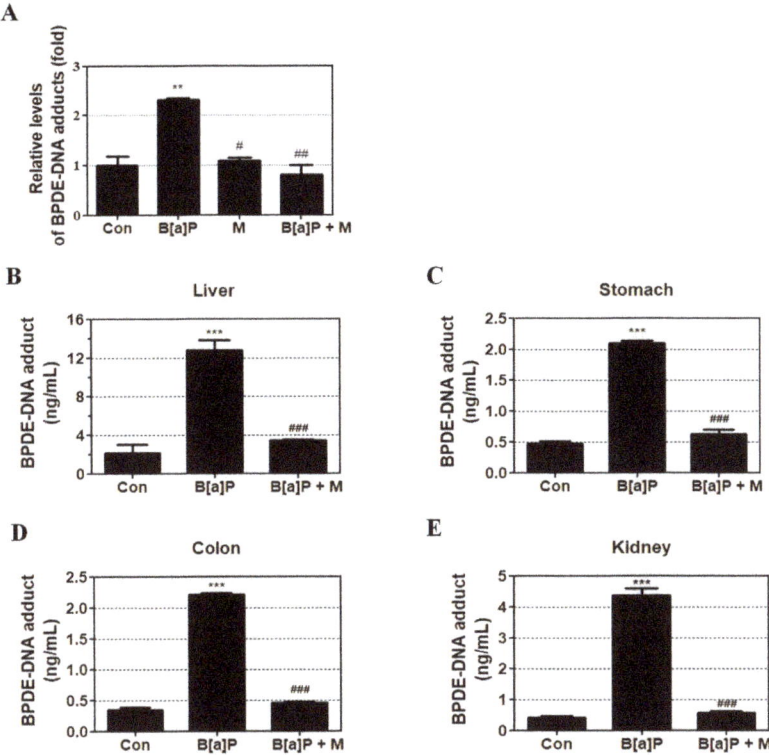

Figure 4. BPDE-DNA adduct concentration in B[a]P and B[a]P + myricetin treated groups. (**A**) Effect of myricetin on BPDE-DNA adduct formation in HepG2 cells following treatment with B[a]P (10 μM) and co-treatment with myricetin (10 μM) for 48 h. (**B–E**) In Sprague-Dawley rats, treatment with B[a]P (2 mg/kg) and co-treatment with myricetin (15 mg/kg) for 55 days. All treatment groups are significantly different when compared with controls (** $p < 0.01$, *** $p < 0.001$) and B[a]P (# $p < 0.05$, ## $p < 0.01$, ### $p < 0.001$). Tukey's multiple comparison test. M: myricetin.

3.4. Regulatory Effect of Myricetin on the Expression of Phase I, II, and III Enzyme

Our results showed that B[a]P induced CYP1A1 and CYP1B1 expression. In contrast, B[a]P + myricetin co-treatment down-regulated CYP1A1, but not CYP1B1, expression in the liver of rats (Figure 5A,B). We confirmed that myricetin co-treatment with B[a]P reduced CYP1A1 expression when compared with B[a]P treatment group (Figure 5C,D). This indicated that myricetin regulated CYP1A1 expression, thereby reducing B[a]P metabolism, which prevented DNA adduct formation.

Next, we measured GST expression in HepG2 cells following B[a]P and B[a]P + myricetin treatment. B[a]P reduced GST expression; however, co-treatment with myricetin recovered this expression when compared with B[a]P treatment alone (Figure 5C,D). In contrast, ABCC2 was not regulated by myricetin. This indicated that myricetin attenuated B[a]P-induced toxicity via reduction of oxidative DNA damage and inhibition of BPDE-DNA adduct formation by inducing GSH conjugated with B[a]P metabolites to recover the GST expression.

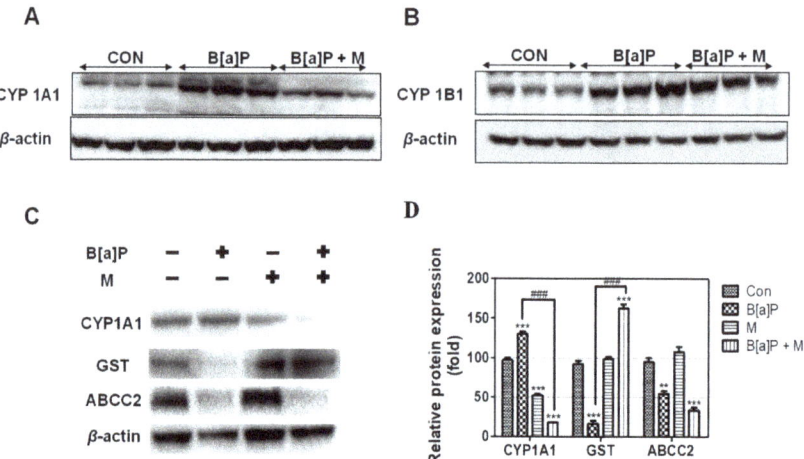

Figure 5. The expression of phase detoxifying enzymes. (**A,B**) The effect of myricetin (15 mg/kg) and B[a]P (2 mg/kg) treatment on CYP1A1 and CYP1B1 enzyme expression in the liver of Sprague-Dawley rats. (**C**) The effect of myricetin (10 μM) and B[a]P (10 μM) treatment on CYP1A1, GST, and ABCC2 enzyme expression in HepG2 cells. (**D**) Quantitative evaluation of relative protein expression of CYP1A1, GST, and ABCC2. All treatment groups are significantly different when compared with controls (** $p < 0.01$, *** $p < 0.001$) and B[a]P (### $p < 0.001$). Tukey's multiple comparison test. M: myricetin.

4. Discussion

B[a]P is carcinogenic, and is formed during food-processing, and in tobacco smoke, waste products, and industry [31,32]. B[a]P is well-known as an ubiquitous environmental agent. Previous studies showed that people were exposed to 8.09–9.20 ng/day of B[a]P [3]. This report indicates that people are exposed to a low dose of B[a]P over their lifetime. Generally, B[a]P accumulated in humans through food; 97% of B[a]P exposure amount is associated with the food chain [2]. This indicates that the exposure of B[a]P is mainly mediated in the gastrointestinal tract such as stomach and colon. Absorbed B[a]P through the gastrointestinal tract passes through the blood vessel to the liver and undergoes the detoxification process. Then, detoxified metabolites are excreted via the urine or bile. Thus, in this study, the liver, kidney, and gastrointestinal tract (stomach and colon) were considered as target organs. After exposure to B[a]P, it is metabolized to BPDE or B[a]P radical cations, which are conjugated with DNA. Previous studies have shown that B[a]P induces genotoxicity by forming BPDE-DNA adducts or 8-OHdG [33]. Additionally, another study shows that the long-term treatment of low-dose B[a]P induces the cancer progression [5]. This means that B[a]P negatively affects the people's health causing dysfunction of hormone, cancers, and autoimmune disease [34]. Previous study shows that inhibition of DNA adduct formation reduces B[a]P mutagenesis and carcinogenesis [35]. Many studies have assessed the effect of flavonoids in reducing the B[a]P-induced toxicity [36–38].

Myricetin, which is present in many foods such as tea, vegetables, and medical plants, is a natural flavonoid that has anti-carcinogenic, -oxidant, and -inflammation effects [39,40]. Generally, the protective effects of myricetin against oxidative stress have been well-studied for a long time. Previous studies have shown that the anti-oxidant effect of myricetin is mediated by its ROS scavenging activity and activation of cellular anti-oxidative mechanisms including nuclear factor erythroid 2-related factor 2 (Nrf2)-linked pathway [41–43]. Myricetin is protective against B[a]P-induced DNA damage via oxidized pyrimidine. In contrast, oxidized purines are not reduced by myricetin [25]. This means that myricetin does not repair after receiving purine-based damage by B[a]P. Therefore, the inhibition of 8-OHdG and BPDE-DNA adducts is important for the attenuation of B[a]P-induced

DNA damage. In this study, we provide new insights into the protective effects of myricetin against B[a]P-induced toxicity.

We confirmed that myricetin recovered cell viability in HepG2 cells, indicating that myricetin could attenuate B[a]P-induced cytotoxicity (Figure 2C). Previous studies have shown that the formation of DNA adducts induces B[a]P genotoxicity via oxidative stress and BPDE. B[a]P is transited to B[a]P-7,8-dione, which enhances ROS production by inducing futile redox cycles [44]. The formation of 8-OHdG is an oxidative DNA damage marker [45]. In addition, B[a]P is sequentially transited to B[a]P-7,8-epoxide, B[a]P-7,8-dihydrodiol, and BPDE, which is a metabolite of B[a]P that causes genotoxicity via the formation of BPDE-DNA adducts [35]. On the other hand, the amount of oxidative DNA damage and the level of BPDE formation are different depending on the types of cell lines and organs [46]. Thus, to evaluate the effect of myricetin on B[a]P-induced toxicity, we analyzed 8-OHdG and BPDE-DNA adducts using HepG2 cells and various organs such as the liver, kidney and gastrointestinal tract (stomach and colon). Our results confirmed that B[a]P induced 8-OHdG and BPDE-DNA adduct formation, respectively. In contrast, co-treatment with myricetin and B[a]P reduced 8-OHdG and BPDE-DNA adduct formation in all organ tissues (Figures 3 and 4). The results indicate that reduction of B[a]P-induced cytotoxicity is induced by myricetin through reducing B[a]P metabolites-DNA adducts formation. To examine whether the side-effects affect the animals by treatment with B[a]P or myricetin, we evaluated the effect of B[a]P and myricetin on body and organ weights. We confirmed that the weights of organs including the liver, stomach, colon, and kidney were not changed in all treatment groups (supplementary information, Figure S1B–E). Moreover, the bodyweight of animals was not significantly different between the treated groups and untreated control groups (supplementary information, Figure S1A). These results indicated that there were no significant side-effects during long-term exposure to B[a]P and myricetin. Therefore, our results show that myricetin attenuates B[a]P-induced genotoxicity mainly by inhibiting oxidative DNA damage and BPDE-DNA adduct formation.

B[a]P-mediated genotoxicity is caused by the interaction of B[a]P metabolites with DNA. Our results show that myricetin reduces B[a]P-induced genotoxicity by reducing the formation of B[a]P metabolites-DNA adduct. We hypothesize that myricetin inhibits the opportunity of B[a]P metabolites conjugated with DNA. Attenuation of B[a]P-DNA adduct formation was considered to be mediated by two factors: (1) reduction in conversion of B[a]P to B[a]P metabolites, and (2) elimination of B[a]P metabolites. Previous studies have showed that the conversion of B[a]P to BPDE requires multi-enzymatic steps [47]. B[a]P is metabolized by CYP 450; its metabolites cause 8-OHdG and BPDE-DNA adduct formation. A report shows that B[a]P metabolism is regulated by CYP1A1 and CYP1B1, which are associated with B[a]P-mediated carcinogenesis [48]. CYP 450 enzymes induce B[a]P conversion to its metabolites, which conjugate with DNA to form carcinogenic DNA adducts [49]. However, our results showed that CYP1A1, but not CYP1B1, expression was decreased by myricetin treatment when compared with B[a]P alone (Figure 5A,B). A previous study has reported that the regulation of BPDE-DNA adduct formation is correlated with CYP1A1 [50]. Furthermore, the attenuation of cellular DNA damage in HepG2 cells is associated with a reduction in oxidative stress via suppression of CYP1A1 [51]. Indeed, CYP1A1 is the most efficient enzyme forming intermediate metabolite of B[a]P-derived DNA adducts in the liver [52]. Taken together with our data, this indicates that myricetin-induced attenuation of B[a]P genotoxicity is caused by reducing the intermediate metabolites of B[a]P-derived DNA adducts via regulation of CYP1A1 expression.

GST is a phase II enzyme that is conjugated with xenobiotics, including B[a]P, which is a well-known detoxification system in the body [53]. One previous study has shown that GST contributes to a reduction in BPDE-DNA adduct formation and 8-OHdG by inducing GSH-conjugation with B[a]P metabolites [54]. Our results showed that B[a]P reduced GST expression, whereas myricetin recovered this effect (Figure 5C,D). These results suggested that myricetin attenuates B[a]P-induced DNA damage by inhibiting 8-OHdG and BPDE-DNA adduct formation via GST expression induction. In contrast, phase III enzymes are not significantly regulated by myricetin (Figure 5C,D). We hypothesize that myricetin regulates other transporter genes or does not affect phase III enzymes. Previous studies have shown that myricetin induces anticancer drug efficiency by modulating drug efflux via transporter gene regulation [55,56]. In addition, many transporter genes have been shown to localize to the basolateral or canalicular membrane, which is associated with the excretion of drugs through the bile or blood [57]. Previous studies have revealed that GSH interacting with BPDE enhances the BPDE solubility in water, which is eliminated by ABCCs [58]. Therefore, further studies are required to assess the excretion mechanism of B[a]P metabolites that are conjugated with phase II enzymes by myricetin. Taken together, myricetin attenuates B[a]P-induced 8-OHdG and BPDE-DNA adduct formation by regulating CYP1A1 and GST expression.

5. Conclusions

This study shows that myricetin reduces B[a]P-induced toxicity by inhibiting BPDE-DNA adduct and 8-OHdG formation. The inhibition of B[a]P-induced genotoxicity is associated with two factors: (1) a reduction of the B[a]P metabolism via reduced CYP1A1 expression, and (2) the elimination of B[a]P metabolites via enhanced GST expression. These results indicate that myricetin inhibits both B[a]P conversion to B[a]P metabolites and B[a]P metabolites conjugated with DNA, thereby inhibiting the formation of 8-OHdG and BPDE-DNA adducts. Our study suggests that myricetin is protective against B[a]P-induced genotoxicity by inhibiting oxidative DNA damage and BPDE-DNA adduct formation.

Supplementary Materials: The following are available online at http://www.mdpi.com/2076-3921/9/5/446/s1, Figure S1: Effect of B[a]P and myricetin on body and organ weights. B[a]P (2 mg/kg) alone or together with myricetin (15 mg/kg) was administered to Sprague-Dawley rats orally for 55 days. (**A**) Body weight changes of the rats during 55 days. (**B–E**) Organ weights of the rats after 55 days. M: myricetin.

Author Contributions: S.-C.J. designed the study, performed the experiments, analyzed the data, and wrote the manuscript. M.K. performed the experiments and analyzed the data. K.S.K. performed the experiments and analyzed the data. H.-S.K. contributed to the writing of the manuscript. J.-S.S. designed the study and contributed to the writing of the manuscript. All authors have read and agreed to the published version of the manuscript.

Funding: This research was supported by a grant (14162MFDS072) from the Ministry of Food and Drug Safety (MFDS, Korea, 2017) and the Dongguk University Research Fund of 2019.

Conflicts of Interest: The authors declare no conflict of interest.

References

1. Fasulo, S.; Marino, S.; Mauceri, A.; Maisano, M.; Giannetto, A.; D'Agata, A.; Parrino, V.; Minutoli, R.; De Domenico, E. A multibiomarker approach in Coris julis living in a natural environment. *Ecotoxicol. Environ. Saf.* **2010**, *73*, 1565–1573. [CrossRef] [PubMed]
2. Hattemer-Frey, H.A.; Travis, C.C. Benzo-a-pyrene: Environmental partitioning and human exposure. *Toxicol. Ind. Health* **1991**, *7*, 141–157. [CrossRef] [PubMed]
3. Alomirah, H.; Al-Zenki, S.; Al-Hooti, S.; Zaghloul, S.; Sawaya, W.; Ahmed, N.; Kannan, K. Concentrations and dietary exposure to polycyclic aromatic hydrocarbons (PAHs) from grilled and smoked foods. *Food Control* **2011**, *22*, 2028–2035. [CrossRef]
4. Sinha, R.; Kulldorff, M.; Gunter, M.J.; Strickland, P.; Rothman, N. Dietary benzo[a]pyrene intake and risk of colorectal adenoma. *Cancer Epidem. Biomar.* **2005**, *14*, 2030–2034. [CrossRef]
5. Ba, Q.; Li, J.; Huang, C.; Qiu, H.; Li, J.; Chu, R.; Zhang, W.; Xie, D.; Wu, Y.; Wang, H. Effects of benzo[a]pyrene exposure on human hepatocellular carcinoma cell angiogenesis, metastasis, and NF-kappaB signaling. *Environ. Health Perspect.* **2015**, *123*, 246–254. [CrossRef] [PubMed]
6. Wu, J.; Zhang, J.; Nie, J.H.; Duan, J.C.; Shi, Y.F.; Feng, L.; Yang, X.Z.; An, Y.; Sun, Z.W. The chronic effect of amorphous silica nanoparticles and benzo [a] pyrene co-exposure at low dose in human bronchial epithelial BEAS-2B cells. *Toxicol. Res. UK* **2019**, *8*, 731–740. [CrossRef] [PubMed]
7. Gelboin, H.V. Benzo [alpha] pyrene metabolism, activation and carcinogenesis: Role and regulation of mixed-function oxidases and related enzymes. *Physiol. Rev.* **1980**, *60*, 1107–1166. [CrossRef]
8. Lobo, V.; Patil, A.; Phatak, A.; Chandra, N. Free radicals, antioxidants and functional foods: Impact on human health. *Pharmacogn. Rev.* **2010**, *4*, 118–126. [CrossRef]

9. Hodek, P.; Koblihova, J.; Kizek, R.; Frei, E.; Arlt, V.M.; Stiborova, M. The relationship between DNA adduct formation by benzo [a] pyrene and expression of its activation enzyme cytochrome P450 1A1 in rat. *Environ. Toxicol. Pharmacol.* **2013**, *36*, 989–996. [CrossRef]
10. Phillips, D.H.; Venitt, S. DNA and protein adducts in human tissues resulting from exposure to tobacco smoke. *Int. J. Cancer* **2012**, *131*, 2733–2753. [CrossRef]
11. Fang, A.H.; Smith, W.A.; Vouros, P.; Gupta, R.C. Identification and characterization of a novel benzo [a] pyrene-derived DNA adduct. *Biochem. Biophys. Res. Commun.* **2001**, *281*, 383–389. [CrossRef] [PubMed]
12. Rose, R.; Hodgson, E. Metabolism of Toxicants. In *A Textbook of Modern Toxicology*; John Wiley & Sons: Hoboken, NJ, USA, 2004. [CrossRef]
13. Zhang, Y. Phase II Enzymes. In *Encyclopedia of Cancer*; Schwab, M., Ed.; Springer: Berlin/Heidelberg, Germany, 2011. [CrossRef]
14. Perumal Vijayaraman, K.; Muruganantham, S.; Subramanian, M.; Shunmugiah, K.P.; Kasi, P.D. Silymarin attenuates benzo(a)pyrene induced toxicity by mitigating ROS production, DNA damage and calcium mediated apoptosis in peripheral blood mononuclear cells (PBMC). *Ecotoxicol. Environ. Saf.* **2012**, *86*, 79–85. [CrossRef] [PubMed]
15. Zhang, L.; Jin, Y.; Chen, M.; Huang, M.; Harvey, R.G.; Blair, I.A.; Penning, T.M. Detoxication of structurally diverse polycyclic aromatic hydrocarbon (PAH) o-quinones by human recombinant catechol-O-methyltransferase (COMT) via O-methylation of PAH catechols. *J. Biol. Chem.* **2011**, *286*, 25644–25654. [CrossRef] [PubMed]
16. Park, J.H.; Mangal, D.; Frey, A.J.; Harvey, R.G.; Blair, I.A.; Penning, T.M. Aryl hydrocarbon receptor facilitates DNA strand breaks and 8-oxo-2′-deoxyguanosine formation by the aldo-keto reductase product benzo [a] pyrene-7,8-dione. *J. Biol. Chem.* **2009**, *284*, 29725–29734. [CrossRef]
17. Hessel, S.; John, A.; Seidel, A.; Lampen, A. Multidrug resistance-associated proteins are involved in the transport of the glutathione conjugates of the ultimate carcinogen of benzo [a] pyrene in human Caco-2 cells. *Arch. Toxicol.* **2013**, *87*, 269–280. [CrossRef]
18. Guo, B.; Xu, Z.; Yan, X.; Buttino, I.; Li, J.; Zhou, C.; Qi, P. Novel ABCB1 and ABCC Transporters Are Involved in the Detoxification of Benzo (α) pyrene in Thick Shell Mussel, Mytilus coruscus. *Front. Mar. Sci.* **2020**, *7*. [CrossRef]
19. Kranz, J.; Hessel, S.; Aretz, J.; Seidel, A.; Petzinger, E.; Geyer, J.; Lampen, A. The role of the efflux carriers Abcg2 and Abcc2 for the hepatobiliary elimination of benzo [a] pyrene and its metabolites in mice. *Chem. Biol. Interact.* **2014**, *224*, 36–41. [CrossRef]
20. Dutta, K.; Ghosh, D.; Nazmi, A.; Kumawat, K.L.; Basu, A. A common carcinogen benzo[a]pyrene causes neuronal death in mouse via microglial activation. *PLoS ONE* **2010**, *5*, e9984. [CrossRef]
21. Sak, K. Cytotoxicity of dietary flavonoids on different human cancer types. *Pharmacogn. Rev.* **2014**, *8*, 122–146. [CrossRef]
22. Adeneye, A.A. Hypoglycemic and hypolipidemic effects of methanol seed extract of Citrus paradisi Macfad (Rutaceae) in alloxan-induced diabetic Wistar rats. *Nig. Q. J. Hosp. Med.* **2008**, *18*, 211–215. [CrossRef]
23. Feng, J.; Chen, X.; Wang, Y.; Du, Y.; Sun, Q.; Zang, W.; Zhao, G. Myricetin inhibits proliferation and induces apoptosis and cell cycle arrest in gastric cancer cells. *Mol. Cell Biochem.* **2015**, *408*, 163–170. [CrossRef] [PubMed]
24. Devi, K.P.; Rajavel, T.; Habtemariam, S.; Nabavi, S.F.; Nabavi, S.M. Molecular mechanisms underlying anticancer effects of myricetin. *Life Sci.* **2015**, *142*, 19–25. [CrossRef] [PubMed]
25. Delgado, M.E.; Haza, A.I.; Arranz, N.; Garcia, A.; Morales, P. Dietary polyphenols protect against N-nitrosamines and benzo (a) pyrene-induced DNA damage (strand breaks and oxidized purines/pyrimidines) in HepG2 human hepatoma cells. *Eur. J. Nutr.* **2008**, *47*, 479–490. [CrossRef] [PubMed]
26. Cai, Y.; Lv, J.; Zhang, W.; Zhang, L. Dietary exposure estimates of 16 polycyclic aromatic hydrocarbons (PAHs) in Xuanwei and Fuyuan, counties in a high lung cancer incidence area in China. *J. Environ. Monit.* **2012**, *14*, 886–892. [CrossRef]
27. Martorell, I.; Nieto, A.; Nadal, M.; Perelló, G.; Marcé, R.M.; Domingo, J.L. Human exposure to polycyclic aromatic hydrocarbons (PAHs) using data from a duplicate diet study in Catalonia, Spain. *Food Chem. Toxicol.* **2012**, *50*, 4103–4108. [CrossRef]
28. Saunders, C.R.; Shockley, D.C.; Knuckles, M.E. Behavioral effects induced by acute exposure to benzo (a) pyrene in F-344 rats. *Neurotox. Res.* **2001**, *3*, 557–579. [CrossRef]

29. Shi, Z.; Dragin, N.; Miller, M.L.; Stringer, K.F.; Johansson, E.; Chen, J.; Uno, S.; Gonzalez, F.J.; Rubio, C.A.; Nebert, D.W. Oral benzo [a] pyrene-induced cancer: Two distinct types in different target organs depend on the mouse Cyp1 genotype. *Int. J. Cancer* **2010**, *127*, 2334–2350. [CrossRef]
30. Jayakumar, J.K.; Nirmala, P.; Praveen Kumar, B.A.; Kumar, A.P. Evaluation of protective effect of myricetin, a bioflavonoid in dimethyl benzanthracene-induced breast cancer in female Wistar rats. *South Asian J. Cancer* **2014**, *3*, 107–111. [CrossRef]
31. Dimitriou, K.; Kassomenos, P. The influence of specific atmospheric circulation types on PM10-bound benzo (a) pyrene inhalation related lung cancer risk in Barcelona, Spain. *Environ. Int.* **2018**, *112*, 107–114. [CrossRef]
32. Ali, N.; Ismail, I.M.I.; Khoder, M.; Shamy, M.; Alghamdi, M.; Al Khalaf, A.; Costa, M. Polycyclic aromatic hydrocarbons (PAHs) in the settled dust of automobile workshops, health and carcinogenic risk evaluation. *Sci. Total Environ.* **2017**, *601–602*, 478–484. [CrossRef]
33. Roh, T.; Kwak, M.Y.; Kwak, E.H.; Kim, D.H.; Han, E.Y.; Bae, J.Y.; Bang du, Y.; Lim, D.S.; Ahn, I.Y.; Jang, D.E.; et al. Chemopreventive mechanisms of methionine on inhibition of benzo (a) pyrene-DNA adducts formation in human hepatocellular carcinoma HepG2 cells. *Toxicol. Lett.* **2012**, *208*, 232–238. [CrossRef] [PubMed]
34. Juhasz, A.L.; Naidu, R. Bioremediation of high molecular weight polycyclic aromatic hydrocarbons: A review of the microbial degradation of benzo [a] pyrene. *Int. Biodeterior. Biodegrad.* **2000**, *45*, 57–88. [CrossRef]
35. Baird, W.M.; Hooven, L.A.; Mahadevan, B. Carcinogenic polycyclic aromatic hydrocarbon-DNA adducts and mechanism of action. *Environ. Mol. Mutagen.* **2005**, *45*, 106–114. [CrossRef] [PubMed]
36. Liu, Y.; Wu, Y.M.; Zhang, P.Y. Protective effects of curcumin and quercetin during benzo (a) pyrene induced lung carcinogenesis in mice. *Eur. Rev. Med. Pharmacol. Sci.* **2015**, *19*, 1736–1743.
37. Shahid, A.; Ali, R.; Ali, N.; Hasan, S.K.; Bernwal, P.; Afzal, S.M.; Vafa, A.; Sultana, S. Modulatory effects of catechin hydrate against genotoxicity, oxidative stress, inflammation and apoptosis induced by benzo (a) pyrene in mice. *Food Chem. Toxicol.* **2016**, *92*, 64–74. [CrossRef]
38. Jee, S.C.; Kim, M.; Sung, J.S. Modulatory Effects of Silymarin on Benzo [a] pyrene-Induced Hepatotoxicity. *Int. J. Mol. Sci.* **2020**, *21*. [CrossRef]
39. Sun, F.; Zheng, X.Y.; Ye, J.; Wu, T.T.; Wang, J.; Chen, W. Potential anticancer activity of myricetin in human T24 bladder cancer cells both in vitro and in vivo. *Nutr. Cancer* **2012**, *64*, 599–606. [CrossRef]
40. Bertin, R.; Chen, Z.; Marin, R.; Donati, M.; Feltrinelli, A.; Montopoli, M.; Zambon, S.; Manzato, E.; Froldi, G. Activity of myricetin and other plant-derived polyhydroxyl compounds in human LDL and human vascular endothelial cells against oxidative stress. *Biomed. Pharmacother.* **2016**, *82*, 472–478. [CrossRef]
41. Su, H.M.; Feng, L.N.; Zheng, X.D.; Chen, W. Myricetin protects against diet-induced obesity and ameliorates oxidative stress in C57BL/6 mice. *J. Zhejiang Univ. Sci. B* **2016**, *17*, 437–446. [CrossRef]
42. Pandey, K.B.; Mishra, N.; Rizvi, S.I. Protective role of myricetin on markers of oxidative stress in human erythrocytes subjected to oxidative stress. *Nat. Prod. Commun.* **2009**, *4*, 221–226. [CrossRef]
43. Rehman, M.U.; Rather, I.A. Myricetin Abrogates Cisplatin-Induced Oxidative Stress, Inflammatory Response, and Goblet Cell Disintegration in Colon of Wistar Rats. *Plants* **2019**, *9*. [CrossRef] [PubMed]
44. Penning, T.M.; Burczynski, M.E.; Hung, C.F.; McCoull, K.D.; Palackal, N.T.; Tsuruda, L.S. Dihydrodiol dehydrogenases and polycyclic aromatic hydrocarbon activation: Generation of reactive and redox active o-quinones. *Chem. Res. Toxicol.* **1999**, *12*, 1–18. [CrossRef] [PubMed]
45. Kasai, H.; Nishimura, S.; Kurokawa, Y.; Hayashi, Y. Oral administration of the renal carcinogen, potassium bromate, specifically produces 8-hydroxydeoxyguanosine in rat target organ DNA. *Carcinogenesis* **1987**, *8*, 1959–1961. [CrossRef]
46. Genies, C.; Maitre, A.; Lefebvre, E.; Jullien, A.; Chopard-Lallier, M.; Douki, T. The extreme variety of genotoxic response to benzo[a]pyrene in three different human cell lines from three different organs. *PLoS ONE* **2013**, *8*, e0078256. [CrossRef] [PubMed]
47. Souza, T.; Jennen, D.; van Delft, J.; van Herwijnen, M.; Kyrtoupolos, S.; Kleinjans, J. New insights into BaP-induced toxicity: Role of major metabolites in transcriptomics and contribution to hepatocarcinogenesis. *Arch. Toxicol.* **2016**, *90*, 1449–1458. [CrossRef]
48. Uppstad, H.; Ovrebo, S.; Haugen, A.; Mollerup, S. Importance of CYP1A1 and CYP1B1 in bioactivation of benzo [a] pyrene in human lung cell lines. *Toxicol. Lett.* **2010**, *192*, 221–228. [CrossRef]
49. Briede, J.J.; Godschalk, R.W.; Emans, M.T.; De Kok, T.M.; Van Agen, E.; Van Maanen, J.; Van Schooten, F.J.; Kleinjans, J.C. In vitro and in vivo studies on oxygen free radical and DNA adduct formation in rat lung and liver during benzo[a]pyrene metabolism. *Free Radic. Res.* **2004**, *38*, 995–1002. [CrossRef]

50. Divi, R.L.; Lindeman, T.L.; Shockley, M.E.; Keshava, C.; Weston, A.; Poirier, M.C. Correlation between CYP1A1 transcript, protein level, enzyme activity and DNA adduct formation in normal human mammary epithelial cell strains exposed to benzo [a] pyrene. *Mutagenesis* **2014**, *29*, 409–417. [CrossRef]
51. Feng, Q.; Torii, Y.; Uchida, K.; Nakamura, Y.; Hara, Y.; Osawa, T. Black tea polyphenols, theaflavins, prevent cellular DNA damage by inhibiting oxidative stress and suppressing cytochrome P450 1A1 in cell cultures. *J. Agric. Food Chem.* **2002**, *50*, 213–220. [CrossRef]
52. Sulc, M.; Indra, R.; Moserova, M.; Schmeiser, H.H.; Frei, E.; Arlt, V.M.; Stiborova, M. The impact of individual cytochrome P450 enzymes on oxidative metabolism of benzo [a] pyrene in human livers. *Environ. Mol. Mutagen.* **2016**, *57*, 229–235. [CrossRef]
53. Frova, C. Glutathione transferases in the genomics era: New insights and perspectives. *Biomol. Eng.* **2006**, *23*, 149–169. [CrossRef]
54. Cai, Y.; Pan, L.; Miao, J. In vitro study of the effect of metabolism enzymes on benzo (a) pyrene-induced DNA damage in the scallop Chlamys farreri. *Environ. Toxicol. Pharmacol.* **2016**, *42*, 92–98. [CrossRef] [PubMed]
55. van Zanden, J.J.; de Mul, A.; Wortelboer, H.M.; Usta, M.; van Bladeren, P.J.; Rietjens, I.M.; Cnubben, N.H. Reversal of in vitro cellular MRP1 and MRP2 mediated vincristine resistance by the flavonoid myricetin. *Biochem. Pharmacol.* **2005**, *69*, 1657–1665. [CrossRef] [PubMed]
56. Lee, W.; Woo, E.R.; Choi, J.S. Effects of myricetin on the bioavailability of carvedilol in rats. *Pharm. Biol.* **2012**, *50*, 516–522. [CrossRef] [PubMed]
57. Pfeifer, N.D.; Hardwick, R.N.; Brouwer, K.L.R. Role of Hepatic Efflux Transporters in Regulating Systemic and Hepatocyte Exposure to Xenobiotics. *Annu. Rev. Pharmacol. Toxicol.* **2014**, *54*, 509–535. [CrossRef]
58. Zhu, S.Q.; Li, L.; Thornton, C.; Carvalho, P.; Avery, B.A.; Willett, K.L. Simultaneous determination of benzo [a] pyrene and eight of its metabolites in Fundulus heteroclitus bile using ultra-performance liquid chromatography with mass spectrometry. *J. Chromatogr. B* **2008**, *863*, 141–149. [CrossRef]

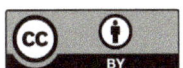

© 2020 by the authors. Licensee MDPI, Basel, Switzerland. This article is an open access article distributed under the terms and conditions of the Creative Commons Attribution (CC BY) license (http://creativecommons.org/licenses/by/4.0/).

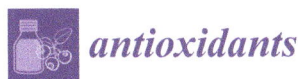

Article

Nitric Oxide Modulation by Folic Acid Fortification

Junsei Taira [1,*] and Takayuki Ogi [2]

1. Department Bioresources Engendering, Okinawa College, National Institute of Technology, 905 Henoko, Nago, Okinawa 905-2192, Japan
2. Okinawa Industrial Technology Center, 12-2 Suzaki, Uruma, Okinawa 904-2234, Japan; ogitkyuk@pref.okinawa.lg.jp
* Correspondence: taira@okinawa-ct.ac.jp; Tel.: +81-980-55-4207

Received: 26 March 2020; Accepted: 4 May 2020; Published: 7 May 2020

Abstract: Folic acid (FA) can be protected the neural tube defects (NTDs) causing nitric oxide (NO) induction, but the alleviation mechanism of the detailed FA function against NO has not yet been clarified. This study focused on elucidation of the interaction of FA and NO. FA suppressed nitrite accumulation as the NO indicator in lipopolysaccharide (LPS)-stimulated RAW264.7 cells, then the expression of the *i*NOS gene due to the LPS treatment was not inhibited by FA, suggesting that FA can modulate against NO or nitrogen radicals. NOR3 (4-ethyl-2-hydroxyamino-5-nitro-3-hexenamide) as the NO donor was used for evaluation of the NO scavenging activity of FA. FA suppressed the nitrite accumulation in a dose-dependent manner. To confirm the reaction product of FA and NO (FA-NO), liquid chromatography–mass spectrometry (LC/MS) was used to measure a similar system containing NOR3 and FA, and then detected the mass numbers of the FA-NO as m/z 470.9 $(M + H)^+$ and m/z 469.1 $(M - H)^-$. In addition, the adducts of the FA-NO derived from ^{14}NO and ^{15}NO gave individual mass numbers of the isotopic ratio of nitrogen for the following products: FA-^{14}NO, m/z 471.14 $(M + H)^+$; m/z 469.17 $(M - H)^-$ and FA-^{15}NO, m/z 472.16 $(M + H)^+$; m/z 470.12 $(M - H)^-$. To clarify the detailed NO scavenging action of FA, an electron spin resonance (ESR) study for radical detecting of the system containing carboxy-PTIO (2-(4-carboxyphenyl)-4,4,5,5-tetramethylimidazoline-1-oxyl-3-oxide) as an NO detection reagent in the presence of NOR3 and FA was performed. The carboxy-PTI (2-carboxyphenyl-4,4,5,5-tetramethylimidazoline-1-oxyl) radical produced from the reaction with NO reduced in the presence of FA showing that FA can directly scavenge NO. These results indicated that NO scavenging activity of FA reduced the accumulation of nitrite in the LPS-stimulated RAW264.7 cells. The NO modulation due to FA would be responsible for the alleviation from the failure in neural tube formation causing a high level of NO production.

Keywords: folic acid; nitric oxide; neural tube defects; RAW264.7 cells; NOR3; ESR; LC/MS

1. Introduction

The falling of neural tube defects (NTDs) in neural tube formation during early embryogenesis includes anencephaly, exencephaly, and spina bifida. Folic acid (FA) is known as a dietary supplement that can be prevent NTDs involving failure of the neural tube (NT) closure in the developing embryo, especially spina bifida and anencephaly in the periconceptional period [1].

Based on this information, the mandatory FA fortification has been associated with a decline in NTD prevalence in many countries [2–4]. A more recent study demonstrated that microglia activation, including the disruption of the endogenous inhibitory system (CD200-CD200R), contributes to injury in spina bifida aperta after birth [5]. Previous study indicated that a moderate level of nitric oxide (NO) and nitric oxide synthase (NOS) play a critical role in normal embryonic development [6]. Physiological concentrations of NO modulate carbon flow through the folate pathway, that is, NO inhibits methionine synthase (MS) involving the interference transfer of the methyl group from the methyl donor, 5-methyl-tetrahydrofolate (5mTHF), to homocysteine during methionine production [7].

In previous studies, the direct effect of FA against NO produced by the NO donor, S-nitroso-N-acetyl-penicillamine (SNAP), on the process of NT closure in the chick embryo ex ovo was examined. NOS involves high NO levels due to the SNAP treatment of the inactivated MS and its activity can only be rescued by FA or vitamin B12, but not by the NOS inhibitor [8,9]. Although FA or vitamin B12 can prevent the NTDs causing the NO induction, the detailed prevention mechanism due to the FA relation to NO has not yet been clarified. Therefore, this study focused on the interaction of FA and NO, and this article describes how FA can directly scavenge NO involved in NTDs.

2. Materials and Methods

2.1. Reagents

4-Ethyl-2-hydroxyamino-5-nitro-3-hexenamide (alternate name: NOR3) and 2-(4-carboxyphenyl)-4,4,5,5-tetramethylimidazoline-1-oxyl-3-oxide (alternate name: carboxy-PTIO) were purchased from Dojindo Molecular Technique Inc. (Kumamoto, Japan). Folic acid (FA), L-arginine, interferon-γ (IFN-γ) and lipopolysaccharide (LPS) were obtained from the FUJI Firm Wako Pure Chemical Corporation (Osaka, Japan). Dulbecco's modified Eagle's medium (DMEM) and fetal bovine serum (FBS) were obtained from Gibco BRL (Grand Island, NY, USA).

2.2. Cell Culture

Raw264.7 cells (mouse macrophages, American type culture collection) were cultured in DMEM in 10% FBS, 100 U/mL penicillin and 100 μg/mL streptomycin at 37 °C in a 5% CO_2 atmosphere.

2.3. Nitrite Assay on RAW264.7 Macrophages

RAW264.7 macrophages in a 96-well microplate were treated with LPS (100 ng/mL), L-arginine (2 mM), and IFN-γ (100 U/mL) with or without the various concentrations of FA (25–200 μM). After culturing for 16 h, the nitrite production as an NO indicator in the medium, was determined by the Griess method as previously reported [10,11].

2.4. iNOS Gene Expression

Reverse transcriptase-polymerase chain reaction (RT-PCR) was carried out according to previously described procedures [12]. Briefly, the LPS-stimulated RAW264.7 macrophages on a 12-well microplate (2.5×10^6 cells/mL) were treated with the FA (200 μM). The total RNA from cells was isolated from the cell lysate and the amplification of the cDNA was performed by the iNOS primers: 5′-CCT TGT TCA GCT ACG CCT TC-3′and 5′-CTG AGG GCT CTG TTG AGG TC-3′ using PCR (GeneAmp® PCR System 9700, Applied Biosystems, Waltham, MA. USA). The PCR product of cDNA (100 ng/μL) was loaded on a DNA chip (Agilent DNA 1000 kit, Agilent Technologies, Santa Clara, CA, USA) and the electrophoresis was performed by a micro DNA analyzer (Agilent 2100 Bioanalyzer, Agilent Technologies, Santa Clara, CA, USA).

2.5. Nitric Oxide (NO) Inhibitory Action

NOR3 as the NO donor was used in the presence of various concentrations of FA (10–200 μM) as previously reported [13]. The reaction mixture containing NOR3 (200 μM), with or without FA in phosphate-buffered saline (PBS) solution, was incubated at room temperature for 60 min. The nitrite accumulation in the reaction mixture was determined using previously reported procedures [10,11]. In addition, the reaction mixture was analyzed by liquid chromatography–mass spectrometry (LC/MS) equipment. The reaction product of FA and NO was measured by LC/MS using a photodiode array detector (Quattromicro API triple-quadruple mass analyzer, Waters Corp., Milford, MA, USA) and monitored at 275 nm on a reversed-phase chromatographic column, YMC Pro C18 (i.d. 3 mm × 10 cm,

YMC Co., Ltd., Kyoto, Japan) at 40 °C. The mobile phase consisting of 1% formic acid and acetonitrile solvent (10%) was carried out at the flow rate of 0.34 mL/min by a linear gradient to 10%, 30% and 100% for 2 min, 3 min and 7 min. The mass spectra were measured under the following conditions: electrospray ionization (ESI) at the cone voltages of 17 volts for the positive ion mode and at 21 volts for the negative ion mode.

2.6. Electron Spin Resonance (ESR) Measurement

The NO scavenging ability of FA was examined in the presence of the carboxy PTIO as the NO detection reagent [14]. The reaction mixture of FA (200 µM), NOR3 (100 µM) and carboxy-PTIO (50 µM) was prepared in PBS and incubated at room temperature for 15 min. An electron spin resonance (ESR) measurement was performed by an ESR spectrometer (JES-FR30, JEOL, Ltd., Tokyo, Japan) operating at the X-band with the modulation frequency of 100 kHz. The reaction mixture was transferred to the capillary (100 × 1.1 mm i.d. (inner diameter)., Drummond Scientific Co., Broomall, PA, USA) and placed in a quartz cell (270 mm long, 5 mm i.d., JEOL DATUM, Ltd., Tokyo, Japan). The ESR signal was measured at 9.4 GHz resonant frequency the following conditions: microwave power; 4 mW; modulation width, 0.1 mT; gain, 500; scan time, 1 min; time constant, 0.3 s.

2.7. Reaction Product of Folic Acid (FA) and NO

The reaction products of FA and NO were prepared as previously reported [11,15]. Milli-Q water (200 mL) was degassed using an ultrasonic device under reduced pressure for 30 min, subsequently a dry nitrogen gas was bubbled for 30 min in a nitrogen gas-filled glove box (762 × 450 × 478 mm, AS-600PC, AS ONE corp., Osaka, Japan). The status of deoxygenation in the aqueous solution was confirmed using an oximeter (MDS-2C, Marubishi Bioengineering Co., Ltd., Tokyo, Japan). This deoxygenated aqueous solution (1 mL) containing FA (4.4 mg), $Na_2S_2O_4$ (20 mg), $Na^{14}NO_2$ or $Na^{15}NO_2$ (40 mg) was incubated in a capped vial at room temperature for 1 h under the anoxic conditions in the glove box. While the similar reaction mixture as control was prepared under the aerobic conditions. Then, the product of NO (FA-^{14}NO and FA-^{15}NO) was immediately analyzed by LC/MS equipment. The reaction product of FA and NO was measured by LC/MS using a photodiode array detector (Xevo-TQD triple-quadrupole mass analyzer, Waters, MA, USA) and monitored at 275 nm on a reversed-phase chromatographic column, Acquity UPLC BEH C18 (i.d. 2.1 mm × 3 cm, 1.7 µm, Waters) at 40 °C. The mobile phase consisting of 0.1% formic acid aqueous solution (100%) and acetonitrile solvent containing 0.1% formic acid was carried out at the flow rate of 0.40 mL/min by a linear gradient to 100%, 5%, 5% for 0.5 min, 3.5 min, 5min. These mass spectra were measured under the following conditions: ESI at the cone voltages of 30 volt in both the positive and negative ion mode.

3. Results

3.1. NO Inhibitory Action

The NO inhibitory action due to FA was evaluated for the NO production in the LPS-stimulated RAW264.7 cells. The nitrite accumulation as the NO indicator increased in the LPS treated cells. When FA was placed in the cells, the nitrite accumulation was inhibited in a dose dependent manner (Figure 1). A previous study showed a similar result that FA inhibited cytotoxicity with apoptosis due to NO [16]. This result indicated that FA has an inhibitory action on the NO production.

3.2. NO Scavenging Activity

The NO scavenging activity due to FA was evaluated using NOR3 as the NO donor. The nitrite accumulation as the NO indicator was examined with or without FA. As shown in Figure 2, FA suppressed the nitrite accumulation in a dose-dependent manner. This result suggested that FA has a potential NO or nitrogen radical scavenging activity. Therefore, the NO scavenging ability due to FA would be responsible for the suppression of the NO production in the LPS-stimulated RAW264.7 cells (Figure 1).

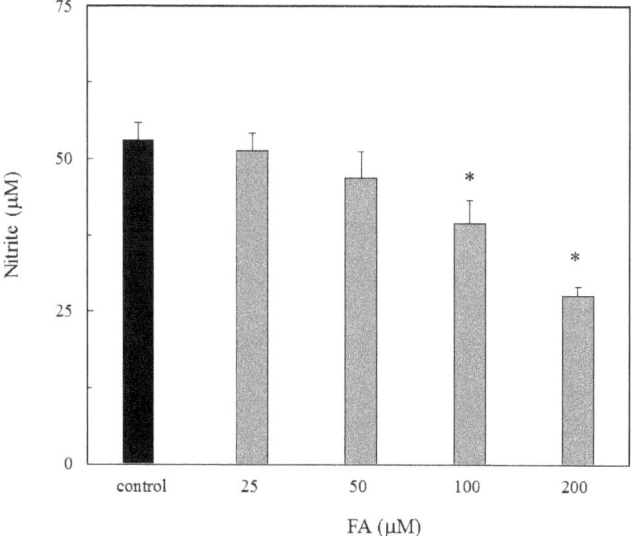

Figure 1. Inhibition of folic acid (FA) for nitric oxide (NO) production in lipopolysaccharide (LPS)-stimulated RAW264.7 macrophages. The various concentrations of FA (25, 50, 100 and 200 µM) were evaluated for the NO production in the LPS-stimulated RAW264.7 macrophages. Data are expressed as mean ± standard deviation (SD) and the significant difference was analyzed by the Student's t-test. *$p < 0.01$ indicates significant difference from the control.

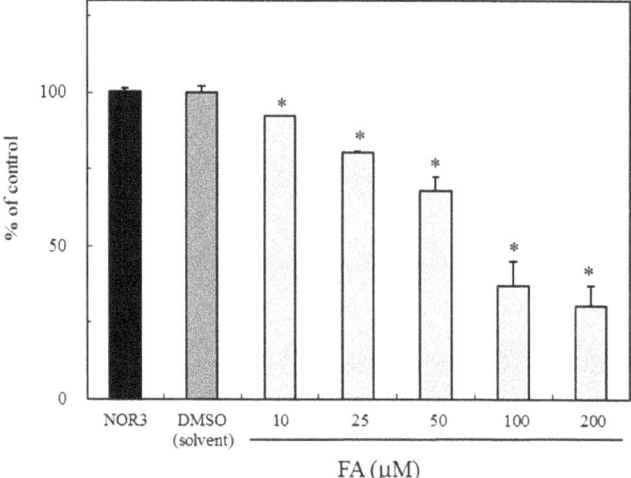

Figure 2. Inhibition of nitrite accumulation due to folic acid (FA). The reaction mixture containing NOR3 (4-ethyl-2-hydroxyamino-5-nitro-3-hexenamide) (200 µM) as the NO donor with or without FA (10, 25, 50, 100 and 200 µM) in phosphate-buffered saline (PBS) solution was incubated at room temperature for 60 min. The nitrite level was used as the NO indicator. Data are expressed as mean ± SD, and the significant difference was analyzed by the Student's t-test. *$p < 0.01$ indicates significant difference from NOR3 without the test compounds.

3.3. Suppression of iNOS Gene Expression

The *i*NOS mRNA gene expression was induced in the LPS-stimulated RAW264.7 cells. The *i*NOS gene expression in the cells was examined with or without FA. As shown in Figure 3, the *i*NOS gene expression by the LPS treatment was not suppressed by the FA treatment. This result suggested that FA can directly scavenge NO or nitrogen radicals which would be responsible for the suppression of the NO production in the LPS-stimulated cells (Figure 1).

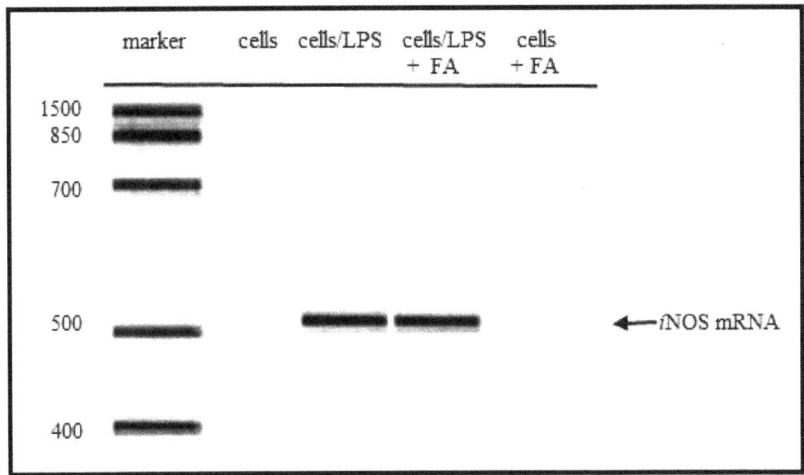

Figure 3. Inhibitory effect of folic acid (FA) for LPS stimulated *i*NOS mRNA expression in LPS-stimulated RAW264.7 macrophages. An *i*NOS mRNA gene expression was induced in the LPS-stimulated RAW264.7 cells. The *i*NOS gene expression in the cells was examined with or without FA (200 µM). Cells, cells without treatment; cells/LPS, cells treated with LPS; cells/LPS + FA, cells treated with LPS and cells + FA, cells treated with FA.

3.4. Determination of FA-NO by Liquid Chromatography–Mass Spectrometry (LC/MS)

To confirm the reaction product of FA and NO (FA-NO), LC/MS was used to measure in the reaction mixture containing NOR3 and FA. The high-performance liquid chromatography (HPLC) chromatogram of the FA-NO produced in the presence of FA and NOR3 indicated in Figure 4. The mass spectrum of the reaction products was detected in both the positive and negative ion mode. The mass numbers of m/z 470.9 $(M + H)^+$ and m/z 469.1 $(M - H)^-$ indicated that the FA-NO was produced by the interaction of FA and NO.

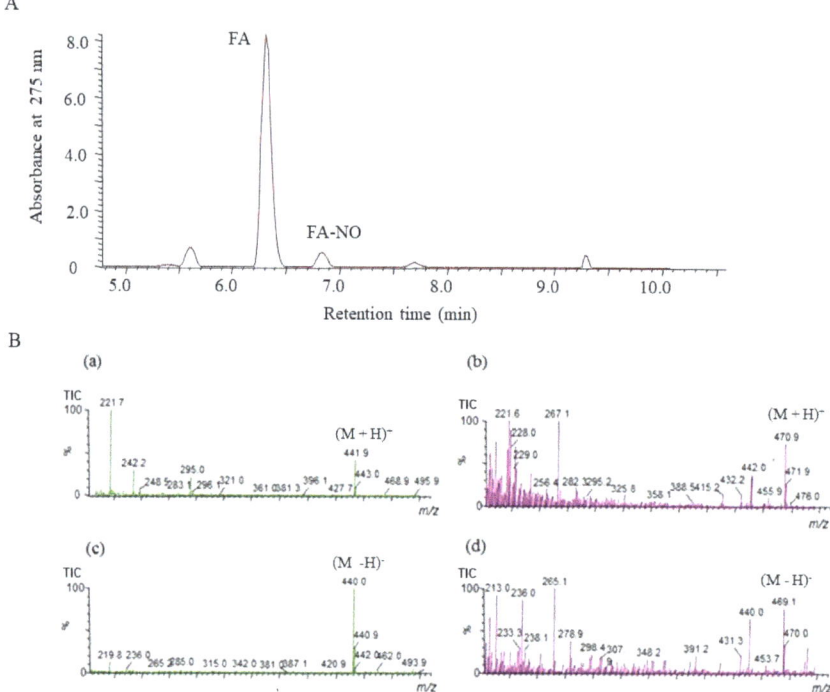

Figure 4. Liquid chromatography–mass spectrometry (LC/MS) chromatogram obtained from reaction mixture containing NOR3 and folic acid (FA). The LC/MS was carried out under the analytical conditions as described in the text. (**A**) Each peak of the high-performance liquid chromatography (HPLC) chromatogram indicated FA and its reaction product with NO, FA-NO. (**B**) These mass spectra indicated (**a**) FA, m/z 441.9 $(M + H)^+$ and (**b**) FA-NO, m/z 470.9 $(M + H)^+$ in the positive ion mode and (**c**) FA, m/z 440.0 $(M - H)^-$ and (**d**) FA-NO, m/z 469.1 $(M - H)^-$ in the negative ion mode of mass spectrometry.

3.5. Products of FA-^{14}NO and FA-^{15}NO

To confirm the ability of the FA scavenging of NO, the product of FA-NO derived from ^{14}NO and ^{15}NO was prepared, and then each mass spectrum was measured by LC/MS. As shown in Figures 5 and 6, each reaction product of ^{14}NO and ^{15}NO with FA under the conditions of aerobic and anoxia was as follows; FA-^{14}NO, m/z 469.17 $(M - H)^-$; m/z 471.14 $(M + H)^+$ for the aerobic conditions and m/z 469.12 $(M - H)^-$; m/z 471.13 $(M + H)^+$ for the anoxic conditions (Figure 5) and also FA-^{15}NO, m/z 470.12 $(M - H)^-$; m/z 472.16 $(M + H)^+$ for the aerobic conditions and m/z 470.21 $(M - H)^-$; m/z 472.14 $(M + H)^+$ for the anoxic conditions (Figure 6). The individual mass number of the FA-NO was clearly distinguished by the difference in the isotopic ratio of nitrogen. In addition, the product of FA-NO in the anoxic conditions was similar yield to that of the aerobic conditions. These results supported the assertion that FA has NO scavenging ability, resulting in the suppression of NO production in the LPS-stimulated RAW264.7 cells (Figure 1).

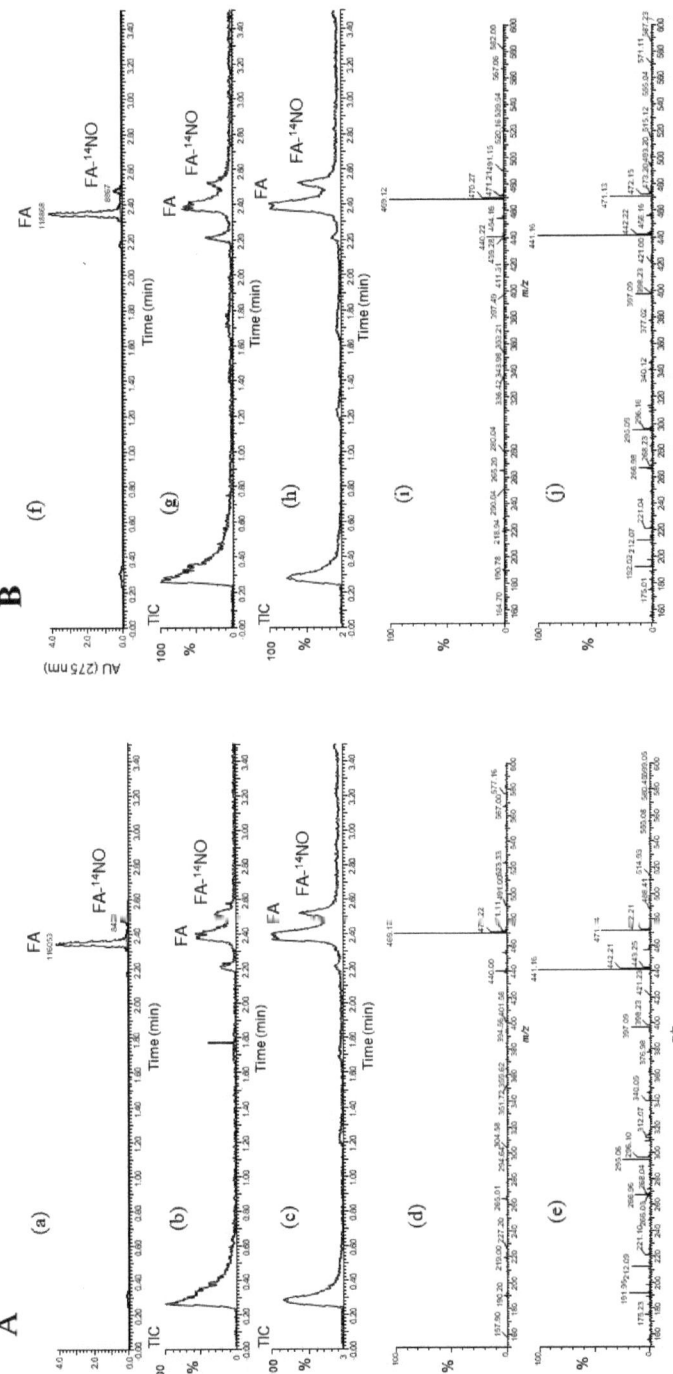

Figure 5. LC/MS chromatogram obtained from the reaction mixture containing folic acid (FA), $Na_2S_2O_4$ and $Na^{14}NO_2$ under the conditions of (**A**) aerobic and (**B**) anoxia. The LC/MS was carried out under the analytical conditions as described in the text. Each peak of LC/MS indicated FA and its reaction product with NO, FA-NO. The HPLC chromatogram indicated FA and its reaction product with NO under the conditions of **A** (**a**) aerobic and **B** (**f**) anoxia. The TIC (total ion chromatogram) and its mass spectra of FA-^{14}NO indicated in the negative and positive ion modes as follows. The aerobic conditions; the TIC of (**b**) and (**c**) for (**d**) m/z 469.17 (M − H)$^-$ and (**e**) m/z 471.14 (M + H)$^+$, and the anoxic conditions; the TIC of (**g**) and (**h**) for (**i**) m/z 469.12 (M − H)$^-$ and (**j**) m/z 471.13 (M + H)$^+$.

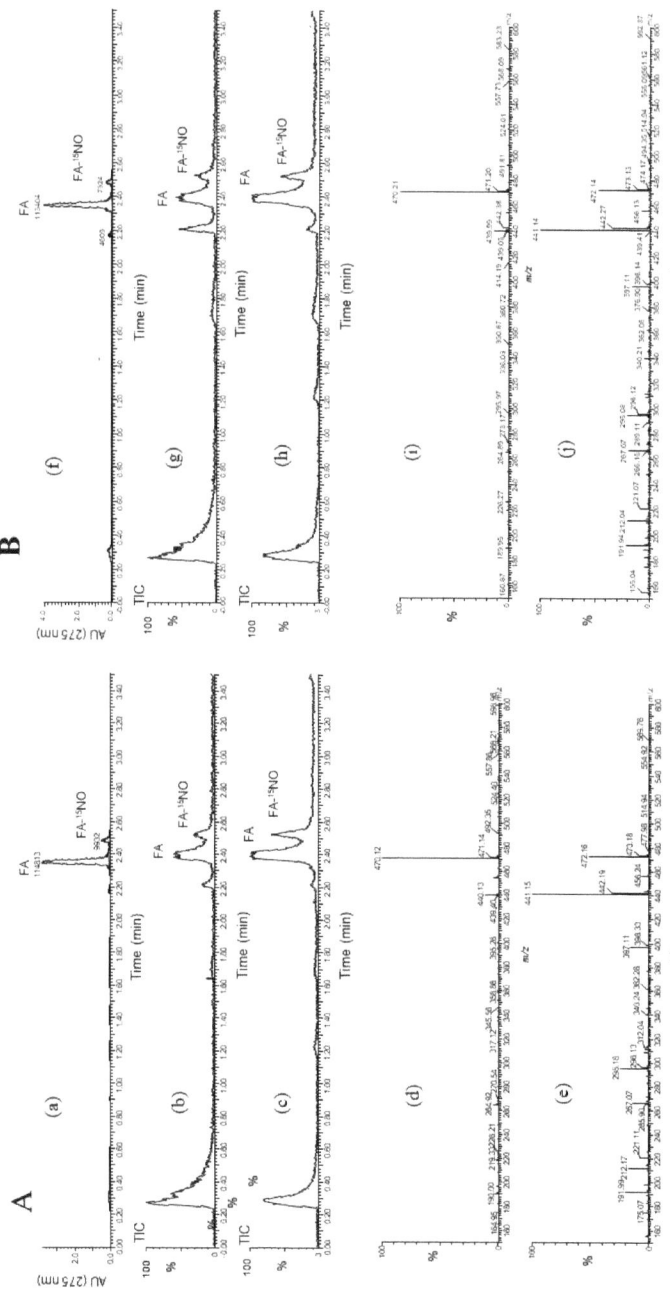

Figure 6. LC/MS chromatogram obtained from the reaction mixture containing folic acid (FA), $Na_2S_2O_4$ and $Na^{15}NO_2$ under the conditions of (**A**) aerobic and (**B**) anoxia. The LC/MS was carried out under the analytical conditions as described in the text. Each peak of LC/MS indicated FA and its reaction product with NO, FA-NO. The HPLC chromatogram indicated FA and its reaction product with NO under conditions that were **A** (**a**) aerobic and **B** (**f**) anoxia. The TIC (total ion chromatogram) and its mass spectra of FA-^{14}NO indicated in the negative and positive ion modes as follows. the aerobic conditions; the TIC of (**b**) and (**c**) for (**d**) m/z 470.12 (M − H)$^-$ and (**e**) m/z 472.16 (M + H)$^+$, and the anoxic conditions; the TIC of (**g**) and (**h**) for (**i**) m/z 470.21 (M − H)$^-$ and (**j**) m/z 472.14 (M + H)$^+$.

3.6. FA Scavenging NO by ESR Study

It is known that nitronyl nitroxide carboxy-PTIO as an NO detection reagent reacts with NO, generate an imino nitroxide, carboxy-PTI radical and NO_2 [17,18]. To clarify the NO scavenging action of FA, an ESR study was performed on the system containing the carboxy-PTIO in the presence of NOR3 and FA. The NO released from NOR3 was detected by carboxy-PTIO, then produced a carboxy-PTI radical as indicated by the arrows in Figure 7. The carboxy-PTI radical was reduced when FA was present in the system, indicating that FA can directly scavenge NO.

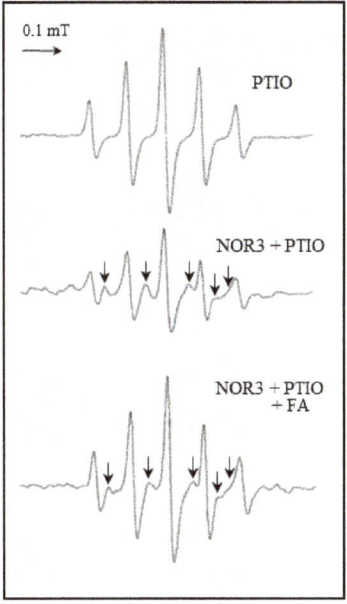

Figure 7. NO savenging activity of folic acid (FA). Electron spin resonance (ESR) spectrum obtained from the reaction mixture containing the carboxy-PTIO (2-phenyl-4,4,5,5-tetramethylimidazoline-1-oxyl-3-oxide, 200 µM) as the NO detection reagent in the presence of NOR3 (200 µM) with or without FA (200 µM). The NO released from NOR3 was detected by carboxy-PTIO, then produced a carboxy-PTI (2-phenyl-4,4,5,5-tetramethylimidazoline-1-oxyl) radical as indicated by the arrows.

4. Discussion

The significance of FA in the prevention of neural tube defects (NTDs) involving the failure of NT closure in the developing embryo is well recognized. NO had been shown to be able to induce NTDs in rat embryos, and biochemical studies showed that NO inhibits methionine synthase (MS) [6,7]. In a previous study, the direct effect of NO produced by the NO donor SNAP on the process of NT closure in the chick embryo ex ovo. was evaluated and the high NO levels by the SNAP treatment inhibited the MS in the methyl transfer reaction of cofactor B12 [8,9]. The alleviation mechanism due to the FA treatment was speculated to be the interference with one-carbon flow through the folate pathway [8]. Previous studies showed that 5-methyl-tetrahydrofolate (5-mTHF), the primary circulating metabolite of FA, improves the endothelial NO synthase (*e*NOS) coupling cofactor tetrahydrobiopterin (BH_4), indicating that the NOS activity regulates the MS activity in the process of NT closure [8]. On the other hand, when the BH_4 is limited, the uncoupled NOS produces the superoxide radical (O_2^-) rather than NO, then produces peroxynitrite by the reaction between O_2^- and NO which causes the endothelial dysfunction [19]. FA has the ability of O_2^- scavenging, which may protect or improve the endothelial function [20–23]. However, the detailed relationship between FA and NO has not yet been clarified. In this study, the effect of FA on the NO production in the LPS-stimulated RAW264.7 cells was examined. The nitrite accumulation in the LPS treatment cells decreased in the presence of FA (Figure 1). An inflammatory cytokine or proinflammatory cytokine including interleukin-1 (IL-1), interleukin-12 (IL-12), and interleukin-18 (IL-18), TNF-α, interferon γ (IFNγ), and granulocyte-macrophage colony stimulating factor (GM-CSF) stimulate the Janus kinase (Jak) and signal transducer and activator of transcription (STAT) pathway (JAK-STAT pathway) as a key role in signal pathways activated by growth factors and cytokines. Expression of *i*NOS and the production of NO in response to LPS/IFN γ are increased through JAK/STAT signaling [24,25]. While the expression of the *i*NOS gene due to the LPS/ IFNγ treatment was not inhibited by the FA treatment, thus the reduction NO due to FA will not be through the JAK-STAT pathway. It is suggested that FA may directly regulate against NO or producing nitrogen radicals during the NO oxidation (Figure 2). The NO-scavenging ability of FA was examined in the reaction with NOR3 as the NO donor. FA suppressed the nitrite accumulation in a dose-dependent manner suggesting that FA provides a direct scavenging ability against NO or nitrogen radicals. The result first showed another possible function of FA which can modulate the nitrogen radicals including NO. Although FA could not suppress the *i*NOS gene expression, the nitrogen radical scavenging function due to FA could suppress for the NO production in the LPS-stimulated cells (Figure 3). To better clarify the function of FA, the FA scavenging NO adduct in the reaction mixture was detected by LC/MS. The mass numbers of m/z 470.9 $(M + H)^+$ and m/z 469.1 $(M - H)^-$ were determined as the adduct of the FA scavenging NO (FA-NO). To obtain more detailed evidence, the FA-NO derived from ^{14}NO and ^{15}NO was measured in both the positive and negative ion mode, and each product of the ^{14}NO or ^{15}NO reaction with FA gave the following mass numbers: FA-^{14}NO, m/z 471.14 $(M + H)^+$; m/z 469.17 $(M - H)^-$ and FA-^{15}NO, m/z 472.16 $(M + H)^+$; m/z 470.12 $(M - H)^-$ (Figures 5A and 6A). The individual mass number of the FA-NO was clearly distinguished by the difference in the isotopic ratio of nitrogen, resulting in the product by the FA reaction with NO. NO reacts with oxygen giving rise to the formation of NO_2 and potentially N_2O_3. To avoid the reactions, the FA reaction with NO in the anoxic conditions was examined, resulting in the product of FA-NO being of a similar yield to that of the aerobic conditions (Figures 5B and 6B). This result suggested that the reactions of FA with NO give rise to folic acid nitrosation.

To clarify the direct NO scavenging action due to FA, an ESR study was performed on the system containing carboxy-PTIO as the NO detection reagent in the presence of NOR3 and FA. The carboxy-PTI radical was then produced from the reaction with NO reduced in the presence of FA (Figure 7). This result strongly supported the assertion that FA can directly scavenge NO and the function of FA suppressed the NO production in the LPS-stimulated cells.

FA can prevent the NTDs causing the NO induction which inhibits MS involving the interference transfer of the methyl group from the 5mTHF to homocysteine in methionine production. This study proposes another alleviation mechanism whereby the NO modulation due to the FA direct scavenging of NO contributes to alleviation from the failure in the NT formation causing the high level of NO production.

5. Conclusions

This study first demonstrated that FA can directly scavenge NO, resulting in the reduction of the accumulation of nitrite in the LPS-stimulated RAW264.7 cells. In addition, the NO modulation due to FA may contribute to alleviation from the failure in neural tube formation causing the high level of NO production.

Author Contributions: All authors (T.O. and J.T.) participated in the experiments and research design of the study. J.T. organized this study including interpretation of the data and wrote the manuscript. All authors have read and agreed to the published version of the manuscript.

Funding: Works described here were supported by Grants from Okinawa Prefecture, Japan.

Conflicts of Interest: The authors declare no conflict of interest.

References

1. Czeizel, A.E.; Dudas, I. Prevention of the first occurrence of neural-tube defects by periconceptional vitamin supplementation. *N. Engl. J. Med.* **1992**, *327*, 1832–1835. [CrossRef] [PubMed]
2. Blencowe, H.; Cousens, S.; Modell, B.; Lawn, J. Folic acid to reduce neonatal mortality from neural tube disorders. *Int. J. Epidemiol.* **2010**, *39*, 110–121. [CrossRef] [PubMed]
3. Crider, K.S.; Bailey, L.B.; Berry, R.J. Folic acid food fortification-its history, effect, concerns, and future directions. *Nutrients* **2011**, *3*, 370–384. [CrossRef] [PubMed]
4. Rosenthal, J.; Casas, J.; Taren, D.; Clinton, J.A.; Alina, F.; Jaime, F. Neural tube defects in Latin America and the impact of fortification: A literature review. *Public Health Nutr.* **2014**, *17*, 537–550. [CrossRef] [PubMed]
5. Oria, M.; Figueira, R.L.; Scorletti, F.; Sbragia, L.; Owens, K.; Li, Z.; Pathak, B.; Corona, M.U.; Marotta, M.; Encinas, J.L.; et al. CD200-CD200R imbalance correlates with microglia and proinflammatory activation in rat spinal cords exposed to amniotic fluid in retinoic acid-induced spina bifida. *Sci. Rep.* **2018**, *8*, 10638–10649. [CrossRef]
6. Lee, Q.P.; Juchau, M.R. Dysmorphogenic effects of nitric oxide (NO) and NO-synthase inhibition: Studies with intra-amniotic injections of sodium nitroprusside and NG-monomethyl-L-arginine. *Teratology* **1994**, *49*, 452–464. [CrossRef]
7. Danishpajo, I.O.; Gudi, T.; Chen, Y.; Kharitonov, V.G.; Sharma, V.S.; Boss, G.R. Nitric oxide inhibits methionine synthase activity in vivo and disrupts carbon flow through the folate pathway. *J. Biol. Chem.* **2002**, *276*, 27296–27303. [CrossRef]
8. Weil, M.; Abeles, R.; Nachmany, A.; Gold, V.; Michael, E. Folic acid rescues nitric oxide-induced neural tube closure defects. *Cell Death Differ.* **2004**, *11*, 361–363. [CrossRef]
9. Nachmany, A.; Goldmm, V.; Tsur, A.; Arad, D.; Weil, M. Neural tube closure depends on nitric oxide synthase activity. *J. Neurochem.* **2006**, *96*, 247–253. [CrossRef]
10. Taira, J.; Nanbu, H.; Ueda, K. Nitric oxide-scavenging compounds in *Agrimonia pilosa* Ledeb on LPS-induced RAW264.7 macrophages. *Food Chem.* **2009**, *115*, 1221–1227. [CrossRef]
11. Taira, J.; Misık, V.; Riesz, P. Nitric oxide formation from hydroxylamine by myoglobin and hydrogen peroxide. *Biochim. Biophys. Acta* **1997**, *1336*, 502–508. [CrossRef]
12. Taira, J.; Ohmine, W.; Nanbub, H.; Ueda, K. Inhibition of LPS-stimulated NO production in RAW264.7 macrophages through *i*NOS suppression and nitrogen radical scavenging by phenolic compounds from *Agrimonia pilosa* Ledeb. *Oxid. Antioxid. Med. Sci.* **2013**, *2*, 21–28. [CrossRef]
13. Taira, J.; Tsuchida, E.; Katoh, M.C.; Uehara, M.; Ogi, T. Antioxidant capacity of betacyanins as radical scavengers for peroxyl radical and nitric oxide. *Food Chem.* **2015**, *166*, 531–536. [CrossRef] [PubMed]
14. Taira, J.; Miyagi, C.; Aniya, Y. Dimerumic acid as an antioxidant from the mold, *Monascus anka*: The inhibition mechanisms against lipid peroxidation and hemeprotein-mediated oxidation. *Biochem. Pharmacol.* **2002**, *63*, 1019–1026. [CrossRef]
15. Yonetani, T.; Yamamoto, H.; Erman, E.J.; Leigh, S.J., Jr.; Reed, H.G.Ž. Electromagnetic properties of hemoproteins. *J. Biol. Chem.* **1972**, *247*, 2447–2455.
16. Taira, J. *Annual Report 2006: Inhibition of Apoptosis in Nitric Oxide Induced PC12 Cells Due to Folic Acid Derivatives*; Okinawa Industrial Tech Center: Okinawa, Japan, 2006; Volume 8, pp. 45–51.
17. Akaike, T.; Yoshida, M.; Miyamoto, Y.; Sato, K.; Kohno, M.; Sasamoto, K.; Miyazaki, K.; Ueda, S.; Maeda, H. Antagonistic action of imidazolineoxyl N-oxides against endothelium-derived relaxing factor/.bul.NO (nitric oxide) through a radical reaction. *Biochemistry* **1993**, *32*, 827–832. [CrossRef]
18. Hogg, N.; Singh, R.J.; Joseph, J.; Neese, F.; Kalyanaraman, B. Reactions of nitric oxide with nitronyl nitroxides and oxygen: Prediction of nitrite and nitrate formation. *Free Radic. Res.* **1995**, *22*, 47–56. [CrossRef]
19. Forstermann, U.; Li, H. Therapeutic effect of enhancing endothelial nitric oxide synthase (eNOS) expression and preventing *e*NOS uncoupling. *Br. J. Pharmacol.* **2011**, *164*, 213–223. [CrossRef]
20. Stanhewicz, A.E.; Kenney, W.L. Role of folic acid in nitric oxide bioavailability and vascular endothelial function. *Nutri. Rev.* **2017**, *75*, 61–70. [CrossRef]
21. Forstermann, U. Janus-faced role of endothelial NO synthase in vascular disease: Uncoupling of oxygen reduction from NO synthesis and its pharmacological reversal. *Biol. Chem.* **2006**, *387*, 1521–1533. [CrossRef]
22. Siragusa, M.; Fleming, I. The eNOS signalosome and its link to endothelial dysfunction. *Pflügers Arch.* **2016**, *468*, 1125–1137. [CrossRef] [PubMed]

23. RaviJoshi, J.; Adhikari, S.; Patro, B.S.; Chatrtropadhyay, S.; Mukherjee, T. Free radical scavenging behavior of folic acid: Evidence for possible antioxidant activity. *Free Radic. Biol. Med.* **2001**, *30*, 12–1390.
24. Horvath, C.M. The Jak-STAT pathway stimulated by interferon gamma. *Sci. STKE* **2004**, *2004*, tr8. [CrossRef] [PubMed]
25. Stempelj, M.; Kedinger, M.; Augenlicht, L.; Klampfer, L. Essential role of the JAK/STAT1 signaling pathway in the expression of inducible nitric-oxide synthase in intestinal epithelial cells and its regulation by butyrate. *J. Biol. Chem.* **2007**, *282*, 9797–9804. [CrossRef] [PubMed]

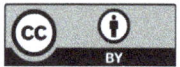

© 2020 by the authors. Licensee MDPI, Basel, Switzerland. This article is an open access article distributed under the terms and conditions of the Creative Commons Attribution (CC BY) license (http://creativecommons.org/licenses/by/4.0/).

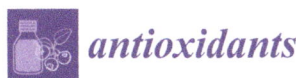

Article

Human Keratinocyte UVB-Protective Effects of a Low Molecular Weight Fucoidan from *Sargassum horneri* Purified by Step Gradient Ethanol Precipitation

Ilekuttige Priyan Shanura Fernando [1], Mawalle Kankanamge Hasitha Madhawa Dias [2], Disanayaka Mudiyanselage Dinesh Madusanka [2], Eui Jeong Han [2], Min Ju Kim [2], You-Jin Jeon [3], Kyounghoon Lee [4], Sun Hee Cheong [1,2], Young Seok Han [5], Sang Rul Park [6] and Ginnae Ahn [1,2,*]

[1] Department of Marine Bio-Food Sciences, Chonnam National University, Yeosu 59626, Korea; shanurabru@gmail.com (I.P.S.F.); sunny3843@chonnam.ac.kr (S.H.C.)
[2] Department of Food Technology and Nutrition, Chonnam National University, Yeosu 59626, Korea; hasithadiasm17636@gmail.com (M.K.H.M.D.); dmdmadusanka88@gmail.com (D.M.D.M.); iosu5772@naver.com (E.J.H.); mijoo92@naver.com (M.J.K.)
[3] Marine Science Institute, Jeju National University, Jeju Self-Governing Province 63333, Korea; youjin2014@gmail.com
[4] Division of Fisheries Science, Chonnam National University, Yeosu 59626, Korea; ricky1106@naver.com
[5] Neo Environmental Business Co., Daewoo Technopark, Doyak-ro, Bucheon 14523, Korea; hanulva@neoenbiz.com
[6] Estuarine & Coastal Ecology Laboratory, Department of Marine Life Sciences, Jeju National University, Jeju 63243, Korea; srpark@jejunu.ac.kr
* Correspondence: gnahn@jnu.ac.kr; Tel.: +82-061-659-7213

Received: 30 March 2020; Accepted: 19 April 2020; Published: 21 April 2020

Abstract: Ultraviolet B (UVB) radiation-induced oxidative skin cell damage is a major cause of photoaging. In the present study, a low molecular weight fucoidan fraction (SHC4) was obtained from *Sargassum horneri* by Celluclast-assisted extraction, followed by step gradient ethanol precipitation. The protective effect of SHC4 was investigated in human keratinocytes against UVB-induced oxidative stress. The purified fucoidan was characterized by Fourier-transform infrared spectroscopy (FTIR), ^{1}H nuclear magnetic resonance (NMR), agarose gel-based molecular weight analysis and monosaccharide composition analysis. SHC4 had a mean molecular weight of 60 kDa, with 37.43% fucose and 28.01 ± 0.50% sulfate content. The structure was mainly composed of α-L-Fucp-(1→4) linked fucose units. SHC4 treatment dose-dependently reduced intracellular reactive oxygen species (ROS) levels and increased the cell viability of UVB exposed HaCaT keratinocytes. Moreover, SHC4 dose-dependently inhibited UVB-induced apoptotic body formation, sub-G_1 accumulation of cells and DNA damage. Inhibition of apoptosis was mediated via the mitochondria-mediated pathway, re-establishing the loss of mitochondrial membrane potential. The UVB protective effect of SHC4 was facilitated by enhancing intracellular antioxidant defense via nuclear factor erythroid 2–related factor 2 (Nrf2)/heme oxygenase-1 (HO-1) signaling. Further studies may promote the use of SHC4 as an active ingredient in cosmetics and nutricosmetics.

Keywords: oxidative stress; ultraviolet B; gradient ethanol precipitation; fucoidan; HaCaT keratinocyte; heme oxygenase-1; nutricosmetic

---

1. Introduction

Ultraviolet B (UVB)-irradiation (280–320 nm) primarily induces cell damage by augmenting intracellular reactive oxygen species (ROS) levels. The radiation easily penetrates the stratum corneum, where it increases the risk of photoaging, with symptoms characterized by thickening of the epidermis, discoloration, skin wrinkling, loss of elasticity and skin cell growth retardation [1]. Recent developments in marine bioresource technology have substantiated the therapeutic potential of marine natural products to be used as cosmeceuticals, functional foods, new drugs and drug leads. Fucoidan is a fucose-rich sulfated polysaccharide found in brown algae that is renowned for its versatile biologic activities. High molecular weight fucoidans closely resemble the structure of heparin and are effective anticoagulants [2]. Nevertheless, low molecular weight fucoidans are reported to possess antioxidant, anti-inflammatory, anticancer and anti-microbial activities [3,4]. Fucoidan mainly contains α-1,3 and α-1,4-linked fucose units with sulfate ester substituents at the 2, 3 and/or 4 positions. However, the chains could also contain monosaccharides such as glucose, mannose, xylose, arabinose and hexuronic acid. The monomer composition, connectivity, branching, sulfation pattern, and molecular weight are species-related [2]. The conventional method of refining fucoidan involves hot water extraction of dry algal powder under mildly acidic pH, followed by ethanol precipitation. The precipitate undergoes additional fractionation via ultrafiltration, size exclusion or anion exchange chromatography. This method lacks efficiency based on the low extraction yield, convenience, time consumption and selectivity over molecular weights.

As fucoidan is mainly localized to the cell wall of brown algae, degradation of the cell wall using enzymes is a well-planned extraction strategy conserving polymer integrity, and thereby its biofunctional properties. The use of enzymes, including Celluclast, Termamyl, Ultraflo, Amyloglucosidase, and Viscozyme, is advisable to obtain fucoidan whose biofunctional properties are preserved [5]. Gradient alcohol precipitation is a fractionation method used for fractionating polysaccharides with gradually narrowed down molecular weight distributions [6]. It is a relatively inexpensive and simple method compared to ultrafiltration and chromatography. The precipitation is achieved by incorporating organic solvents such as methanol, ethanol, isopropanol, 1-butanol and acetone or concentrated inorganic salts such as ammonium sulfate $((NH_4)_2SO_4)$ and polymerizing agents such as polyethylene glycol (PEG). The use of this method has been previously reported for fractionating fucoidan [7]. The present study was undertaken as a part of a project to investigate possible industrial uses of *S. horneri* as a sustainable approach for managing its large biomass. The extraction of fucoidan enriched crude polysaccharides followed an optimized green approach using enzymes, while the fractionation followed a step gradient ethanol precipitation.

2. Materials and Methods

Fucoidan standard, KBr (FTIR grade), deuterium oxide, 2′,7′-dichlorodihydrofluorescein diacetate (DCFH2-DA) and 3-(4,5-dimethylthiazol-2-yl)-2,5-diphenyltetrazolium bromide (MTT), o-Toluidine blue, trifluoroacetic acid and 2-mercaptoethanolwere purchased from Sigma-Aldrich (St. Louis, MO, USA). Celluclast was obtained from Novozyme Co. (Bagsvaerd, Denmark). Chloroform, methanol and ethanol were of analytical grade. Dulbecco's Modified Eagle Medium (DMEM), fetal bovine serum (FBS) and penicillin/streptomycin mixture were purchased from GIBCO INC., (Grand Island, NY, USA). Primary and ary antibodies were purchased from Cell Signalling Technology, Inc. (Beverly, MA, USA) and Santa Cruz Biotechnology (Santa Cruz, CA, USA).

2.1. Preparation of Fucoidan Fraction

2.1.1. Extraction of Fucoidan Enriched Polysaccharide

Washed and dried *S. horneri* samples collected off Jeju coast were provided to us by Seojin Biotech Company limited. The samples were pulverized using an MF 10 basic, IKA microfine grinder (Werke, Germany). Depigmentation was carried out using a solvent system of chloroform and methanol 1:1. Next, the dried powder was soaked in a solution of ethanol containing 10% formaldehyde for 3 h at 40 °C. The dried powder was washed twice with 80% ethanol. After evaporating off any remaining solvent, the sample powder was suspended in 5 L of deionized water at a 1:10 (kg/L) ratio. The pH was adjusted to 4.5 by adding diluted HCl while equilibrating at 50 °C in a shaking incubator for 1 h.

Celluclast was added at a 0.5% sample ratio and kept for 8 h under continuous agitation at 50 °C. The mixture was filtered through a muslin cloth. Celluclast was heat-denatured at 100 °C for 10 min. The extract was neutralized at room temperature by adding diluted NaOH and centrifuged at 5000× g for 20 min to remove unfiltered particles. The supernatant (4.5 L) was frozen and lyophilized to reduce the volume to 1 L.

2.1.2. Step Gradient Ethanol Precipitation

The ratio of ethanol was determined following optimization studies. As the first step in gradient ethanol precipitation, 250 mL of ethanol was gently added to 1 L of the extract while stirring. The mixture was incubated at 4 °C for 12 h, allowing it to equilibrate while precipitating the polysaccharides (Figure 1). After, the mixture was centrifuged at 5000× g for 20 min at 4 °C to obtain the first precipitate designated as SHC1. Sequentially the second, third and fourth precipitates were collected by, respectively adding 500 mL, 1 L and 2 L of ethanol to the supernatant after each precipitation step. All precipitates were dually washed with 95% ethanol (homogenization) and centrifuged to recover the polymer. Finally, the precipitates were dissolved in deionized water and dialyzed using 3.5-kD molecular weight cutoff dialysis membranes (Spectra/Por, Los Angeles, CA, USA). Polysaccharide fractions were lyophilized and stored at −20 °C for proceeding experiments.

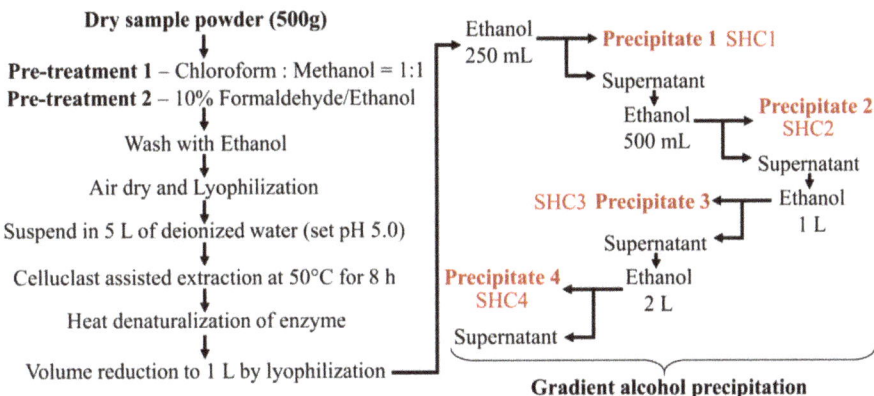

Figure 1. The procedure of sample pretreatment, enzyme-assisted extraction, and fractionation by gradient ethanol precipitation.

2.2. Analysis of Molecular Weight (MW) Distribution

Approximate molecular weight distribution, homogeneity, and separation efficiency of the polysaccharide fractions were analyzed by an agarose gel electrophoresis method [3]. Briefly, markers and samples (1 mg mL^{-1}) were electrophoresed in 1% agarose gels in Tris-Borate-EDTA running buffer (pH 8.3) at 100 V for 20 min. The gel was stained with 0.02% toluidine blue and 0.5% Triton X-100 in 3% acetic acid and de-stained with 3% acetic acid.

2.3. Fourier-Transform Infrared Spectroscopy (FTIR) and Monosaccharide Composition Analysis

Polysaccharide powders were cast into KBr pellets and analyzed by a VERTEX 70v FTIR spectrometer (Bruker, Germany) [3]. For the monosaccharide composition analysis, polysaccharides were hydrolyzed with 4 M of trifluoroacetic acid and separated on a CarboPac PA1 column integrated to a Dionex ED50 Detector (HPAEC-PAD) (Dionex, Sunnyvale, CA, USA). A standardized monosaccharide mixture was used as the reference standard [3].

2.4. H^1 Nuclear Magnetic Resonance (NMR) Analysis

The selected polysaccharide fraction, SHC4, was deuterium exchanged by co-lyophilizing with deuterium oxide, dissolved in deuterium oxide, and analyzed by a JNM-ECX400, 400 MHz spectrometer (JEOL, Tokyo, Japan).

2.5. In Vivo Cell Culture

2.5.1. Cell Maintenance

HaCaT keratinocytes (Korean Cell Line Bank, Seoul, Korea) were maintained in DMEM containing 10% FBS and 1% penicillin-streptomycin. Cells were sub-cultured once every two days. Exponentially growing cells were used for seeding (2×10^5 cells mL^{-1}). After 24 h, wells were treated with different sample concentrations and further incubated for 24 h. Cytotoxicity was measured by MTT assay. Briefly, cells were incubated with MTT for 4 h, dissolved in dimethyl sulfoxide (DMSO), and the absorbance readings were taken at 540 nm using a SpectraMax® M2 system (Molecular Devices, Sunnyvale, CA, USA).

2.5.2. UVB Exposure and Oxidative Stress Analysis

HaCaT keratinocytes were incubated for 2 h with different concentrations of samples. The cell culture media was withdrawn from the wells, once washed, and then filled with PBS. Wells except the control were exposed to UVB (50 mJ cm^{-2}) by a UVP CL-1000L ultraviolet cross-linker (Upland, CA, USA). Immediately after the irradiation, PBS was withdrawn, once washed, and replaced with serum-free culture media. Intracellular ROS levels were measured after incubating for an hour (DCFH2-DA assay) and cell viability was measured by MTT assay after incubating for 24 h [1]. SHC4 that indicated superior antioxidant and cytoprotective effects were further verified by DCFH2-DA staining of cells and analysis by fluorescence microscopy (EVOS FL Auto 2 Imaging, ThermoFisher Scientific, CA, USA) and flow cytometry (CytoFLEX, Beckman Coulter, PA, USA) based on methods described in our previous publications [8].

2.5.3. Analysis of Nuclear Morphology

Cells were stained with either Hoechst 33342 or mixture of acridine orange and ethidium bromide according to the method described in our previous publication [9]. Nuclear morphologies were visualized on an EVOS FL Auto 2 Imaging microscope (Thermo-Fisher, Waltham, MA, USA).

2.5.4. Western Blot Analysis

HaCaT cells after initial sample treatment and UVB-exposure were used for the experiments following a 24 h incubation period. Western blot analysis was done following our previously reported method [10]. A nuclear and cytoplasmic extraction kit, NE-PER® (Thermo Scientific, Rockford, IL, USA), was used to isolate cytosolic and nucleic proteins. Proteins were standardized using a BCA^{TM} protein assay kit (Pierce, Rockford, IL, USA). Electrophoresis was carried out using 10% SDS-polyacrylamide gels. SuperSignal™ West Femto Maximum Sensitivity Substrate (Thermo, Burlington, ON, Canada) was used for the detection of protein bands on a Core Bio DavinchChemi imaging system (Seoul, Korea).

2.5.5. Cell Cycle Analysis

Harvested cells were permeabilized in 70% ethanol for 30 min, incubated in PBS containing EDTA, RNase and propidium iodide at 37 °C for 30 min, and analyzed by a Beckman Coulter CytoFLEX flow cytometer (Brea, CA, USA). A dual-region gating approach, initial FS vs. SS to remove derbies and FL3-area vs. FL3-hight to eliminate doublets, was applied. Sub-G$_1$ apoptotic cell population percentages were used for data compression.

2.5.6. JC-1 Assay

Mitochondria membrane potential was ratiometrically measured by flow cytometry using MitoProbe JC-1 Assay Kit (Thermo Fisher Scientific, Waltham, MA, USA) following the manufacturer's instructions. Cultured cells were initially subjected to sample treatment and UVB-exposure. After 4 h, cells were harvested for the assay.

2.5.7. Comet Assay

DNA damage in individual cells was evaluated by alkaline comet assay following the procedure outlined in our previous publication [9]. Briefly, cells were harvested and suspended in low-melting agarose at 37 °C and gently applied on the surface of agarose coated slides. The slides were overnight immersed in alkaline lysis buffer at 4 °C. Electrophoresis was performed at 4 °C in an alkaline running buffer. Finally, the slides were submerged in a chilled neutralization buffer and stained with ethidium bromide. Comet tails were pictured on an EVOS FL Auto 2 Imaging microscope and tail DNA contents were quantified using OpenComet plugin in NIH Image J software (US National Institutes of Health, Bethesda, MD, USA).

2.6. Statistical Analysis

The data from experiments are presented as mean ± standard error (SE). Statistical comparisons were carried out by one-way analysis of variance by Duncan's test using PASW Statistics 19.0 software (SPSS, Chicago, IL, USA). The level of significance was set at * $p < 0.05$ and ** $p < 0.01$.

3. Results

3.1. Extraction Efficiency and Proximate Compositions

The enzyme (Celluclast)-assisted extraction yield of *S. horneri* powder was 20.30 ± 0.32%. Yields corresponding to precipitated polysaccharides during step gradient ethanol precipitation are provided in Table 1. The highest yield was observed from fraction SHC2, obtained by incorporating 500 mL of ethanol. The proximate chemical compositions of the subsequent fractions indicated a gradual increase in the degree of sulfation in polysaccharides. The polyphenol, protein and ash content were comparatively low in all fractions, demonstrating the efficiency of the procedure in obtaining sulfated polysaccharides.

Table 1. Yield and proximate composition of the major components in the fractions.

	Yield (%)	SHC1	SHC2	SHC3	SHC4
		5.25	16.75	4.26	3.81
Sulfated polysaccharide content (%)	Polysaccharide	72.02 ± 0.46	62.29 ± 0.09	54.34 ± 0.00	45.96 ± 0.36
	Sulfate	13.85 ± 0.47	19.26 ± 0.11	23.64 ± 0.48	28.01 ± 0.50
Polyphenol content (%)		3.06 ± 0.44	2.59 ± 0.15	1.91 ± 0.30	1.24 ± 0.21
Protein content (%)		0.54 ± 0.03	0.68 ± 0.01	0.44 ± 0.02	0.50 ± 0.01
Ash content (%)		1.85 ± 0.11	0.88 ± 0.09	0.70 ± 0.12	0.54 ± 0.02

SHC1-SHC4 denote different polysaccharide fractions obtained via step gradient ethanol precipitation. Data represent the mean ± standard deviation of triplicate determinants ($n = 3$).

3.2. Molecular Weights Distribution of Polysaccharide Fractions and Their Vibrational Spectra

Agarose gel electrophoresis has previously been used to estimate the weight distributions of anionic polysaccharides [11,12]. The heterogeneous nature of polysaccharides results in a weight distribution rather than a single band. As Figure 2A indicates, the molecular weight distributions of the polysaccharide fractions are gradually reduced in subsequent fractions. The approximate weight distributions were calculated using the Image J software based on the mean values of weight distributions of the molecular weight markers. Accordingly, the mean molecular weights of the fractions, SHC1, SHC2, SHC3 and SHC4, were estimated to be 230, 205, 90 and 60 kDa, respectively. The fingerprint region of the polysaccharide vibrational spectra (wavenumbers 2000–500 cm^{-1}) is depicted in Figure 2B. The peak at 840 cm^{-1} represented C-O-S bending vibrations of axial sulfate substituents on the carbon at the 4 position (C-4) of fucose units. The prominent, broad peak between 1200–970 cm^{-1} occurred from the overlapping of peaks corresponding to C-C and C-O stretching vibrations of pyranoid rings and C-O-C stretching of glycosidic bonds, which are common to all polysaccharides. The major peak between 1220–1270 cm^{-1} and its minor encounter at 585 cm^{-1} were attributed to the O=S=O stretching vibrations of sulfates, which is a characteristic feature of sulfated polysaccharides such as fucoidans. The intense peak at the 1620 cm^{-1} region corresponds to the bending vibration of O-H moieties [13–15].

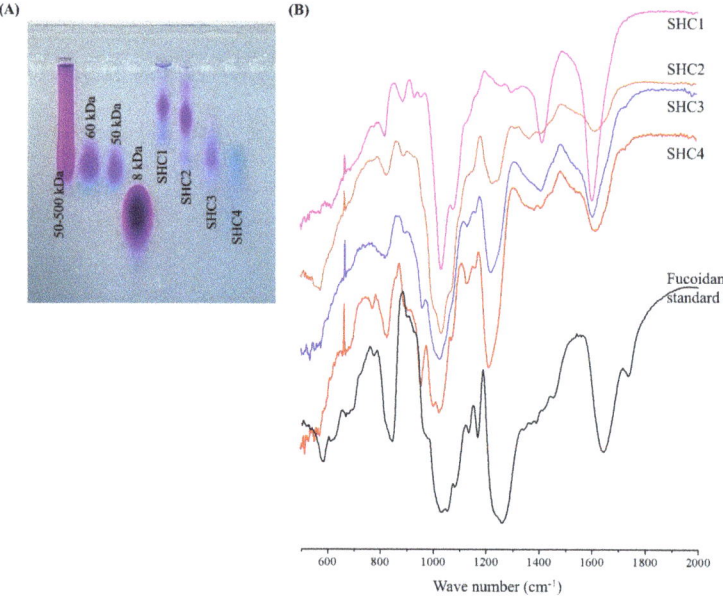

Figure 2. Characterization of polysaccharide fractions (SHC1–SHC4) obtained by step gradient ethanol precipitation. (**A**) Molecular weights (MW) distribution analysis of polysaccharide fractions compared to 50–500-kDa, 60-kDa, 50-kDa and 8-kDa MW standards and (**B**) vibrational spectra of polysaccharide fractions compared to commercial fucoidan standard.

3.3. SHC4 Increased the Protective Effects against UVB-Induced Oxidative Stress

The cytotoxicity of polysaccharide fractions within 25–200 µg mL^{-1} concentrations was examined prior to the evaluation of their bioactivities. None of the fractions indicated a significant decrease in cell proliferation within the tested concentration range (Figure 3A). Hence, the above concentrations were considered safe for the subsequent analysis of UVB protective effects. Based on DCFH2-DA and MTT assays, UVB irradiation significantly increased the intracellular ROS generation and inhibited cell proliferation (Figure 3B). All fucoidan fractions dose-dependently attenuated the effects of UVB irradiation. The best UVB protective effects were observed from the SHC4 fraction (25–100 µg mL^{-1}): it significantly reduced UVB-induced intracellular ROS levels and increased cell proliferation. The 200 µg mL^{-1} concentration of SHC4 deviated from the dose-dependent response observed for the 25–100 µg mL^{-1} concentration range. Due to the increase seen in intracellular ROS levels and the affiliated inhibition of cell viability, the 200 µg mL^{-1} concentration was not used in subsequent analysis. Fluorescence-activated cell sorting (FACS) analysis using the DCFH2-DA fluoroprobe was considered reliable compared to the DCFH2-DA assay as it would omit the error caused by the decrease in fluorescence intensity due to cell death. As Figure 3C indicates, UV irradiation causes the peak to shift to higher intensity (Y-axis—FITC A) compared to the control. The effects were dose-dependently recovered with increasing concentrations of SHC4. Fluorescence microscopy analysis of DCFH2-DA fluoroprobe-treated cells indicated increased green fluorescence for ROS in UV-exposed cells compared to the control (Figure 3D), whereas the fluorescence was dose-dependently decreased with SHC4 treatment. Results of each ROS assay showed a moderate correlation, indicating the antioxidant effects of SHC4.

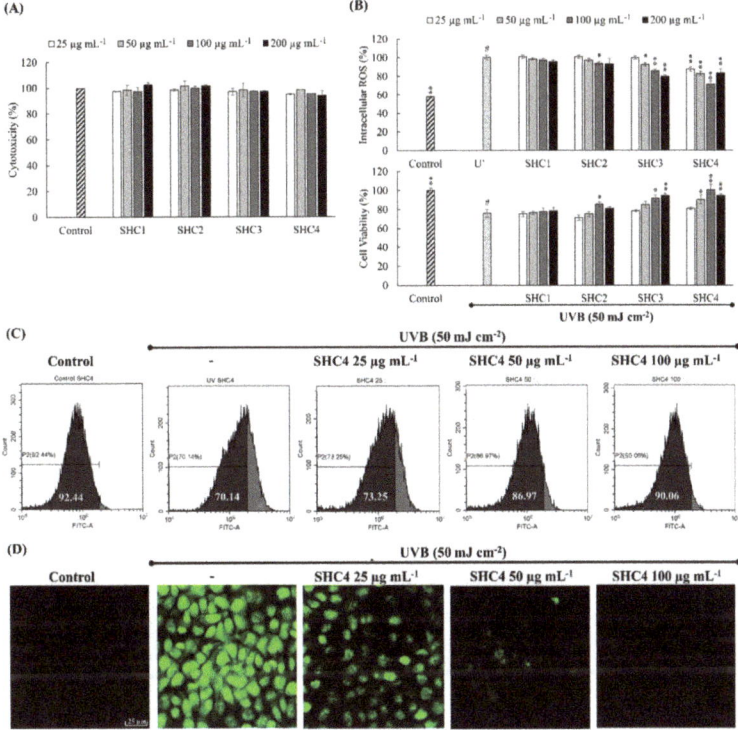

Figure 3. Protective effects of low molecular weight fucoidan fraction (SHC4) against ultraviolet B (UVB)-induced oxidative stress in HaCaT keratinocytes. (**A**) Cytotoxicity dose responses of polysaccharide fractions. (**B**) Analysis of intracellular reactive oxygen species (ROS) levels and cell viability after UVB exposure. Analysis of intracellular ROS levels by (**C**) flow cytometry and (**D**) fluorescence microscopy. HaCaT cells were treated with different doses of polysaccharide fractions for 2 h and exposed to UVB radiation. Measurement of intracellular ROS were performed 1 h after UVB exposure. Data represent the mean ± standard deviation of triplicate determinants ($n = 3$). * $p < 0.05$ and ** $p < 0.01$ are significantly different compared with group indicated by "#".

3.4. Characterization of SHC4 by NMR and Monosaccharide Composition Analysis

Integrated with FTIR spectra, monosaccharide composition analysis and NMR spectra provide reliable evidence to characterize fucoidans. The NMR spectrum of SHC4 (Figure 4A) was obtained with a relatively low resolution, mainly because of the heterogeneous nature of the polymer. However, we were able to identify some characteristic peaks in the spectrum, signifying fucoidans. The intense signals obtained between 1.1–1.2 ppm represented protons of methyl groups in fucopyranose.

Based on previous records, the occurrence of peaks in the 1.1–1.2 ppm area is attributable to an α-L-Fucp-(1→4) connectivity pattern [16]. The proton signals between 2.0–2.2 ppm represent alcoholic protons [16], while signals between 3.5–4.0 ppm were attributed to H2-H6 sugar residues. The prominent signal at 4.6 ppm, 1[H] can be attributed to protons at the anomeric center of 3-linked d-galactopyranosyl residues [16,17]. The signal at 6.25 ppm indicates α-anomeric protons of l-fucopyranosyl units [15]. The obtained results were similar to findings recorded from other brown seaweeds [3,15–17]. HPAEC-PAD analysis of monosaccharide composition (Figure 4B) proposed higher fucose (81.45%) and mannose (8.63%) content, which suggested that SHC4 was a mannofucan.

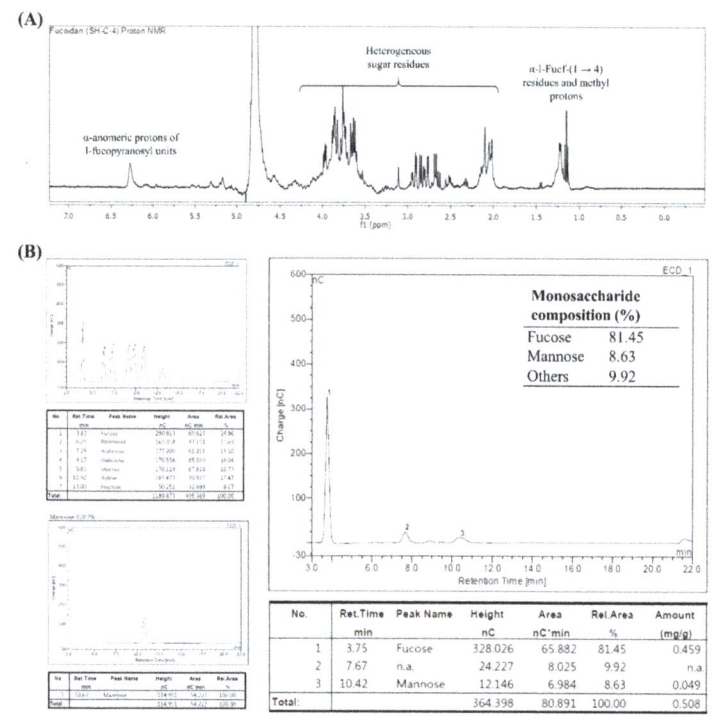

Figure 4. Characterization of fraction SHC4 by nuclear magnetic resonance (NMR) and monosaccharide composition analysis. SHC4 (**A**) ^{1}H NMR spectrum and (**B**) monosaccharide composition analysis.

3.5. SHC4 Reduced UVB-Induced Apoptotic Body Formation and DNA Damage

Cell death due to UVB-induced oxidative stress is reported to proceed via apoptosis [18]. Thus, we assessed apoptotic body formation and DNA damage. Hoechst 33,342 and nuclear double staining with ethidium bromide and acridine orange are the methods of choice for studying nuclear morphology. Hoechst 33,342 binds specifically to DNA, allowing the identification of apoptotic nuclei with DNA fragmentation and chromatin condensation [19]. A prompt increase of chromatin condensation and DNA fragmentation was seen in UVB-stimulated cells compared to the control (Figure 5A). The occurrence of orange-colored nuclear fragments in UVB-exposed cells upon nuclear double staining was indicative of late apoptotic events. SHC4 treatment dose-dependently suppressed the formation of apoptotic bodies, demonstrating its protective effects. According to Figure 5C, the increase in the Sub-G_1 population (23.88%) further indicates UVB-induced apoptosis compared to non-irradiated controls (0.83%). SHC4 treatment dose-dependently reduced the Sub-G_1 population. Additionally, DNA damage was examined by comet assay (Figure 5D). The increased tail DNA content was an indication of UVB-induced DNA damage. SHC4 treatment dose-dependently reduced UVB-induced cell damage.

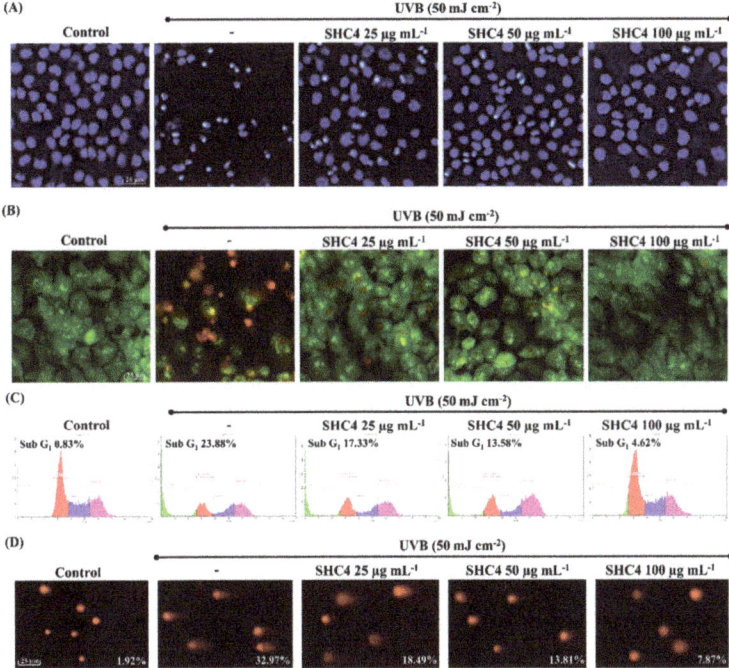

Figure 5. Effects of SHC4 on ultraviolet B (UVB)-induced apoptotic body formation and DNA damage. Nuclear morphology analysis of apoptotic body formation by (**A**) Hoechst 33342 and (**B**) nuclear double staining with ethidium bromide and acridine orange. (**C**) Cell cycle analysis of Sub-G_1 apoptotic cell accumulation. (**D**) Analysis of DNA damage by comet assay. Comet-tail DNA contents were quantified using OpenComet plugin in ImageJ software. HaCaT cells were treated with different doses of polysaccharide fractions for 2 h and exposed to UVB radiation. Cells were harvested for experiments 1 h after UVB exposure. Repeatability of results was validated with three independent determinations ($n = 3$).

3.6. SHC4 Exerted Its Protective Effects against UVB-Induced Oxidative Stress by Inhibiting Mitochondria-Mediated Apoptosis Signaling

The loss of the mitochondrial membrane potential due to pro- and anti-apoptotic Bcl-2 family proteins cause a subsequent discharge of caspase activators inducing apoptosis. The collapse of the mitochondrial inner transmembrane potential ($\Delta\Psi m$) causes the opening of permeability transition pores resulting in an inward flux of water, which causes swelling and disruption of the outer membrane [20]. Based on a flow cytometry JC-1 assay (Figure 6A), a higher proportion of JC-1 aggregates with 530 nm emission (unhealthy mitochondria) were observed in UVB-exposed cells (78.77%), which was analogous to carbonyl cyanide m-chlorophenyl hydrazone (CCCP) treated cells. CCCP is a potent disruptor of the mitochondrial membrane potential. The membrane potential was dose-dependently attenuated following SCOC4 treatment, as evidenced by the increased emission at 590 nm and decreased emission at 530 nm. Key molecular mediators of the mitochondria-mediated apoptosis pathway were studied by western blot analysis (Figure 6B). An immediate increase was observed for BAX, caspases-3 and 9, p53, cleaved P poly (ADP-ribose) polymerase (PARP) and cytochrome C upon UVB-stimulation, whereas the anti-apoptotic proteins, Bcl-xL and Bcl2 levels were decreased. SHC4 dose-dependently attenuated levels of molecular mediators, exhibiting its protective effects. Intracellular antioxidant enzymes, such as heme oxygenase-1 (HO-1), glutathione peroxidase (GPx), catalase (CAT) and superoxide dismutase (SOD) play a crucial role in maintaining the redox balance in cells. Compounds that can upregulate the transcription of the above antioxidant enzymes offer protective effects against oxidative stress, which can lead to apoptosis [21]. According to Figure 6C, UVB exposure slightly increases Nrf2 levels in the nucleus as well as HO-1 levels in the cytosol. SHC4 treatment further induced Nrf2 and HO-1 levels in UVB exposed keratinocytes in a dose-dependent manner.

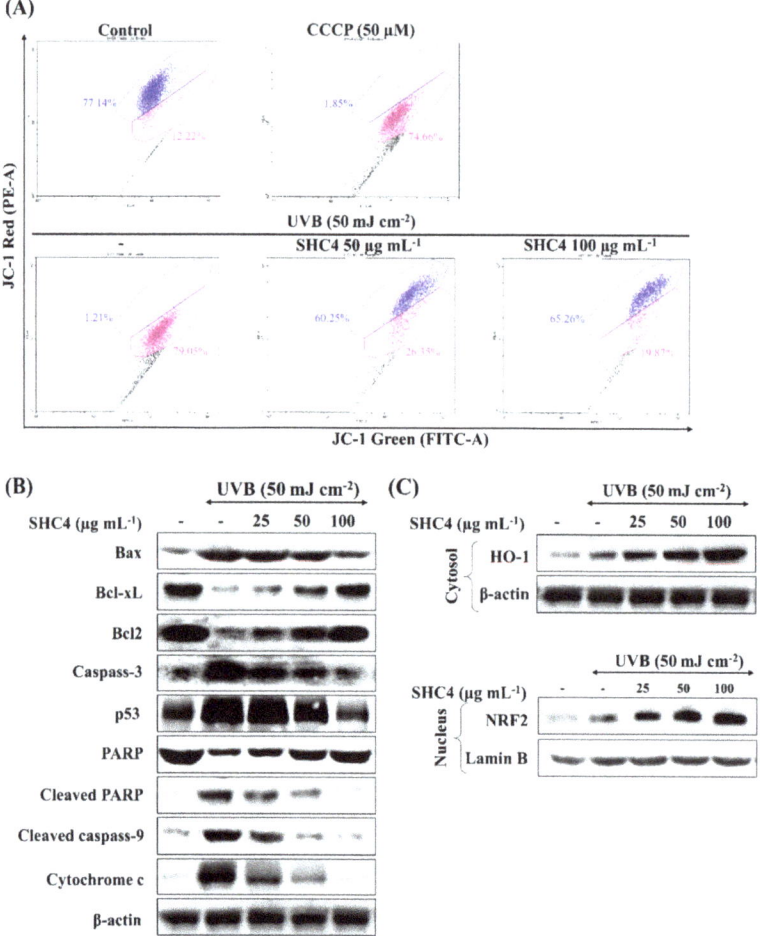

Figure 6. Western blot analysis of the protective effects of SHC4 against UVB-induced apoptosis mediators. Analysis of the UVB protective effects of SHC4 on (**A**) changes in mitochondria inner transmembrane potential by JC-1 assay, (**B**) mediation of mitochondria-mediated apoptotic pathway proteins against UVB-induced apoptosis and (**C**) effects on intracellular antioxidant enzymes. HaCaT cells were treated with different doses of SHC4 for 2 h and exposed to UVB radiation. Cells were, respectively harvested after 4 h and 24 h for the JC-1 assay and western blot analysis. Repeatability of results was validated with three independent determinations (n = 3).

4. Discussion

The edible brown seaweed *Sargassum horneri* has long been acknowledged for its biofunctional effects. It is abundant along the Jeju island coasts in South Korea. Currently, the native *S. horneri* population is threatened by the massive invasion of *S. horneri* from the east coast of China [22]. This not only threatens the coastal ecosystem but also reduces the attraction for tourists. Climate changes have contributed to warmer temperatures and increased rainfall, which increase fertilizer runoff from paddy fields and the aquaculture industry, adding nutrients to coastal areas. The drastic change observed in *S. horneri* growth pattern is an example of how human activities alter the environmental balance. Other than clearing up the coasts, the utilization of *S. horneri* in the food industry and for obtaining functional ingredients such as polyphenols, fucoidan and alginic acid could be an effective and beneficial strategy.

Celluclast is a food-grade cellulase that hydrolyzes cell wall cellulose, resulting in a higher extraction yield of plant materials. The water-based extract under pH 4.5 may contain ions and polar metabolites such as phenols, soluble polysaccharides and proteins. Alternatively, extraction at acidic pH greatly reduces alginate contamination. Based on preliminary investigations, the addition of $CaCl_2$ was not required as the formation of calcium alginate was negligible. Pretreatment with a mixture of chloroform and methanol (1:1) is reported to reduce lipophilic contaminants [23]. The chloroform and methanol (1:1) extract is currently studied for its potential bioactive natural products. Pretreatment with 10% formaldehyde in ethanol is reported to reduce the polyphenolic contamination of polysaccharides [23]. Otherwise, the contamination could lead to unreliable observations when assessing the bioactivities of polysaccharides. Further, washing with 80% ethanol not only removes any remaining formaldehyde but also removes polar compounds, such as phenolic acids. The reduced levels of polyphenol, protein and ash content (a measure of mineral content) in polysaccharide fractions obtained by step gradient ethanol precipitation suggested the efficacy of the reported method. The current pretreatment and extraction strategy was developed based on observations by several previous studies and preliminary analysis [3,11,14,24].

Crude fucoidan is generally obtained by adding a large volume of ethanol to the water-based extract. Subsequent fractionation is done by filtering precipitated polysaccharides through a series of molecular weight cutoff membranes (ultrafiltration) or by chromatography using size exclusion or anion exchange columns [23]. Ultrafiltration and chromatography are not suitable for industrial-scale preparations considering the investment, cost of equipment and operation delays. The step gradient ethanol precipitation method offers convenience over conventional fucoidan purification techniques. However, the technique has not widely been used for fractionating fucoidans except for that in one reported study [7]. The gradient alcohol precipitation method is commonly used in dextran fractionation and less frequently for purifying other polysaccharides such as starch, hemicellulose, glucan, fructan, pectin, arabinan and pullulan [6]. Based on agarose gel electrophoresis, four different fractions with approximate molecular weight distributions of 230, 205, 90 and 60 kDa were successfully obtained using step gradient ethanol precipitation. The high yield of the SHC2 fraction suggested that most fucoidans in *S. horneri* had a molecular weight range of approximately 205 kDa. Furthermore, low molecular weight polysaccharide fractions indicated a higher degree of sulfation. This further relates to the solubility of polysaccharides, where the ionic characteristics of polysaccharides increase with an increased degree of sulfation. Hence, the step gradient ethanol precipitation method could be said to separate fucoidans based on both the molecular weight and solubility.

The structural features of the fucoidan heteropolysaccharide vary considerably depending on seaweed species and environmental conditions. These features include monosaccharide composition, connectivity, chain length, degree of sulfation and connectivity of sulfate groups. Due to its heterogeneous nature, a full-scale analysis of connectivity remains challenging. Based on the present observations, the fractions were identified as fucoidans by FTIR and chemical composition analysis. Though it is not a generally accepted explanation, we propose that fucoidans could be ranked based on their quality, with the major parameters including the amount of fucose and degree of sulfation.

According to many studies, the fucose amount is directly proportional to the degree of sulfation, which suggests that most sulfate groups remain attached to fucose units in fucoidan [3]. The fucoidan fraction that had the most prominent antioxidant effects, SHC4, was found to contain 45.96 ± 0.36% polysaccharides, of which, 81.45% was fucose, which corresponded to 37.43% of the fraction weight with a sulfate content of 28.01 ± 0.50%. ^{1}H NMR data revealed the presence of α-L-Fucp-(1→4) residues, which are a major feature of fucoidans. Hence, we designated SHC4 as a high-quality fucoidan. The lack of data on monosaccharide and sulfate group connectivity patterns is a limitation of the present study. The connectivity "methylation analysis" requires the fucoidan to be further fractionated, obtaining a less heterogeneous polymer mix.

Fucoidan is renowned for its potential antioxidant properties among a wide range of bioactivities [23]. The dose-dependent reduction of intracellular ROS levels in all fractions indicated the protective effect of fucoidans. Considering the slope observed for each fraction dose, the rate of the intracellular ROS reduction increased in succession, with the SHC4 fraction showing the most reduction. This suggested that low molecular weight and high-quality fucoidans had superior antioxidant properties. The increments observed for cell viability suggested that the protective effects of SHC4 were within the 25–100 μg mL^{-1} concentration range. The minor reduction in cell viability at 200 μg mL^{-1} concentration could be associated with toxic effects of sulfated polysaccharides under high concentrations. Further bioassays were conducted to assess the protective effects of SHC4 against UVB-induced oxidative stress and apoptosis. There was a reduction in UVB-induced apoptotic body formation, accumulation of Sub-G$_1$ apoptotic cells and DNA damage, clarifying the potential antioxidant activity of SHC4. Further studies were then performed to understand the effects of SHC4 on the regulation of apoptosis.

The mitochondria-mediated apoptosis pathway is considered a major signaling route mediating apoptosis; the underlying mechanism can vary based on the type of cell, stimulus and other factors. Oxidative stress resulting from multiple factors, including the induction of UVB-radiation is reported to activate the mitochondria-mediated apoptosis pathway [18]. The pathway is initiated with the permeabilization of the mitochondrial outer membrane. The permeabilization is controlled by Bcl-2 family proteins, which includes anti-apoptotic proteins (Bcl-2 and Bcl-xL) and pro-apoptotic proteins (Bax, Bak, Bok, Bad, Bid, Bik, Bim, Bmf, Puma and Noxa). Their primary function is disrupting the functions of the Bcl-2 family proteins, thereby promoting the release of apoptogenic proteins present in the intermembrane space. Released apoptogenic proteins include cytochrome c, apoptosis-inducing factor (AIF) and endonuclease G. Cytochrome c with pro-caspase 9 and apoptosis protease activating factor (APAF-1) form an 'apoptosome'. The apoptosome promotes caspase 9 activation, in turn activating effector caspases, which collectively execute apoptosis. Both AIF and endonuclease G contribute to DNA fragmentation and chromosomal condensation, features that are a hallmark of apoptosis [25]. Apart from the aforementioned mediators, permeabilization of the mitochondrial outer membrane causes the release of numerous proteins that antagonize the activation of caspases. Pro-apoptotic stimuli inducing p53 further aggravate mitochondrial pathway-mediated apoptosis. p53 plays a crucial role in ultraviolet-induced apoptosis in HaCaT keratinocytes [26]. Under physiological conditions, p53 is maintained at a low concentration, inhibiting its transcriptional activity. Activation and post-translational stabilization of p53 drives the expression of pro-apoptotic factors, provoking death pathways. Caspases, consisting of initiator and effector caspases, are proteases that mediate cell death. Initiator caspases, such as caspase-9, activate death receptors, whereas effector caspases directly mediate the cleavage of numerous cytoplasmic and nuclear substrates. Cytochrome c activates caspase-9 and subsequently activates downstream effector caspases such as caspase-3, −6 and −7 [9]. The cleavage of PARP, a nuclear enzyme that maintains DNA stability, repair and transcription, is another crucial feature of apoptosis. Effector caspases cause the cleavage of PARP, thereby inhibiting its catalytic activity [9]. The present observations clarified the effect of UVB on the initiation of mitochondria-mediated apoptosis proteins and the dose-dependent attenuation effects of SHC4. There could be numerous alternative pathways, other than the prominent mitochondria-mediated apoptosis that regulate oxidative stress-induced cell death. Hence, further studies could broaden the understanding of the effects of fucoidan on UVB-induced apoptosis.

Based on previous studies, fucoidans are reported to upregulate gene expression of HO-1 and SOD-1 in HaCaT keratinocytes via upregulating the transcription factor Nrf2 [21]. Similar results were observed during the present analysis, where SHC4 treatment caused a dose-dependent increase of HO-1 production in the cytosol and Nrf2 levels in the nucleus. This suggested that the protective effects of fucoidan against UVB-induced oxidative stress were mediated by Nrf2/HO-1 signaling.

5. Conclusions

Based on the present analysis, step gradient ethanol precipitation was identified as a desirable approach to obtain fucoidan fractions with different molecular weight distributions. The fucoidan fraction with a mean molecular weight of 60 kDa from *S. horneri* was mainly composed of α-L-Fucp-(1→4) linked fucose units with 37.43% fucose content and a 28.01 ± 0.50% sulfate content. The above fucoidan fraction, SHC4, demonstrated significant protective effects against UVB-induced photodamage in dermic keratinocytes by enhancing intracellular antioxidant defense. In the future, SHC4 could be studied for developing cosmetics with UV protective effects.

Author Contributions: Conceptualization, I.P.S.F. and G.A.; Methodology, I.P.S.F.; Software, I.P.S.F.; Validation, I.P.S.F., E.J.H. and M.J.K.; Formal analysis, I.P.S.F.; Investigation, I.P.S.F., D.M.D.M. and M.K.H.M.D.; Resources, G.A., K.L., Y.S.H. and Y.-J.J.; Data curation, E.J.H. and M.J.K.; Writing—Original draft preparation, I.P.S.F.; Writing—Review and editing, G.A.; Visualization, D.M.D.M. and M.K.H.M.D.; Supervision, G.A.; Project administration, S.H.C., S.R.P. and G.A.; Funding acquisition, S.H.C., S.R.P. and G.A. All authors have read and agreed to the published version of the manuscript.

Funding: This work (Grants No. M01201920180359) was supported by the Korea Institute of Marine Science & Technology Promotion (KIMST).

Conflicts of Interest: The authors declare no conflict of interest.

References

1. Wang, L.; Kim, H.S.; Oh, J.Y.; Je, J.G.; Jeon, Y.-J.; Ryu, B. Protective effect of diphlorethohydroxycarmalol isolated from ishige okamurae against uvb-induced damage in vitro in human dermal fibroblasts and in vivo in zebrafish. *Food Chem. Toxicol.* **2019**, *136*, 110963. [CrossRef] [PubMed]
2. Athukorala, Y.; Jung, W.-K.; Vasanthan, T.; Jeon, Y.-J. An anticoagulative polysaccharide from an enzymatic hydrolysate of ecklonia cava. *Carbohydr. Polym.* **2006**, *66*, 184–191. [CrossRef]
3. Fernando, I.P.S.; Sanjeewa, K.K.A.; Samarakoon, K.W.; Lee, W.W.; Kim, H.-S.; Kang, N.; Ranasinghe, P.; Lee, H.-S.; Jeon, Y.-J. A fucoidan fraction purified from chnoospora minima; a potential inhibitor of lps-induced inflammatory responses. *Int. J. Biol. Macromol.* **2017**, *104*, 1185–1193. [CrossRef] [PubMed]
4. Fernando, I.P.S.; Kim, K.-N.; Kim, D.; Jeon, Y.-J. Algal polysaccharides: Potential bioactive substances for cosmeceutical applications. *Crit. Rev. Biotechnol.* **2018**, *39*, 99–113. [CrossRef]
5. Heo, S.-J.; Park, P.-J.; Park, E.-J.; Kim, S.-K.; Jeon, Y.-J. Antioxidant activity of enzymatic extracts from a brown seaweed ecklonia cava by electron spin resonance spectrometry and comet assay. *Eur. Food Res. Technol.* **2005**, *221*, 41–47. [CrossRef]
6. Hu, X.; Goff, H.D. Fractionation of polysaccharides by gradient non-solvent precipitation: A review. *Trends Food Sci. Technol.* **2018**, *81*, 108–115. [CrossRef]
7. Xin, L.; Bin, L.; Xiao-Lei, W.; Zhen-Liang, S.; Chang-Yun, W. Extraction, fractionation, and chemical characterisation of fucoidans from the brown seaweed sargassum pallidum. *Czech J. Food Sci.* **2016**, *34*, 406–413. [CrossRef]
8. Fernando, I.P.S.; Jayawardena, T.U.; Kim, H.-S.; Vaas, A.P.J.P.; De Silva, H.I.C.; Nanayakkara, C.M.; Abeytunga, D.T.U.; Lee, W.; Ahn, G.; Lee, D.-S.; et al. A keratinocyte and integrated fibroblast culture model for studying particulate matter-induced skin lesions and therapeutic intervention of fucosterol. *Life Sci.* **2019**, *233*, 116714. [CrossRef]

9. Fernando, I.P.S.; Sanjeewa, K.K.A.; Ann, Y.-S.; Ko, C.-I.; Lee, S.-H.; Lee, W.W.; Jeon, Y.-J. Apoptotic and antiproliferative effects of stigmast-5-en-3-ol from dendronephthya gigantea on human leukemia hl-60 and human breast cancer mcf-7 cells. *Toxicol. In Vitro* **2018**, *52*, 297–305. [CrossRef]
10. Park, S.Y.; Fernando, I.P.S.; Han, E.J.; Kim, M.J.; Jung, K.; Kang, D.S.; Ahn, C.B.; Ahn, G. In vivo hepatoprotective effects of a peptide fraction from krill protein hydrolysates against alcohol-induced oxidative damage. *Mar. Drugs* **2019**, *17*, 690. [CrossRef]
11. Fernando, I.P.S.; Sanjeewa, K.K.A.; Samarakoon, K.W.; Kim, H.-S.; Gunasekara, U.K.D.S.S.; Park, Y.-J.; Abeytunga, D.T.U.; Lee, W.W.; Jeon, Y.-J. The potential of fucoidans from chnoospora minima and sargassum polycystum in cosmetics: Antioxidant, anti-inflammatory, skin-whitening, and antiwrinkle activities. *J. Appl. Phycol.* **2018**, *30*, 3223–3232. [CrossRef]
12. Fernando, I.P.S.; Jayawardena, T.U.; Sanjeewa, K.K.A.; Wang, L.; Jeon, Y.-J.; Lee, W.W. Anti-inflammatory potential of alginic acid from sargassum horneri against urban aerosol-induced inflammatory responses in keratinocytes and macrophages. *Ecotoxicol. Environ. Saf.* **2018**, *160*, 24–31. [CrossRef] [PubMed]
13. Jayawardena, T.U.; Fernando, I.S.; Lee, W.W.; Sanjeewa, K.A.; Kim, H.-S.; Lee, D.-S.; Jeon, Y.-J. Isolation and purification of fucoidan fraction in turbinaria ornata from the maldives; inflammation inhibitory potential under lps stimulated conditions in in-vitro and in-vivo models. *Int. J. Biol. Macromol.* **2019**, *131*, 614–623. [CrossRef] [PubMed]
14. Fernando, I.P.S.; Sanjeewa, K.K.A.; Samarakoon, K.W.; Lee, W.W.; Kim, H.-S.; Kim, E.-A.; Gunasekara, U.K.D.S.S.; Abeytunga, D.T.U.; Nanayakkara, C.; Silva, E.D.d.; et al. Ftir characterization and antioxidant activity of water soluble crude polysaccharides of sri lankan marine algae. *Algae* **2017**, *32*, 75–86. [CrossRef]
15. Vinoth Kumar, T.; Lakshmanasenthil, S.; Geetharamani, D.; Marudhupandi, T.; Suja, G.; Suganya, P. Fucoidan—A α-d-glucosidase inhibitor from sargassum wightii with relevance to type 2 diabetes mellitus therapy. *Int. J. Biol. Macromol.* **2015**, *72*, 1044–1047. [CrossRef] [PubMed]
16. Palanisamy, S.; Vinosha, M.; Marudhupandi, T.; Rajasekar, P.; Prabhu, N.M. In vitro antioxidant and antibacterial activity of sulfated polysaccharides isolated from spatoglossum asperum. *Carbohydr. Polym.* **2017**, *170*, 296–304. [CrossRef]
17. Palanisamy, S.; Vinosha, M.; Marudhupandi, T.; Rajasekar, P.; Prabhu, N.M. Isolation of fucoidan from sargassum polycystum brown algae: Structural characterization, in vitro antioxidant and anticancer activity. *Int. J. Biol. Macromol.* **2017**, *102*, 405–412. [CrossRef]
18. Baek, J.Y.; Park, S.; Park, J.; Jang, J.Y.; Wang, S.B.; Kim, S.R.; Woo, H.A.; Lim, K.M.; Chang, T.-S. Protective role of mitochondrial peroxiredoxin iii against uvb-induced apoptosis of epidermal keratinocytes. *J. Investig. Dermatol.* **2017**, *137*, 1333–1342. [CrossRef]
19. Kijima, M.; Mizuta, R. Histone h1 quantity determines the efficiencies of apoptotic DNA fragmentation and chromatin condensation. *Biomed. Res.* **2019**, *40*, 51–56. [CrossRef]
20. Green, D.R.; Reed, J.C. Mitochondria and apoptosis. *Science.* **1998**, *281*, 1309–1312. [CrossRef]
21. Ryu, M.J.; Chung, H.S. Fucoidan reduces oxidative stress by regulating the gene expression of ho1 and sod1 through the nrf2/erk signaling pathway in hacat cells. *Mol. Med. Rep.* **2016**, *14*, 3255–3260. [CrossRef] [PubMed]
22. Kim, H.-S.; Sanjeewa, K.; Fernando, I.; Ryu, B.; Yang, H.-W.; Ahn, G.; Kang, M.C.; Heo, S.-J.; Je, J.-G.; Jeon, Y.-J. A comparative study of sargassum horneri korea and china strains collected along the coast of jeju island south korea: Its components and bioactive properties. *Algae* **2018**, *33*, 341–349. [CrossRef]
23. Fernando, I.P.S.; Kim, D.; Nah, J.-W.; Jeon, Y.-J. Advances in functionalizing fucoidans and alginates (bio)polymers by structural modifications: A review. *Chem. Eng. J.* **2019**, *355*, 33–48. [CrossRef]
24. Sanjeewa, K.K.A.; Fernando, I.P.S.; Kim, E.-A.; Ahn, G.; Jee, Y.; Jeon, Y.-J. Anti-inflammatory activity of a sulfated polysaccharide isolated from an enzymatic digest of brown seaweed sargassum horneri in raw 264.7 cells. *Nutr. Res. Pract.* **2017**, *11*, 3. [CrossRef] [PubMed]

25. Gupta, S. Molecular signaling in death receptor and mitochondrial pathways of apoptosis. *Int. J. Oncol.* **2003**, *22*, 15–20. [CrossRef]
26. Henseleit, U.; Zhang, J.; Wanner, R.; Haase, I.; Kolde, G.; Rosenbach, T. Role of p53 in uvb-induced apoptosis in human hacat keratinocytes. *J. Investig. Dermatol.* **1997**, *109*, 722–727. [CrossRef]

© 2020 by the authors. Licensee MDPI, Basel, Switzerland. This article is an open access article distributed under the terms and conditions of the Creative Commons Attribution (CC BY) license (http://creativecommons.org/licenses/by/4.0/).

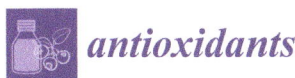

Article

Computational Study of *Ortho*-Substituent Effects on Antioxidant Activities of Phenolic Dendritic Antioxidants

Choon Young Lee [1],*, Ajit Sharma [1], Julius Semenya [1], Charles Anamoah [1], Kelli N. Chapman [1] and Veronica Barone [2],*

[1] Department of Chemistry and Biochemistry, Central Michigan University, Mount Pleasant, MI 48859, USA; sharm1a@cmich.edu (A.S.); semen1j@cmich.edu (J.S.); anamo1c@cmich.edu (C.A.); chapm1kn@cmich.edu (K.N.C.)
[2] Department of Physics and Science of Advanced Materials Program, Central Michigan University, Mount Pleasant, MI 48859, USA
* Correspondence: lee1cy@cmich.edu (C.Y.L.); baron1v@cmich.edu (V.B.)

Received: 7 February 2020; Accepted: 19 February 2020; Published: 25 February 2020

Abstract: Antioxidants are an important component of our ability to combat free radicals, an excess of which leads to oxidative stress that is related to aging and numerous human diseases. Oxidative damage also shortens the shelf-life of foods and other commodities. Understanding the structure–activity relationship of antioxidants and their mechanisms of action is important for designing more potent antioxidants for potential use as therapeutic agents as well as preservatives. We report the first computational study on the electronic effects of *ortho*-substituents in dendritic tri-phenolic antioxidants, comprising a common phenol moiety and two other phenol units with electron-donating or electron-withdrawing substituents. Among the three proposed antioxidant mechanisms, sequential proton loss electron transfer (SPLET) was found to be the preferred mechanism in methanol for the dendritic antioxidants based on calculations using Gaussian 16. We then computed the total enthalpy values by cumulatively running SPLET for all three rings to estimate electronic effects of substituents on overall antioxidant activity of each dendritic antioxidant and establish their structure–activity relationships. Our results show that the electron-donating o-OCH_3 group has a beneficial effect while the electron-withdrawing o-NO_2 group has a negative effect on the antioxidant activity of the dendritic antioxidant. The o-Br and o-Cl groups did not show any appreciable effects. These results indicate that electron-donating groups such as o-methoxy are useful for designing potent dendritic antioxidants while the nitro and halogens do not add value to the radical scavenging antioxidant activity. We also found that the half-maximal inhibitory concentration (IC50) values of 2,2-diphenyl-1-picrylhydrazyl (DPPH) better correlate with the second step (electron transfer enthalpy, ETE) than the first step (proton affinity, PA) of the SPLET mechanism, implying that ETE is the better measure for estimating overall radical scavenging antioxidant activities.

Keywords: antioxidant; dendrimer; electronic effect; hydrogen atom transfer (HAT); single electron transfer-proton transfer (SET-PT); sequential proton loss electron transfer (SPLET); DPPH

1. Introduction

The use of antioxidants to combat oxidative damage caused by excess free radicals is important for food, medical, cosmetics and other industries. Hence, synthesis of new potent antioxidants to tackle specific oxidative problems in these areas is very much needed. Phenolic antioxidants have attracted much attention in recent years, since many natural antioxidants contain the phenolic moiety.

Recently, we reported a new class of phenolic antioxidants that we called dendritic antioxidants. Syringaldehyde and vanillin, very weak natural antioxidants, were used as building blocks to assemble potent phenolic antioxidant dendrimers with half-maximal inhibitory concentration (IC50) values significantly smaller than the building blocks. For example, dendrimers with 4, 6 and 8 syringol units had 27-, 100-, and 170-fold higher scavenging activities, respectively, than the syringaldehyde building block [1–3]. Besides enhancing radical scavenging, the dendritic architecture allowed metal chelation, thereby preventing potentially deleterious pro-oxidant effects of the antioxidants. We have also previously shown the ability of these dendritic antioxidants to protect biomolecules such as DNA and low-density lipoproteins from radical damage. Dendritic antioxidants offer several advantages similar to dendrimers. For example, their size, solubility, chelation ability, and antioxidant activity may be precisely manipulated by using appropriate cores and building blocks. Therefore, understanding the structure–activity relationship of dendritic antioxidants and their mechanism of action is paramount.

Substituents, such as electron-donating groups (EDGs) and electron-withdrawing groups (EWGs) on the phenol ring significantly affect the antioxidant activity of a phenolic antioxidant [3–5]. Several computational and experimental studies suggest that EDGs (e.g., OH, NH_2, OCH_3, CH_3) decrease O–H bond dissociation enthalpy (BDE) of the phenol, which implies increased antioxidant activity [6–10]. On the other hand, EWGs showed varying results. Some computational studies reveal that EWGs, such as NO_2, CN, CF_3, F, Cl, and Br increase BDE of the phenol (lower antioxidant activity) [9,10]. However, experimental studies on halogens report different activities depending on the position relative to the phenol OH or the number of halogen substituents. For example, 6-chromanol with di-o-Cl substitution showed lower galvinoxyl radical scavenging activity but better than mono-o-Cl and tri-Cl substitution (two o-Cl groups and one m-Cl) compared to the unsubstituted 6-chromanol [5]. Hydroxycinnamic acids with mono-o-Br showed no effect in 2,2-diphenyl-1-picrylhydrazyl (DPPH) radical scavenging activity [4].

Antioxidant action for free radical scavenging can occur in several different ways, but the ultimate outcome is the donation of a hydrogen atom (H•) to the radical. The hydrogen atom transfer can occur in multiple different ways. It can be (1) direct H• atom transfer to radicals, (2) electron transfer, followed by H^+ loss, or (3) proton loss, followed by electron transfer. The proposed mechanism for (1) is the hydrogen atom transfer (HAT) mechanism in which the hydrogen atom (H•) is transferred from the phenolic OH to the radical. In the HAT mechanism, the BDE is the most important parameter in estimating the antioxidant activity. The mechanism for (2) is the single electron transfer-proton transfer (SET-PT), in which an electron is first transferred from PhOH to the radical. The PhOH then becomes a phenoxy radical cation (PhOH•$^+$), which in turn deprotonates during the second step to form a phenoxy radical (PhO•). In the SET-PT mechanism, the radical transfer in the 1st step is measured as the ionization potential (IP) and the deprotonation in the 2nd step corresponds to the proton dissociation enthalpy (PDE). The proposed mechanism for (3) is the sequential proton loss electron transfer (SPLET), which also proceeds via two steps. The 1st step involves the deprotonation of PhOH, forming a phenoxide ion (PhO$^-$). Subsequently, the PhO$^-$ ion transfers an electron to the radical and becomes a phenoxy radical (PhO•). The enthalpy of the 1st step is denoted as the proton affinity (PA) and the 2nd step corresponds to the electron transfer enthalpy (ETE). HAT has been reported to be the most favorable antioxidant mechanism in non-polar solvents or in gas phase, while SET-PT and SPLET are the more prevalent mechanisms in polar solvents [9–15]

Computational studies of the electronic effects on dendritic antioxidants with multiple free radical scavenging sites have not been reported before. In order to study the effects of EDGs and EWGs on dendritic antioxidants, we performed computational studies using the Density Functional Theory (DFT) calculations for a series of small phenol-based dendritic antioxidants (in methanol), each containing either an EDG or an EWG that is $ortho$ to the phenolic OH group.

2. Materials and Methods

All calculations were performed using Gaussian 16 [16]. Geometry optimizations as well as frequency calculations were obtained using the B3LYP functional and the 6-311++G** basis set. Several conformations were used as initial structures to find the minimum energy conformation due to the flexibility of the studied compounds. All structures have been relaxed without symmetry constraints until maximum forces and displacements were smaller than 4.5×10^{-4} Hartree/Bohr and 1.8×10^{-3} Bohr, respectively. The requested convergence of the root mean square (RMS) variation of the density matrix elements and the total energy per cell in the self-consistent field procedure is 10^{-8} a.u. and 10^{-6} Hartree, respectively. To model the solvent effect of methanol, the Polarizable Continuum Model/Solvation Model Density (PCM/SMD) from Truhlar et al. was used in all calculations, including geometry optimizations [17].

For the different mechanisms studied here, the enthalpies are defined as follows:

1. Bond Dissociation Enthalpy: $H(PhO\bullet) + H(H\bullet) - H(PhOH)$
2. Ionization Potential: $H(PhOH\bullet^+) + H(e^-) - H(PhOH)$
3. Proton Dissociation Enthalpy: $H(PhO\bullet) + H(H^+) - H(PhOH\bullet^+)$
4. Proton Affinity: $H(PhO^-) + H(H^+) - H(PhOH)$
5. Electron Transfer Enthalpy: $H(PhO\bullet) + H(e^-) - H(PhO^-)$

From these definitions, it becomes clear that in order to find the total enthalpies of each mechanism we need the enthalpies for the electron, proton, and the H atom in methanol. As reported before, the solvation enthalpy of the H atom in most organic solvents is about 5 kJ/mol and we therefore adopted this value for methanol [17]. Methanol solvation enthalpies of the proton (−1071 kJ/mol) and the electron (−77 kJ/mol) have been calculated here at the same level of theory as the main compounds (B3LYP/6-311++G**). These values are obtained by performing the calculation of a methanol molecule in methanol (PCM/SMD model) and then the methanol molecule after addition of a proton (or addition of an electron) in methanol (PCM/SMD model) as indicated by:

6. Proton solvation enthalpy: $H(H^+(CH_3OH)(methanol)) - H(H^+(gas)) - H((CH_3OH)(methanol))$
7. Electron solvation enthalpy: $H(CH_3OH^-(methanol)) - H(e^-(gas)) - H(CH_3OH(methanol))$

where the enthalpy of a proton in the gas phase is taken as $\frac{5}{2}RT$.

3. Results and Discussion

3.1. Geometry Optimization

For each compound in Figure 1, we performed geometry optimizations. Structural relaxation of all compounds was carried out to find their minimum energy conformation as detailed under Materials and Methods. Our calculations indicate that in the optimized lowest energy conformation, the three phenol rings of each dendritic antioxidant were almost perpendicular to each other, indicating the absence of π-π stacking interaction between the phenol rings and no steric hindrance between the *ortho*-substituents.

The *o*-OCH$_3$ group of the common phenol ring (in the reference and compounds 1–5) was oriented in the same plane as the aromatic ring. It has been reported that in such an orientation, the 2p-type lone pair of electrons on the oxygen is parallel to the aromatic p-orbitals, thereby efficiently overlapping the aromatic π-electron cloud of PhOH [18]. This orientation stabilizes the incipient phenoxy radical (PhO•) and weakens the OH bond of PhOH [18]. The methyl of the OCH$_3$ groups orients away from the OH group and the H of the phenol-OH points towards the oxygen of *o*-OCH$_3$, forming an intramolecular hydrogen bond. If there are two OCH$_3$ groups *ortho* to the phenolic OH (such as in compound 2), both groups are in the same plane as the phenol ring with the methyl groups orienting away from the OH. It was also observed that *o*-NO$_2$, *o*-Br, and *o*-Cl groups formed an H-bond with the H of phenolic OH in the energy-minimized conformation.

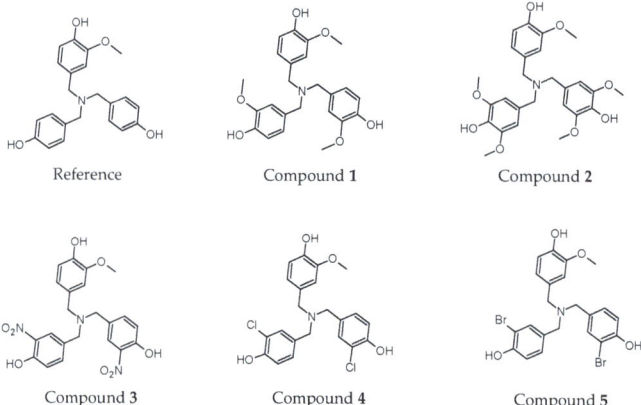

Figure 1. Structures of reference and target compounds 1–5.

3.2. Enthalpy Calculations

To the best of our knowledge, this is the first computational study on the mechanism of action of dendritic antioxidants with multiple free radical scavenging sites.

We determined the enthalpy for each individual ring present on the dendritic antioxidants. To distinguish the enthalpy of each phenol O–H in the target compounds, X, X' and Y notations were used (Figure 2). X and X' represent equivalent phenol rings with either an EDG or EWG *ortho* to the phenolic OH. Y denotes the common ring with one *o*-OCH$_3$ group.

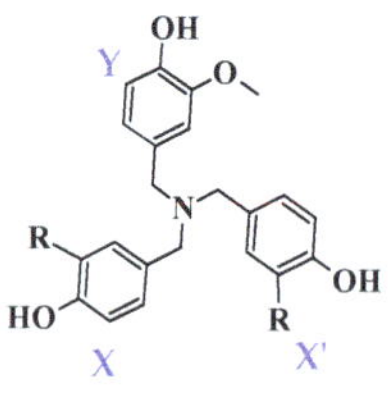

Figure 2. General structure of the compounds and notation (X, X' and Y) for the phenol rings. R = H, electron-donating or electron-withdrawing group.

In this study, only compound **2** contains PhOH with two *ortho* substituents (OCH$_3$). The enthalpy of **2** can be affected by not only electronic but also steric effects. The additional OCH$_3$ group might help stabilize the incipient phenoxy radical electronically but might also confer a slight negative impact via steric effect. Since all other compounds have only one *ortho* substituent on each ring, a direct comparison of compound **2** with others might not be fair, but to get further insights into the effect of multiple electron-donating groups on antioxidant activity, we decided to design the compound and calculate its enthalpy nonetheless.

In most computational studies involving the electronic effects of substituents on antioxidant activities, the 1st step of each proposed mechanism, BDE (HAT), IP (1st step of SET-PT), and PA (1st step of SPLET), was reported to be the thermodynamically significant [9–11]. In some cases, the 2nd step of SET-PT and SPLET is not even calculated. To understand the antioxidant mechanisms (in methanol) more thoroughly, we calculated the enthalpy of the energy minimized structure of each dendritic molecule for all steps in the three proposed mechanisms (HAT, SET-PT, and SPLET) at the B3LYP/6-311G** level of theory. For the HAT mechanism (Table 1), we calculated the enthalpy for each ring independently as if only one ring in the molecule reacted with the radical: three values in the first column, one for the common phenol ring with *o*-OCH$_3$ (Y) and the other two for the two equivalent phenol rings (X, X′) where R is either an o-EDG or o-EWG. In the second column of each compound, the enthalpy values for the two equivalent phenol rings (X, X′) were averaged. In the case of SET-PT, only one value is given for each step for each compound (Table 2) since the loss of an electron is a global property and will most likely occur at the phenol ring with the highest electron density in an antioxidant with multiple phenol OH groups. For SPLET (Tables 3 and 4), we present three values in the first column and two in the second column as we did for HAT (calculated raw data is shown in Table S1 in Supplementary Information).

Table 1. Calculated O–H bond dissociation enthalpy (BDE) values (kJ/mol) of the phenol rings (X, X′, and Y) in methanol.

Compound	Reference (H)		Compound 1 (one OCH$_3$)		Compound 2 (two OCH$_3$)		Compound 3 (NO$_2$)		Compound 4 (Cl)		Compound 5 (Br)	
Phenol ring	BDE	<BDE>	BDE	<BDE>	BDE	<BDE>	BDE	<BDE>	BDE	<BDE>	BDE	<BDE>
X	345	345	328	329	311	311	379	377	342	342	342	342
X′	345		329		311		375		342		341	
Y	328	328	330		329	329	330	330	329	329	330	330

Table 2. Calculated ionization potential (IP) and proton dissociation enthalpy (PDE) values (kJ/mol) in methanol.

Compound	Reference (H)	Compound 1 (one OCH$_3$)	Compound 2 (two OCH$_3$)	Compound 3 (NO$_2$)	Compound 4 (Cl)	Compound 5 (Br)
IP	430	427	440	448	439	437
PDE	57 (Y) [a]	60	30 (X/X′) [a]	41 (Y) [a]	50 (Y) [a]	51 (Y) [a]

[a] In parenthesis, we indicated the ring where the proton dissociation occurs.

Table 3. Calculated proton affinity (PA) values (kJ/mol) of the phenol rings (X, X′ and Y) in methanol.

Compound	Reference (H)		Compound 1 (one OCH$_3$)		Compound 2 (two OCH$_3$)		Compound 3 (NO$_2$)		Compound 4 (Cl)		Compound 5 (Br)	
Phenol ring	PA	<PA>	PA	<PA>	PA	<PA>	PA	<PA>	PA	<PA>	PA	<PA>
X	150	150	153	154	151	151	116	117	132	132	136	136
X′	150		155		151		119		132		137	
Y	152	152	154		152	152	152	152	152	152	152	152

Table 4. Calculated electron transfer enthalpy (ETE) values (kJ/mol) of the phenol rings (X, X′ and Y) in methanol.

Compound	Reference (H)		Compound 1 (one OCH$_3$)		Compound 2 (two OCH$_3$)		Compound 3 (NO$_2$)		Compound 4 (Cl)		Compound 5 (Br)	
Phenol ring	ETE	<ETE>	ETE	<ETE>	ETE	<ETE>	ETE	<ETE>	ETE	<ETE>	ETE	<ETE>
X	355	354	333	334	319	319	422	419	370	369	364	364
X′	354		333		319		415		368		364	
Y	335	335	334		336	336	337	337	336	336	337	337

3.2.1. HAT Mechanism

In MeOH, o-OCH$_3$ (EDG) decreased BDE$_{O-H}$ whereas o-NO$_2$ (EWG) increased BDE$_{O-H}$. Ortho-halogens (Cl and Br) showed similar BDE$_{O-H}$ compared to the unsubstituted reference (Table 1).

3.2.2. SET-PT Mechanism

The IP values of all compounds (except for **2**) are most likely derived from their common phenol ring (Y) with one o-OCH$_3$ because the ring has the highest electron density. In the case of compound **2**, its IP value could be derived from either of the two phenol rings (with two o-OCH$_3$) since they are electron richer than the phenol ring with one o-OCH$_3$.

Unexpectedly, compound **2** showed higher IP and lower PDE values than the reference and compound **1** (Table 2). Since **2** is the only one with two *o*-substituents, direct comparison with others might be misleading. Without considering compound **2**, *o*-OCH$_3$ (EDG) decreased IP whereas EWGs (*o*-NO$_2$, *o*-Cl, and *o*-Br) increased IP. The *ortho*-OCH$_3$ group increased PDE whereas the *o*-NO$_2$, *o*-Cl, and *o*-Br groups decreased PDE compared to the reference. It should be noted that the differences in IP and PDE values between the compounds are very small, implying they might be derived from the same ring, probably Y.

3.2.3. SPLET Mechanism

Our results show that *o*-OCH$_3$ (EDG) slightly increased PA whereas *o*-NO$_2$ (EWG) significantly decreased PA (Table 3). *Ortho*-OCH$_3$ decreased ETE considerably while *o*-NO$_2$ increased ETE substantially compared to the reference (Table 4). *Ortho*-halogens (*o*-Cl and *o*-Br) exhibited slightly lower PA and slightly higher ETE values compared to the unsubstituted reference.

3.3. Thermodynamically Favorable Antioxidant Mechanism for Dendritic Antioxidants

Thermodynamically favorable processes should be determined by calculating the change in the free energy of a reaction (ΔG). The entropy component (−TΔS) in the proposed mechanisms is negligible, meaning that ΔG largely depends on the enthalpy (ΔH). Therefore, it is reasonable to determine the most preferred mechanism from enthalpy values [9,11].

In methanol, the SET-PT is clearly the least favored mechanism due to the large enthalpy of the first step. The SPLET mechanism has an overall low enthalpy in the first step but the enthalpy of the second step is comparable to the BDE in the HAT mechanism. However, the second step in SPLET is not isolated and occurs simultaneously with the reduction of the radical (in this case DPPH•) (reaction 2a + 2b in Scheme 1) as stated in the original papers that introduced the SPLET mechanism [13,19]. The authors state that based on studies between phenolic antioxidant and the DPPH radical in hydroxylic solvents like methanol or ethanol, the deprotonation step (1st step of SPLET) is equilibrium (reaction 1 in Scheme 1) and electron transfer from PhO$^-$ to the DPPH radical is fast (reaction 2a + 2b in Scheme 1) [13,14,19]. Many studies consider the first step as thermodynamically significant, perhaps based on these reports, and thus the enthalpy of only the 1st step is used to determine the major operating mechanism or in assessing the antioxidant potential. However, we wish to include the role of the DPPH radical in determining the major antioxidant mechanism. If we consider the electron transfer from PhO$^-$ (reaction 2a, Scheme 1) to the DPPH radical (reaction 2b, Scheme 1) to be concurrently occurring in the second step, the overall enthalpy of the second step can be reduced by −303 kJ/mol (reaction 2b), thus significantly favoring the SPLET mechanism over HAT in methanol. We note that the enthalpy for DPPH reduction was obtained at the same level of theory as all other calculations following reaction 2b (Scheme 1).

$$\text{PhOH} \rightleftharpoons \text{PhO}^- + \text{H}^+ \quad (\text{PA, 1st step}) \quad \text{------------------------} \quad (1)$$

$$\text{PhO}^- \longrightarrow \text{PhO}\bullet + e^- \quad (\text{ETE, 2nd step}) \quad \text{----------------------} \quad (2a)$$

$$\text{DPPH}\bullet + e^- \longrightarrow \text{DPPH}^- \quad (\Delta H_{\text{DPPH}\bullet} = -303 \text{ kJ/mol}) \quad \text{----------------} \quad (2b)$$

$$\text{PhO}^- + \text{DPPH}\bullet \xrightarrow{\text{Fast}} \text{PhO}\bullet + \text{DPPH}^- \quad (\text{net ETE}) \quad \text{------------------} \quad (2a + 2b)$$

Scheme 1. Reaction between antioxidant (PhOH) and the DPPH radical via the SPLET mechanism.

Our computational study indicates that although both HAT and SPLET mechanisms are possible, SPLET is the more prevalent mechanism for dendritic antioxidants in the presence of the DPPH radical in methanol. This result is consistent with previous studies reporting that SPLET is the major operating mechanism in polar ionizing solvents, while HAT is more favorable in nonpolar solvents or in gas [9–11,13,14]. However, it should be cautioned that the SPLET process between dendritic antioxidants and DPPH• in methanol should not be extrapolated to other radicals or solvents.

Values of pKa depend on the PA of phenol O–H: the higher the PA, the more difficult it is to deprotonate, meaning a higher pKa. Based on the pKa values calculated using the ChemAxon pKa calculator (Table S2 in Supplementary Information), the phenol rings in the dendritic antioxidants have pKa values of less than 11.0, indicating that they are weakly acidic. It was shown that phenols with pKa values below 12.5 can undergo the SPLET process with radicals derived from molecules with low pKa values, e.g., DPPH• and ROO• [19].

3.4. Prediction of Overall Antioxidant Activity of Dendritic Antioxidants

Since our dendritic antioxidants have three potential radical scavenging sites, it is important to know whether all three phenol rings can undergo the SPLET mechanism and contribute to the antioxidant activity or whether their enthalpy becomes too high after one or two radical scavenging and stops. Hence, we determined the cumulative total enthalpy (ΔH_{cum}) using SPLET as the major operating mechanism in methanol to estimate the overall antioxidant activity of our dendritic compounds. Starting from the phenol ring which had the lowest PA value based on the PA order determined in the SPLET mechanism (Table 3), H$^+$ was removed and then an electron was removed immediately after to form a PhO• radical. The process was repeated based on the PA enthalpy order of the PhOH rings and continued cumulatively until all three PhOH rings became PhO• radicals. Figure 3 shows a scheme of the changes in the reference compound after each step. The ΔH_{cum} of each compound was determined by adding the PA values of steps 1–3 and the ETE values of steps 1–3. These cumulative enthalpy calculations enable us to determine potential enthalpy cooperative effects of the rings in the dendritic antioxidants.

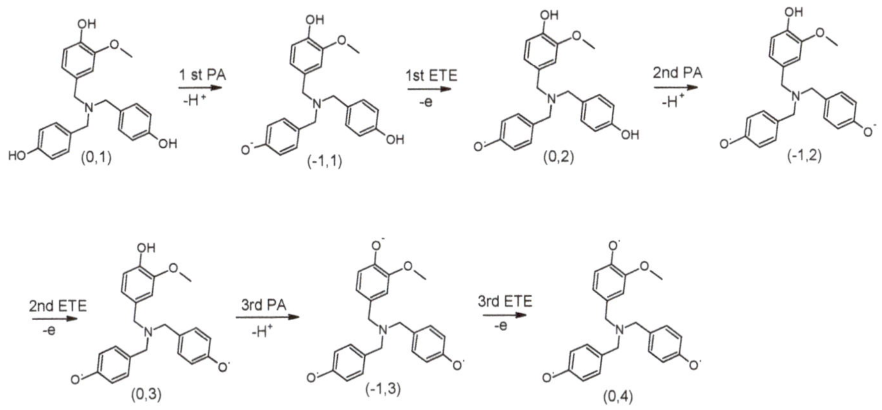

Figure 3. Scheme of the reference compound undergoing consecutive sequential proton loss electron transfer (SPLET) mechanisms. The order was determined based on the computed PA values shown in Table 3. At each step, charge and spin multiplicity of the resulting molecule are indicated in parenthesis (charge, spin multiplicity).

In the SPLET mechanism, the 1st step corresponds to the PA. EWGs decrease PA whereas EDGs increase PA. This means PhO$^-$ formation occurs more readily with PhOH containing an EWG and the resulting PhO$^-$ will undergo fast e-transfer to the radical. This may lead to the misconception that a PhOH with an EWG is a better antioxidant than the one with an EDG (higher PA). Based on our experience, antioxidants containing EDGs are better antioxidants than those containing EWGs. In our laboratory, syringaldehyde (4-hydroxy-3,5-dimethoxybenzaldehyde) and vanillin (4-hydroxy-3-methoxybenzaldehyde), each containing an aldehyde group, were used to synthesize dendritic antioxidants via reductive amination. Syringaldehyde and vanillin are very weak antioxidants by themselves, but dendrimers derived from them showed significantly higher antioxidant activities (as determined by the DPPH assay [20]). For example, antioxidant dendrimers containing eight syringaldehyde or vanillin derivatized units showed over 170- and 70-fold increase in DPPH radical scavenging activity rather than 8-fold compared to syringaldehyde and vanillin starting material, respectively [3]. The dramatic increase was caused in part by the replacement of the electron-withdrawing aldehyde (in the starting material) with an electron-donating benzyl group (in the dendrimer). Based on this observation, EDGs are more beneficial than EWGs for antioxidant activity. Although EDGs contribute to increasing PA in polar solvents, they will decrease ETE, thus helping electron transfer from the antioxidant to the radical occur more efficiently. Hence, we argue that the 2nd step (ETE) needs to be considered in determining the full antioxidant potential of our dendritic antioxidants since EDGs reduce ETE considerably. In addition, to emulate each phenol ring reacting with a radical (DPPH• was used in this study), the enthalpy change of the DPPH radical that is undergoing reduction by an electron from PhOH ring was considered. Therefore, the net enthalpy of the 2nd step of each PhOH ring was determined by combining ETE of PhOH (reaction 2a in Scheme 1) with ΔH of DPPH•, which is −303 kJ/mol (reaction 2b in Scheme 1).

In the reference compound, the phenol rings with no substituent (X and X′) had a lower PA than the common ring (Y) and thereby are expected to lose H^+ before the common ring. Thus, the H^+ was removed from one of the phenol rings with no substituent (X) and formed a $PhO^−$ ion. The 1st PA enthalpy was 150 kJ/mol. In turn, an electron was removed to form a PhO• radical. The 1st ETE was 355 kJ/mol to which the ETE of DPPH• (−303 kJ/mol) was added, giving a net ETE of 52 kJ/mol. The process was repeated for the 2nd phenol ring (X′) to determine the 2nd PA and ETE, which were 147 kJ/mol and 56 kJ/mol, respectively. The 3rd PA and ETE, which originate in the common ring, were 128 kJ/mol and 61 kJ/mol, respectively.

Compound **1** has the same three phenol rings with one o-EDG (OCH_3) on each ring. Each phenol ring underwent the SPLET process one by one. The 1st, 2nd, and 3rd PA/ETE were 154/30, 150/37, 147/41 kJ/mol, respectively. Our results show a slight decrease in PA values as more H^+ is removed. In contrast, ETE increases as the reaction progresses.

In the case of compound **2**, the first H^+ was removed from one of the rings with two o-OCH_3 (X or X′), because it had a lower PA than the common ring (Y). The 1st, 2nd, and 3rd PA/ETE were 151/16, 149/19, 148/40 kJ/mol, respectively. Its ETE values are substantially lower than those of the reference compound and **1**. By looking at the order of overall ETE values (compound **2** < compound **1** < reference compound), we can see the importance of EDG on the electron-donating potential of the antioxidants.

In compound **3**, the two phenol rings containing o-NO_2 had the lowest PA values. Therefore, the first proton was removed from one of the PhOH rings with NO_2. The 1st PA was determined to be 116 kJ/mol. Then, an electron was removed to form a PhO• radical (1st ETE = 119 kJ/mol). The same process was repeated for the 2nd phenol ring with the NO_2 group. The 2nd PA and ETE were 116 kJ/mol, and 116 kJ/mol, respectively. The common ring underwent SPLET last. Its PA and ETE were 69 kJ/mol and 119 kJ/mol, respectively. Calculations were also done for compounds **4** and **5** to determine their PA and ETE in the same manner. The 1st, 2nd, and 3rd PA/ETE of compound **4** were 132/66, 130/70, 114/73 kJ/mol, respectively. The 1st, 2nd, and 3rd PA/ETE of compound **5** were 136/61, 133/66, 118/70 kJ/mol, respectively (calculated raw data is shown in Table S3 in Supplementary Information).

Figure 4 summarizes how each step affects the enthalpy of the following step, according to DFT. Overall, PA values gradually decrease while ETE values increase as more and more phenol rings undergo radical scavenging. This means that the enthalpy values in the later steps are affected by the phenol ring(s), which underwent deprotonation and ETE earlier. None of the steps showed a significant increase in the corresponding enthalpy values, suggesting that the multiple SPLET process can occur and all three PhOH rings in our dendritic antioxidants are able to scavenge free radicals.

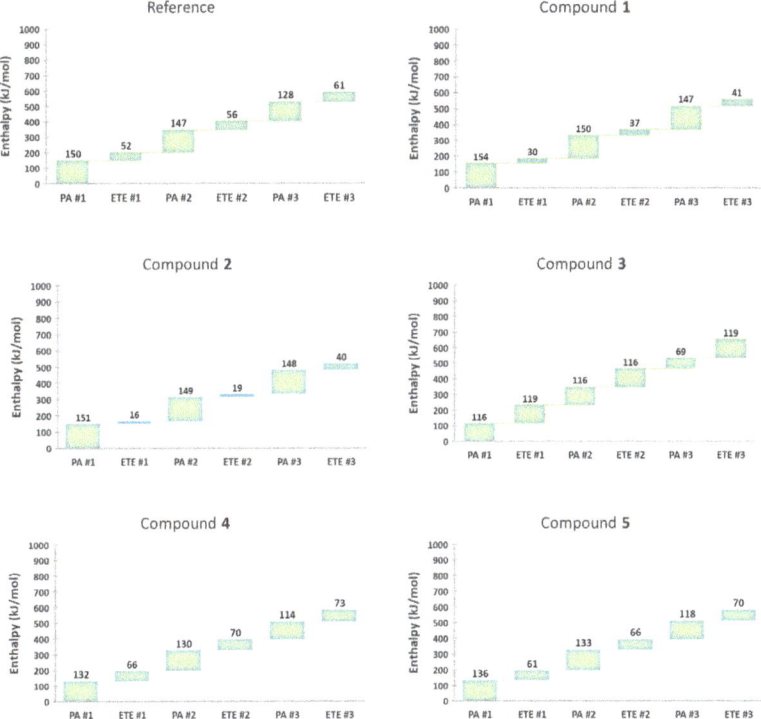

Figure 4. Enthalpy value of each step in a multiple SPLET process for the compounds studied. Each ETE value has been decreased by 303 kJ/mol ($\Delta H_{DPPH\bullet} = -303$ kJ/mol) to account for the reaction with the DPPH radical.

The ΔH_{cum} of each compound, determined by cumulatively adding PA and ETE of all three rings with consideration of the $\Delta H_{DPPH\bullet}$ is shown in Figure 5. The overall enthalpy order is compound **2** (523 kJ/mol) < compound **1** (559 kJ/mol) < compound **5** (584 kJ/mol) ≈ compound **4** (585 kJ/mol) < reference compound (594 kJ/mol) < compound **3** (655 kJ/mol).

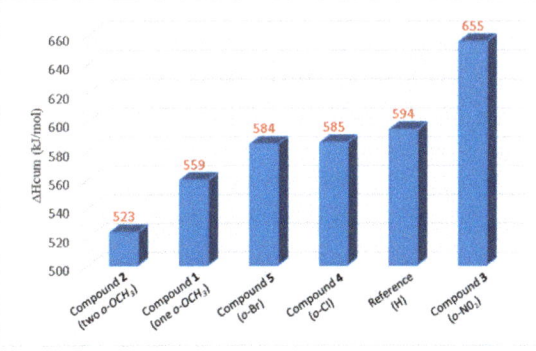

Figure 5. The cumulative total enthalpy (ΔH_{cum}) of consecutive SPLET mechanisms.

If the $\Delta H_{DPPH\bullet}$ is not considered, the overall ΔH_{cum} order is compound **2** (1432 kJ/mol) < compound **1** (1468 kJ/mol) < compound **5** (1493 kJ/mol) ≈ compound **4** (1494 kJ/mol) < reference compound (1503 kJ/mol) < compound **3** (1564 kJ/mol). It is worth mentioning that the cumulative total enthalpy values (ΔH_{cum}) are slightly higher than the summed-up enthalpy (ΔH_{tot} = PA in Table 3 + ETE in Table 4) of the three rings in each compound: compound **2** (1428 kJ/mol) < compound **1** (1462 kJ/mol) < compound **5** (1490 kJ/mol) = compound **4** (1490 kJ/mol) < reference compound (1496 kJ/mol) < compound **3** (1561 kJ/mol). Nonetheless, the order remains the same. The difference in the ΔH_{cum} and ΔH_{tot} indicates that the phenol rings in the dendritic antioxidants are mutually dependent on each other.

Based on these results, compound **2** (two o-OCH$_3$) had the lowest total enthalpy, followed by **1** (one o-OCH$_3$), suggesting that PhOH with EDG will have higher antioxidant activity compared to the unsubstituted PhOH; the more EDG on PhOH, the better the antioxidant. Compound **3** (containing o-NO$_2$) showed a higher total enthalpy compared to the reference compound. This suggests that PhOH with EWG will have poorer antioxidant activity than the unsubstituted PhOH. Compounds containing o-halogens (Cl and Br) had slightly lower enthalpy than the reference. However, the enthalpy values are very close to each other, suggesting that halogens do not have a significant effect on the overall antioxidant activity.

In order to determine if the dendritic antioxidants composed of 3 phenol rings are more active radical scavengers than their starting materials and fragments, we determined PA, ETE and ΔH of vanillin and syringaldehyde (starting materials) as well as the fragments of compound **1**, 4-(aminomethyl)-2-methoxyphenol (Y') and 4-methyl-2-methoxyphenol (Y") and fragments of compound **2**, 4-(aminomethyl)-2,6-dimethoxyphenol (X') and 4-methyl-2,6-dimethoxyphenol (X") (Table 5).

Table 5. PA, ETE and ΔH of starting materials and fragments of compounds **1** and **2**.

	Molecule	PA (kJ/mol)	ETE (kJ/mol)	ΔH (kJ/mol)
	Compound **1**	451	1017	1468
Starting material	Vanillin (Y)	120	386	1518 [a]
Fragment 1	4-(Aminomethyl)-2-methoxyphenol (Y')	151	335	1458 [b]
Fragment 2	4-Methyl-2-methoxyphenol (Y")	155	328	1449 [c]
	Compound **2**	448	984	1432
Starting Material	Syringaldehyde (X)	118	371	1484 [d]
Fragment 1	4-(Aminomethyl)-2,6-dimethoxyphenol (X')	152	317	1424 [e]
Fragment 2	4-Methyl-2,6-dimethoxyphenol (X")	155	310	1413 [f]

[a] ΔH = 3 equiv. PA (Y) + 3 equiv. ETE (Y), [b] ΔH = 3 equiv. PA (Y') + 3 equiv. ETE (Y'), [c] ΔH = 3 equiv. PA (Y") + 3 equiv. ETE (Y"), [d] ΔH = 2 equiv. PA (X) + 1 equiv. PA (Y) + 2 equiv. ETE (X) + 1 equiv. ETE (Y), [e] ΔH = 2 equiv. PA (X') + 1 equiv. PA (Y') + 2 equiv. ETE (X') + 1 equiv. ETE (Y'), [f] ΔH = 2 equiv. PA (X") + 1 equiv. PA (Y") + 2 equiv. ETE (X") + 1 equiv. ETE (Y").

Compound **1** has three rings derived from vanillin. Therefore, the PA and ETE of vanillin were tripled (3 equivalents) and then added together to determine the total enthalpy (ΔH). ΔH of vanillin (1518 kJ/mol) was higher than that (1468 kJ/mol) of compound **1**. In the case of compound **2**, it can be considered to be derived from 2 equivalents of syringaldehyde (X) and 1 equivalent of vanillin (Y). Therefore, both PA and ETE were calculated by using the formula, 2X+Y, giving a PA of 356 kJ/mol and an ETE of 1128 kJ/mol. The total enthalpy (ΔH) of the starting material (1484 kJ/mol) was higher than that of compound **2** (1432 kJ/mol). The higher enthalpy values of the starting materials are likely due to the presence of the electron-withdrawing aldehyde group on both molecules.

Both compounds **1** and **2** had lower PA but higher ETE and ΔH, compared to their respective fragments. This trend suggests that radical scavenging of antioxidants with multiple radical scavenging sites is a multistep cumulative process, which results in a gradual decrease in PA and increase in ETE as more radical scavenging sites are used up. The higher ΔH of dendritic antioxidants is understandable because their radical scavenging is a cumulative process. By the time the 2nd and 3rd phenol rings undergo the SPLET process, the antioxidant already has one phenoxy and two phenoxy radicals, respectively, which are higher in energy than the ground state (neutral phenol).

3.5. Correlation of Enthalpy Values with DPPH IC50

It is important to know how well theoretically computed enthalpy values of dendritic antioxidants correlate with their experimental DPPH radical scavenging activities [21]. We first determined the cumulative total PA (PA_{cum}) and ETE (ETE_{cum}) by adding up the PA and ETE of steps 1–3 shown in Figure 4, respectively. Then, PA_{cum}, and ETE_{cum} were added to determine ΔH_{cum} (Table 6). To see the enhancing/decreasing effect, the enthalpy differences between each compound and the reference were determined ($\Delta(\Delta H_{cum})$, ΔPA_{cum}, and ΔETE_{cum}) and $\Delta IC50$ values were determined the same way. These differences are depicted in Figure 6. Based on these graphs, we observe that the trend of $\Delta IC50$ resembles that of $\Delta(\Delta H_{cum})$ most closely, followed by ΔETE_{cum}.

Table 6. The cumulative enthalpy values, ΔH_{cum}, PA_{cum}, and ETE_{cum}, for dendritic antioxidants and the experimental DPPH IC50 values.

Compound	ΔH_{cum} (kJ/mol)	PA_{cum} (kJ/mol)	ETE_{cum} (kJ/mol)	IC50 (µM) [a]
Reference compound	594	425	169	34.9
Compound 1 (one OCH_3)	559	451	108	10.2
Compound 2 (two OCH_3)	523	448	75	8.0
Compound 3 (NO_2)	655	301	354	55.9
Compound 4 (Cl)	585	376	209	34.9
Compound 5 (Br)	584	387	197	30.4

[a] Data from [21].

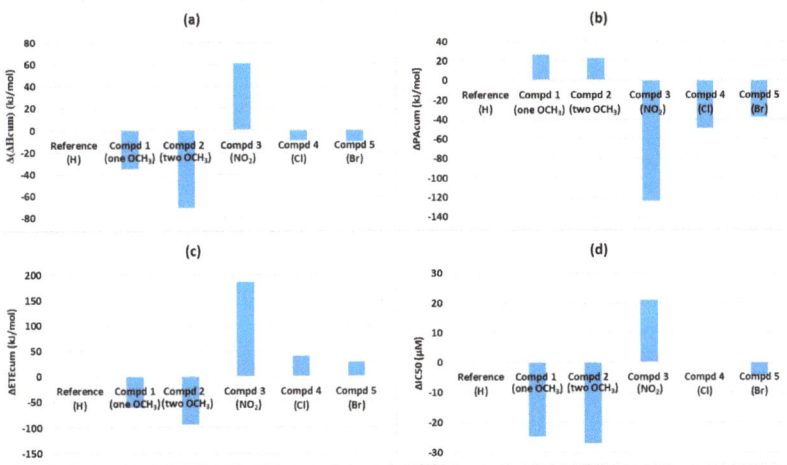

Figure 6. Graphical representation of the enthalpy deviation of each compound from the value of the reference compound: (a) $\Delta(\Delta H_{cum})$, (b) ΔPA_{cum}, (c) ΔETE_{cum} and (d) $\Delta IC50$.

We also determined the Pearson correlation coefficients (r) between the IC50 and ΔH_{cum}/ PA_{cum}/ ETE_{cum} values to determine which parameter of the SPLET mechanism better correlates with the IC50 values. Although the IC50 order looks slightly different from the order of ΔH_{cum} (Table 6), their correlation was quite impressive: r = 0.9596 with a 95% confidence interval (0.6692, 0.9957) based on Fischer's Z-transformation (Figure 7a). The PA_{cum} showed a strong negative correlation with IC50: r =

−0.9189 with a 95% confidence interval (−0.9912, −0.4222) (Figure 7b). The r of IC50 to ETE$_{cum}$ was 0.9623 with a 95% confidence interval (0.6882, 0.9960) (Figure 7c).

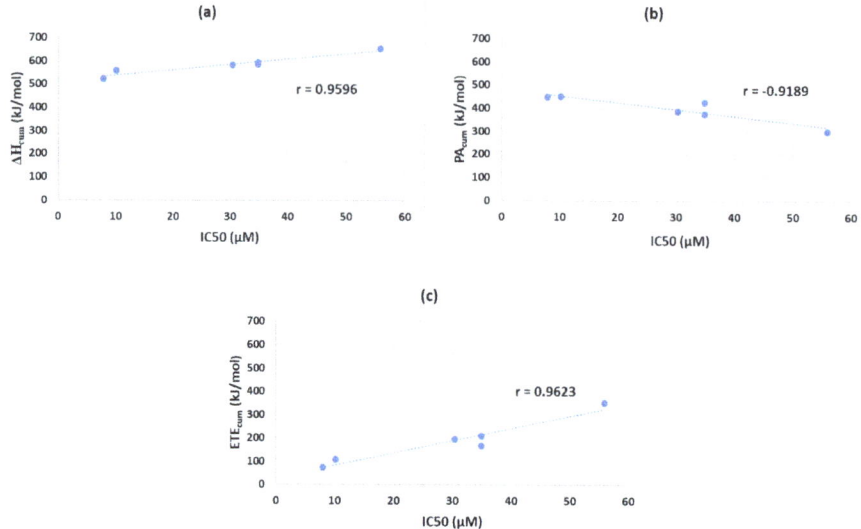

Figure 7. Correlation between IC50 and ΔH$_{cum}$ (**a**), IC50 and PA$_{cum}$ (**b**), and IC50 and ETE$_{cum}$ (**c**).

These r values, based on the collected data, indicate that the IC50 correlates better with ΔH$_{cum}$ and ETE$_{cum}$ as opposed to PA$_{cum}$. These results suggest that between ETE and PA, the ETE might be a more significant measure in estimating the antioxidant potential than PA. From our study, it is clear that o-EDGs like OCH$_3$ increase antioxidant activity whereas o-EWGs such as NO$_2$ decrease it and the trend is more consistent with ETE. Some studies reported compounds containing EWGs to be better antioxidants in the SPLET mechanism than their counterparts with EDGs because of the lower PA values obtained from EWG containing compounds [11]. Their interpretation is reasonable if we consider the findings in the original papers that proposed the SPLET mechanism: the 1st step (PA) of SPLET is equilibrium and PhOH is converted to PhO$^-$ with the help of ionizing solvents. Once, the PhO$^-$ is formed in the 1st step, the 2nd step (ETE) occurs rapidly in the presence of DPPH radicals [13,14]. It was also reported that rate constants of PhOHs/DPPH•reactions in alcohols were increased by the addition of a base, indicating that PhO$^-$ formation is important in SPLET [19]. The formation of PhO$^-$ is directly related to the acidity of the PhOH: the more acidic PhOH is, the faster PhO$^-$ forms. Based on these reports, phenols containing EWGs seem to be better antioxidants than unsubstituted ones and those containing EDGs. This is because phenols with EWGs can form PhO$^-$ more readily and enter the SPLET mechanism faster. The comparison of IC50 values between our o-NO$_2$ (55 μM) and o-OCH$_3$ (8 μM) containing antioxidants (both having similar intramolecular and intermolecular H-bonding properties in ionizing solvents like methanol) suggest that faster formation of PhO$^-$ (lower PA of o-NO$_2$) does not necessarily result in better antioxidant activities. The negative effect of o-NO$_2$ on the antioxidant activity was shown not only by our study but also other experimental studies [22]. Thus, we propose that the 2nd step (ETE) of SPLET should be considered in assessing the full antioxidant potential of phenolic antioxidants. In agreement with our proposal, Li et al. showed that the introduction of o-NH$_2$ will be more beneficial for the antioxidant activity than o-NO$_2$ although their o-NO$_2$ containing compound had lower PA value than the o-NH$_2$ counterpart [10].

4. Conclusions

Enthalpy values for model dendritic antioxidants with either an o-EDG or o-EWG were determined for each step of the three proposed mechanisms (HAT, SET-PT and SPLET) in methanol using DFT calculations. Based on our results, o-OCH$_3$ (o-EDG) decreases BDE, IP (1st step of SET-PT), and ETE (2nd step of SPLET) and increases PDE (2nd step of SET-PT) and PA (1st step of SPLET) while o-NO$_2$ (EWG) showed the opposite effects. SPLET was found to be the preferred mechanism in methanol when DPPH• was used as the radical.

To compare relative antioxidant activity between the dendritic compounds, the total enthalpy of each compound was determined by cumulatively running SPLET for all three PhOH rings and adding all the enthalpy values. The results showed that o-OCH$_3$ (EDG) increases the antioxidant activity whereas o-NO$_2$ (EWG) decreases it. In comparison, *ortho*-halogens (Br and Cl) showed negligibly lower enthalpy values compared to the unsubstituted PhOH. Correlation of the DPPH radical scavenging activities with each step in SPLET revealed that the experimental IC50 values better correlate with ETE (the 2nd step) rather than PA (the 1st step), implying that ETE is a more important factor in estimating the role of substituents on antioxidant activity than PA.

Supplementary Materials: The following are available online at http://www.mdpi.com/2076-3921/9/3/189/s1. Table S1. DFT calculations in methanol; Table S2. Values of pKa obtained using ChemAxon pKa calculator; Table S3. Multistep DFT calculations in methanol.

Author Contributions: Conceptualization, C.Y.L.; calculations, V.B.; data curation, J.S., C.A., K.N.C. and V.B.; formal analysis, C.Y.L., A.S. and V.B.; writing—original draft, C.Y.L.; writing—review and editing, C.Y.L. and A.S. All authors have read and agreed to the published version of the manuscript.

Funding: This research received no external funding.

Conflicts of Interest: The authors declare no conflict of interest.

References

1. Lee, C.Y.; Sharma, A.; Cheong, J.E.; Nelson, J.L. Synthesis and Antioxidant Properties of Dendritic Polyphenols. *Bioorg. Med. Chem. Lett.* **2009**, *19*, 6326–6330. [CrossRef]
2. Lee, C.Y.; Sharma, A.; Uzarski, R.L.; Cheong, J.E.; Xu, H.; Held, R.A.; Upadhaya, S.K.; Nelson, J.L. Potent Antioxidant Dendrimers Lacking Pro-Oxidant Activity. *Free Radic. Biol. Med.* **2011**, *50*, 918–925. [CrossRef]
3. Lee, C.Y.; Nanah, C.N.; Held, R.A.; Clark, A.R.; Huynh, U.G.T.; Maraskine, M.C.; Uzarski, R.L.; McCracken, J.; Sharma, A. Effect of Electron Donating Groups on Polyphenol-Based Antioxidant Dendrimers. *Biochimie* **2015**, *111*, 125–134. [CrossRef]
4. Gaspar, A.; Garrido, E.M.; Esteves, M.; Quezada, E.; Milhazes, N.; Garrido, J.; Borges, F. New Insights into the Antioxidant Activity of Hydroxycinnamic Acids: Synthesis and Physicochemical Characterization of Novel Halogenated Derivatives. *Eur. J. Med. Chem.* **2009**, *44*, 2092–2099. [CrossRef]
5. Inami, K.; Iizuka, Y.; Furukawa, M.; Nakanishi, I.; Ohkubo, K.; Fukuhara, K.; Fukuzumi, S.; Mochizuki, M. Chlorine Atom Substitution Influences Radical Scavenging Activity of 6-Chromanol. *Bioorg. Med. Chem.* **2012**, *20*, 4049–4055. [CrossRef] [PubMed]
6. Bordwell, F.G.; Cheng, J.P. Substituent Effects on the Stabilities of Phenoxyl Radicals and the Acidities of Phenoxyl Radical Cations. *J. Am. Chem. Soc.* **1991**, *113*, 1736–1743. [CrossRef]
7. Wright, J.S.; Johnson, E.R.; DiLabio, G.A. Predicting the Activity of Phenolic Antioxidants: Theoretical Method, Analysis of Substituent Effects, and Application to Major Families of Antioxidants. *J. Am. Chem. Soc.* **2001**, *123*, 1173–1183. [CrossRef] [PubMed]
8. De Heer, M.I.; Korth, H.G.; Mulder, P. Poly Methoxy Phenols in Solution: O–H Bond Dissociation Enthalpies, Structures, and Hydrogen Bonding. *J. Org. Chem.* **1999**, *64*, 6969–6975. [CrossRef]
9. Najafi, M.; Najafi, M.; Najafi, H. Theoretical Study of the Substituent and Solvent Effects on the Reaction Enthalpies of the Antioxidant Mechanisms of Tyrosol Derivatives. *Bull. Chem. Soc. Jpn.* **2013**, *86*, 497–509. [CrossRef]
10. Wang, L.; Yang, F.; Zhao, X.; Li, Y. Effects of Nitro- and Amino-Group on the Antioxidant Activity of Genistein: A Theoretical Study. *Food Chem.* **2019**, *275*, 339–345. [CrossRef]

11. Zheng, Y.-Z.; Chen, D.-F.; Deng, G.; Guo, R. The Substituent Effect on the Radical Scavenging Activity of Apigenin. *Molecules* **2018**, *23*, 1989. [CrossRef] [PubMed]
12. Najafi, M.; Mood, K.H.; Zahedi, M.; Klein, E. DFT/B3LYP Study of the Substituent Effect on the Reaction Enthalpies of the Individual Steps of Single Electron Transfer-Proton Transfer and Sequential Proton Loss Electron Transfer Mechanisms of Chroman Derivatives Antioxidant Action. *Comput. Theor. Chem.* **2011**, *969*, 1–12. [CrossRef]
13. Litwinienko, G.; Ingold, K.U. Abnormal Solvent Effects on Hydrogen Atom Abstraction. 2. Resolution of the Curcumin Antioxidant Controversy. The Role of Sequential Proton Loss Electron Transfer. *J. Org. Chem.* **2004**, *69*, 5888–5896. [CrossRef] [PubMed]
14. Foti, M.; Daquino, C.; Geraci, C. Electron-Transfer Reaction of Cinnamic Acids and Their Methyl Esters with the DPPH• Radical in Alcoholic Solutions. *J. Org. Chem.* **2004**, *69*, 2309–2314. [CrossRef]
15. Stepanić, V.; Matijašić, M.; Horvat, T.; Verbanac, D.; Chlupáćová, M.K.; Saso, L.; Žarković, N. Antioxidant Activities of Alkyl Substituted Pyrazine Derivatives of Chalcones—In vitro and in Silico Study. *Antioxidants* **2019**, *8*, 90. [CrossRef]
16. Frisch, M.J.; Trucks, G.W.; Schlegel, H.B.; Scuseria, G.E.; Robb, M.A.; Cheeseman, J.R.; Scalmani, G.; Barone, V.; Mennucci, B.; Petersson, G.A.; et al. *Gaussian 16, Revision B.03*; Gaussian, Inc.: Wallingford, CT, USA, 2016.
17. Marenich, A.V.; Cramer, C.; Truhlar, D. Universal Solvation Model Based on Solute Electron Density and on a Continuum Model of the Solvent Defined by the Bulk Dielectric Constant and Atomic Surface Tensions. *J. Phys. Chem. B* **2009**, *113*, 6378–6396. [CrossRef] [PubMed]
18. Burton, G.W.; Doba, T.; Gabe, E.J.; Hughes, L.; Lee, F.L.; Prasad, L.; Ingoldo, K.U. Autoxidation of Biological Molecules. 4. Maximizing the Antioxidant Activity of Phenols. *J. Am. Chem. Soc.* **1985**, *107*, 7053–7065. [CrossRef]
19. Litwinienko, G.; Ingold, K.U. Abnormal Solvent Effects on Hydrogen Atom Abstractions. 1. The Reactions of Phenols with 2, 2-Diphenyl-1-Picrylhydrazyl (Dpph•) in Alcohols. *J. Org. Chem.* **2003**, *68*, 3433–3438. [CrossRef] [PubMed]
20. Brand-Williams, W.; Cuvelier, M.E.; Berset, C. Use of Free Radical Method to Evaluate Antioxidant Activity. *LWT Food Sci Technol. LWT Food Sci. Technol.* **1995**, *28*, 25–30. [CrossRef]
21. Lee, C.Y.; Anamoah, C.; Semenya, J.; Chapman, K.N.; Knoll, A.N.; Brinkman, F.; Malone, J.I.; Sharma, A. Electronic (Donating or Withdrawing) Effects of Ortho-Phenolic Substituents in Dendritic Antioxidants. *Tetrahedron Lett.* **2020**. [CrossRef]
22. Grenier, J.L.; Cotelle, N.; Cotelle, P.; Catteau, J.P. Antioxidant Properties of Nitrocaffeic Acids. *Bioorg. Med. Chem. Lett.* **1996**, *6*, 431–434. [CrossRef]

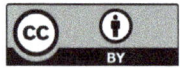

© 2020 by the authors. Licensee MDPI, Basel, Switzerland. This article is an open access article distributed under the terms and conditions of the Creative Commons Attribution (CC BY) license (http://creativecommons.org/licenses/by/4.0/).

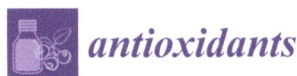

Article

The Effect of Nano-Epigallocatechin-Gallate on Oxidative Stress and Matrix Metalloproteinases in Experimental Diabetes Mellitus

Adriana Elena Bulboaca [1], Paul-Mihai Boarescu [1,*], Alina Silvia Porfire [2,*], Gabriela Dogaru [3,*], Cristina Barbalata [2], Madalina Valeanu [4], Constantin Munteanu [5], Ruxandra Mioara Râjnoveanu [6], Cristina Ariadna Nicula [7] and Ioana Cristina Stanescu [8]

1. Department of Pathophysiology, Iuliu Hațieganu University of Medicine and Pharmacy Cluj-Napoca, Victor Babeș Street, no. 2-4, 400012 Cluj-Napoca, Romania; adriana.bulboaca@umfcluj.ro
2. Department of Pharmaceutical Technology and Biopharmaceutics, Iuliu Hațieganu University of Medicine and Pharmacy Cluj-Napoca, Victor Babeș Street, no. 41, 400012 Cluj-Napoca, Romania; barbalata.cristina@umfcluj.ro
3. Department of Physical Medicine and Rehabilitation, Iuliu Hațieganu University of Medicine and Pharmacy Cluj-Napoca, Viilor Street, no. 46-50, 400347 Cluj-Napoca, Romania
4. Department of Medical Informatics and Biostatistics, Iuliu Hațieganu University of Medicine and Pharmacy Cluj-Napoca, Louis Pasteur Street, no. 6, 400349 Cluj-Napoca, Romania; mvaleanu@umfcluj.ro
5. Department of Medical Rehabilitation, "BagdasarArseni" Emergency Clinical Hospital Bucharest, Berceni Street, no. 12, 041915 Cluj-Napoca, Romania; office@bioclima.ro
6. Department of Pneumology, Iuliu Hațieganu University of Medicine and Pharmacy Cluj-Napoca, B.P. Hasdeu Street, no. 6, 400371 Cluj-Napoca, Romania; andra_redro@yahoo.com
7. Department of Ophthalmology, Iuliu Hațieganu University of Medicine and Pharmacy Cluj-Napoca, Clinicilor Street, no. 3-5, 400006 Cluj-Napoca, Romania; niculacristina65@yahoo.com
8. Department of Neurology, Iuliu Hațieganu University of Medicine and Pharmacy Cluj-Napoca, Victor Babeș Street, no. 43, 400012 Cluj-Napoca, Romania; ioana.stanescu.umfcluj@gmail.com
* Correspondence: boarescu.paul@umfcluj.ro (P.-M.B.); aporfire@umfcluj.ro (A.S.P.); dogarugabrielaumf@gmail.com (G.D.); Tel.: +40-752-921-725 (P.-M.B.); +40-264-595-770 (A.S.P.); +40-724-231-022 (G.D.)

Received: 11 January 2020; Accepted: 18 February 2020; Published: 20 February 2020

Abstract: Background: The antioxidant properties of epigallocatechin-gallate (EGCG), a green tea compound, have been already studied in various diseases. Improving the bioavailability of EGCG by nanoformulation may contribute to a more effective treatment of diabetes mellitus (DM) metabolic consequences and vascular complications. The aim of this study was to test the comparative effect of liposomal EGCG with EGCG solution in experimental DM induced by streptozotocin (STZ) in rats. Method: 28 Wistar-Bratislava rats were randomly divided into four groups (7 animals/group): group 1—control group, with intraperitoneal (i.p.) administration of 1 mL saline solution (C); group 2—STZ administration by i.p. route (60 mg/100 g body weight, bw) (STZ); group 3—STZ administration as before + i.p. administration of EGCG solution (EGCG), 2.5 mg/100 g b.w. as pretreatment; group 4—STZ administration as before + i.p. administration of liposomal EGCG, 2.5 mg/100 g b.w. (L-EGCG). The comparative effects of EGCG and L-EGCG were studied on: (i) oxidative stress parameters such as malondialdehyde (MDA), indirect nitric oxide (NOx) synthesis, and total oxidative status (TOS); (ii) antioxidant status assessed by total antioxidant capacity of plasma (TAC), thiols, and catalase; (iii) matrix-metalloproteinase-2 (MMP-2) and -9 (MMP-9). Results: L-EGCG has a better efficiency regarding the improvement of oxidative stress parameters (highly statistically significant with p-values < 0.001 for MDA, NOx, and TOS) and for antioxidant capacity of plasma (highly significant $p < 0.001$ for thiols and significant for catalase and TAC with $p < 0.05$). MMP-2 and -9 were also significantly reduced in the L-EGCG-treated group compared with the EGCG group ($p < 0.001$). Conclusions: the liposomal nanoformulation of EGCG may serve as an adjuvant therapy in DM due to its unique modulatory effect on oxidative stress/antioxidant biomarkers and MMP-2 and -9.

Keywords: epigallocatechin-gallate; liposomes; diabetes mellitus; oxidative stress

1. Introduction

Consuming green tea has been linked to human health and longevity for centuries. In particular, green tea catechins are involved in many biological processes such as antioxidant activity and modulation of various cellular lipid and protein metabolisms [1]. Green tea contains a great amount of polyphenols (flavonols, flavones, and flavanols) with similar structure, possessing lots of therapeutic active components including catechin, epicatechin, epicatechin-3-gallate, and epigallocatechin-3-gallate (EGCG) [2]. EGCG is the most active and abundant compound (65% of total catechin content) [3,4].

Green tea therapeutic effects have been studied intensively, proving beneficial in various diseases such as cancer [5], hyperlipidemia [6,7], cardiovascular diseases [8,9], neurodegenerative diseases [10,11], and infectious diseases [12,13]. Some reports also suggest that daily consumption of tea catechins may help in controlling type 1 [14] and type 2 diabetes mellitus [1]. It has been demonstrated that green tea consumption reduces fasting glucose levels, an effect mediated by EGCG [15]. Lipophilic EGCG has been shown to reduce glycemia and serum lipids in experimental diabetes mellitus induced by streptozotocin (STZ) in rats [16].

Type 1 diabetes mellitus (DM) is associated with an autoimmune-mediated destruction of pancreatic beta cells, leading to absolute insulin deficiency [17]. One of the most used experimental models for testing various therapies addressing type 1 DM is based on STZ administration. STZ induces type 1 DM, with destruction of pancreatic beta cells and associated insulin deficiency, as a result of its cytotoxic effect, mediated by increased synthesis of reactive oxygen species (ROS) and subsequent inflammation [18–20]. A protective effect of EGCG on pancreatic beta cells has been already demonstrated in experimental studies [21]; meanwhile, oral chronic administration of EGCG proved to have hypoglycemic and hypolipidemic effects and to reduce oxidative stress in streptozotocin-diabetic rats [22]. EGCG can exert antioxidant, anti-inflammatory, antiangiogenetic, and antifibrotic effects [2]. The catechol or galloyl groups from catechins act as scavengers for metal ions, reducing further production of free radicals [23]. Another essential effect is represented by the scavenging activity for free radicals, through phenoxyl compounds [24]. EGCG treatment can also reduce oxidative stress by increasing the level of antioxidant enzymes, such as superoxide dismutase (SOD), glutathione peroxidase (GP), and catalase (CAT), emerging in an antiapoptotic consequence [25].

Matrix metalloproteinases (MMPs) are a family of enzymes (peptidases) involved in degradation and remodeling of extracellular matrix (ECM) [26]. Recent studies reveal that MMPs can regulate chemokines and cytokines synthesis, thus participating in innate immunity processes, inflammation, and angiogenesis [27]. MMPs can be generated by various cell types, such as endothelial cells and mononuclear cells of the immune system [28]. Pathological induction of MMP synthesis is associated with an imbalance between synthesis and degradation of ECM proteins leading to ECM degradation [29]. High glucose ambience influences the MMPs' increased synthesis and low tissue inhibitors of MMPs (TIMP) activity [30]. Increased levels of MMP-2 and MMP-9 are observed in type 1 diabetic patients and animal models, such as STZ-induced diabetes mellitus in rats [31,32], and are associated with microvascular complications of DM [28].

Analyzing the EGCG therapeutic properties and pharmacokinetic parameters, considerable individual differences and variations between results were noted [33]. EGCG is highly lipophilic, which explains its low bioavailability (0.2% to 2% of the total load ingested by healthy people), mainly because a large amount of the ingested EGCG is degraded by local microbiota and does not enter into the blood circulation [34]. Improvement of bioavailability and stability of EGCG can be obtained by encapsulation in nanoparticles [35]. Catechin nanoemulsions proved to be stable for long periods of time (120 days at 4 °C) [36]. Liposomes, assembled from phospholipid bilayers similar to cell membranes, are one of the nanoparticles frequently used for drug delivery [23]. Their biphasic character makes them suitable for being carriers for both hydrophilic (in the central aqueous compartment) and hydrophobic (in lipid bilayers) compounds [37,38]. Nanoformulation by encapsulation in liposomes could also facilitate the solubility for hydrophobic particles [4]. Through all of these properties, liposomes can offer an enhanced bioavailability, stability, and shelf life for sensitive ingredients [39].

The aim of this study was to investigate the effect of two forms of EGCG (EGCG solution and liposomal EGCG) on oxidative stress parameters, antioxidant capacity, serum MMP-2 and -9, and pancreatic and liver function in STZ-induced diabetes mellitus in rats.

2. Materials and Methods

2.1. Materials

The substances used for liposomal preparation were: Epigallocatechin-gallate (EGCG) derived from green tea (Sigma-Aldrich, Steinheim, Germany); 1,2-dipalmitoyl-sn-glycero-3-phosphocholine (DPPC): N-(carbonyl-methoxypolyethylenglycol-2000)-1,2-distearoylsn-glycero-3-phosphoethanolamine Na-salt (MPEG-2000-DSPE) (Lipoid GmbH, Ludwigshafen am Rhein, Germany); and cholesterol (CHO) obtained from sheep wool (Sigma-Aldrich, Steinheim, Germany). All other solvents and reactive substances were obtained from Sigma-Aldrich, Steinheim, Germany, and had an analytical degree of purity.

2.2. Experimental Model

The study was approved by the Ethic Committee of the University and by the National Sanitary Veterinary Authority number 137/13.11.2018. Twenty-eight male Wistar-Bratislava rats were procured from the Centre of Experimental Medicine, University of Medicine and Pharmacy, Cluj-Napoca, Romania. The rats weighed 200–250 g, were kept in polypropylene cages, with day–night regimen, at constant temperature (24 ± 2 °C) and humidity ($60 \pm 5\%$). Free access to food (standardized pellets from Cantacuzino Institute, Bucharest, Romania) and water was provided to all animals. The animals were randomly divided into 4 groups (7 rats/group). The groups were organized as follows:

group 1—control group (C)—with intraperitoneal (i.p.) administration of 1 mL saline solution,
group 2—STZ administration by i.p. route (STZ),
group 3—STZ administration as before + i.p. administration of EGCG solution (EGCG),
group 4—STZ administration as before + i.p. administration of liposomal EGCG (L-EGCG).

Each medication was dissolved in saline solution (0.9% sodium chloride) and the volume administered i.p. was 1 mL [19]. The following doses were used: STZ—60 mg/100 g body weight (b.w.) [40]; EGCG in saline solution or in liposomal form were freshly prepared and were administrated i.p. in a dose of 2.5 mg/100 g b.w./day as pretreatment, two consecutive days before STZ administration [41]. Intraperitoneal administration was preferred as a method that improves EGCG bioavailability, compared to low bioavailability with oral administration [42].

Blood samples were taken at 48 h after STZ administration, under ketamine anesthesia (5 mg/100 g bw, i.p. route) from retro-orbital sinus, followed by rat euthanasia by cervical dislocation [43]. Rats with glucose higher or equal to 200 mg/dL were considered to have diabetes mellitus [20].

2.3. Preparation and Physicochemical Characterization of EGCG-Loaded Liposomes

For the preparation of liposomes, we used a modified film hydration method [44,45]. The lipid double-layer components, having a 70 mM concentration (DPPC:MPEG-2000-DSPE:CHO = 4.75:0.25:1 molar ratio), were dissolved in ethanol in a round-bottomed glass flask. Ethanol was evaporated at 45 °C under low pressure; the lipid film product was hydrated with a solution of EGCG diluted in highly purified water, pH = 5.00, at the same temperature. The resulted liposomal dispersion was then extruded through polycarbonate membranes with 200 nm final pore dimension, with LiposoFastLF-50 equipment (Avestin Europe GmbH, Mannheim, Germany). Unencapsulated

EGCG particles were removed by dialysis method, using Slide-A-Lyzer filters (cassettes) with 10 kDa molecular weight cut-off.

To assess the amount of liposomal-loaded EGCG, we used a spectrophotometric method—the reaction with Folin–Ciocâlteu reagent (Merck, Darmstadt, Germany) [46]. During this procedure, a dilution of liposomal dispersion with methanol 1:10 (v/v) was made, and a UV-VIS spectrophotometer (Specord 200 Plus, Analytik Jena, Überlingen, Germany) measured the absorbance value.

The size and polydispersity index of liposomes were assessed by dynamic light scattering method (with a 90° scattering angle), and the zeta potential was measured by laser Doppler electrophoresis; a Zetasizer Nano ZS analyzer was used for both assessments (Malvern Instruments Co., Malvern, UK).

The mean liposomal concentration of the L-EGCG solution was about 900 μg/mL, and encapsulation efficiency was over 80%. Liposomal vesicles' mean size was 170 nm, and polydispersity index was less than 0.2, meaning that the vesicles' size and uniformity were appropriate to ensure a prolonged circulation in the blood. Aggregative stability was ensured by values of 51.83 mV of the zeta potential.

2.4. Oxidative Stress and Antioxidant Parameters Assessment

Parameters associated with oxidative stress and antioxidant status were determined from collected blood samples. The parameters used to assess oxidative stress were: malondialdehyde (MDA) [47], indirect nitric oxide (NOx) synthesis assessment [48], and total oxidative status (TOS) [49]. Antioxidant status parameters were represented by total antioxidant capacity of plasma (TAC) [50], thiols [51], and catalase [52]. All measurements were performed using a Jasco V-350 UV-VIS spectrophotometer (Jasco International Co, Ltd., Tokyo, Japan). Matrix metalloproteinases (MMPs) were appraised from serum using a rat ELISA kit (Boster Biological technology, Pleasanton, CA, USA) and a Stat Fax 303 ELISA reader (Quantikine, McKinley Place NE, MN, USA).

2.5. Assessment of Beta Pancreatic Cells and Hepatic Cells Function

Glycemia was measured at 48 h after DM induction, as it was previously observed that STZ induces significant beta cell death at 48 after administration [53]. Glycemia was also used as a parameter for pancreatic function changes induced by experimental diabetes mellitus. Hepatic cytolysis was assessed by serum levels of aspartate aminotransferase (AST) and alanine aminotransferase (ALT) measured by a standardized technique (Vita Lab Flexor E, Spankeren, The Netherlands) [40].

2.6. Data Analysis

The SPSS software package version 21.0 (SPSS Inc., Chicago, IL, USA) was used for statistical analysis and graphic representations. The acceptable error threshold was $p = 0.05$. In order to describe the continuous quantitative data, we used the arithmetic mean and the standard deviation (SD). The distribution of investigated markers in groups was plotted as individual values (circles) and median (line), as recommended by Weissgerber and coauthors [54]. The Kruskal–Wallis ANOVA was used to test the differences in the investigated markers. The Mann–Whitney test was used in post hoc analysis when significant differences were identified by the Kruskal–Wallis ANOVA test.

3. Results

No rat died during the experiment, so the analysis was conducted on all seven rats in each group. All P values for comparison between groups are presented in Supplementary Table S1.

In our experimental model, diabetes mellitus was successfully induced by STZ: all rats that received STZ were definitely diabetic, proven by glycemia >200 mg/dL and values significantly higher in diabetic rats compared to control group: 401.81(11.31) mg/dL versus 84.27 (2.87) mg/dL, respectively (expressed as mean and standard deviation), with a p-value < 0.001. Also, hepatic damage was detected in the STZ group, quantified by significant elevation of transaminases AST and ALT (Table 1).

Table 1. Values of oxidative stress parameters, antioxidants levels, glycemia, hepatic enzymes, and matrix metalloproteinases in the four groups, expressed as mean and standard deviation.

Parameter	Control (n = 7)	STZ (n = 7)	STZ + EGCG (n = 7)	STZ + L-EGCG (n = 7)
MDA [nmol/mL]	2.52(0.24)	20.94(1.67)	19.83(1.1)	14.1(1.67)
NOx [µmol/L]	24.35(2.24)	64.34(2.26)	60.63(2.65)	40.36(2.89)
TOS [µmol/L]	17.19(1.05)	74.22(2.63)	66.68(3.45)	44.84(3.06)
Thiols [mmol /L]	213.4(6.64)	112.33(6.02)	131.1(3.17)	145.64(5.14)
Catalase [U/mL]	20.12(1.87)	10.87(0.87)	12.81(1.69)	15.8(2.42)
TAC [mEq/L]	1.41(0.09)	0.64(0.06)	0.83(0.14)	1.07(0.13)
Glycemia [mg/dL]	84.27(2.87)	401.81(11.31)	391.1(10.55)	365.3(6.56)
AST [U/L]	26.03(2.16)	150.37(9.16)	141.5(9.45)	80.67(8.88)
ALT [U/L]	24.63(2.25)	204.58(9.8)	193.17(6.57)	64.18(3.42)
MMP-2 [ng/mL]	86.14(5.96)	221(7.19)	217.71(7.23)	156(6.73)
MMP-9 [ng/mL]	19.57(1.27)	37(2.24)	36.29(2.56)	28.14(2.19)

MDA = malondialdehyde; NOx = indirect nitric oxide; TOS = total oxidative status; AST= aspartate aminotransferase; ALT = alanine aminotransferase; MMP-2 = matrix metalloproteinase 2; MMP-9 = matrix metalloproteinase 9; STZ = streptozotocin control; STZ + EGCG = STZ and EGCG solution i.p. as pretreatment; STZ + L-EGCG = STZ and liposomal EGCG i.p. as pretreatment.

Oxidative stress parameters (MDA, NOx, and TOS) significantly increased after induction of DM (p-values <0.001 in all items, Figure 1a–c, Table 1). MMP-2 and MMP-9 levels were significantly higher in the STZ-induced DM group compared with control group (p-values <0.001, Figure 4a,b, Table 1). Serum antioxidant capacity, measured by thiol, catalase, and TAC levels, was significantly reduced in diabetic rats compared to control animals (p-values < 0.001 in all items, Figure 2a–c, Table 1).

In the diabetic group pretreated with EGCG, oxidative stress parameters NOx and TOS were significantly reduced compared to the untreated STZ group (with p-values of 0.017 and <0.001, respectively, Figure 1b,c).

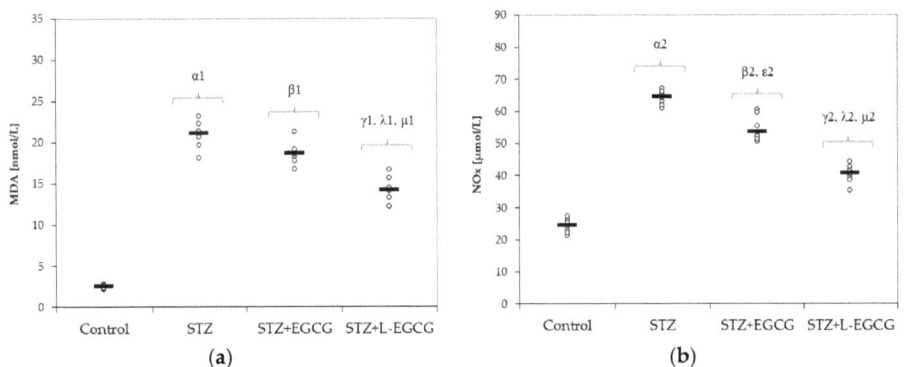

(a)   (b)

Figure 1. *Cont.*

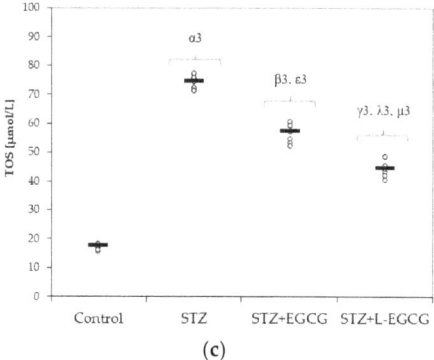

(c)

Figure 1. Distribution of oxidative stress intensity by groups: (**a**) MDA (malondialdehyde), (**b**) NOx (indirect nitric oxide), (**c**) TOS (total oxidative status) on all study groups (7 rats/group). STZ = streptozotocin control; STZ + EGCG = STZ and EGCG solution i.p. as pretreatment; STZ + L-EGCG = STZ and liposomal EGCG i.p. as pretreatment. The symbol–number codes correspond to the p-values < 0.05 as follows: α—STZ compared to control; β—STZ + EGCG compared to control; ε—STZ + EGCG compared to STZ; γ—STZ + L-EGCG compared to control; λ—STZ + L-EGCG compared to STZ; μ—STZ + L-EGCG compared to STZ + EGCG.

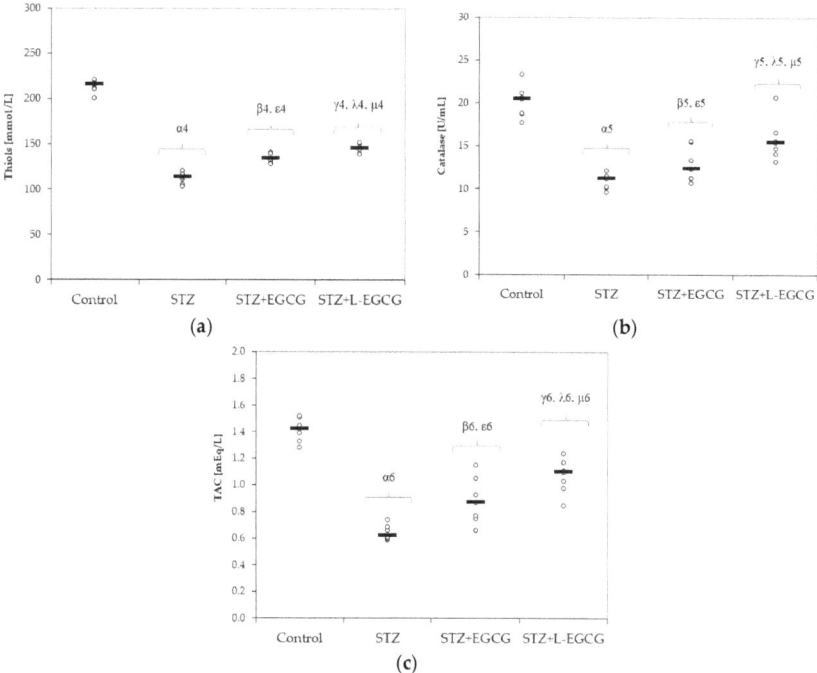

Figure 2. Distribution of plasmatic antioxidant capacity by groups: (**a**) Thiols, (**b**) Catalase, (**c**) TAC (total antioxidant capacity) on all study groups (7 rats/group). STZ = streptozotocin control; STZ + EGCG = STZ and EGCG solution i.p. as pretreatment; STZ + L-EGCG = STZ and liposomal EGCG i.p. as pretreatment. The symbol–number codes correspond to the p-values < 0.05 as follows: α—STZ compared to control; β—STZ + EGCG compared to control; ε—STZ + EGCG compared to STZ; γ—STZ + L-EGCG compared to control; λ—STZ + L-EGCG compared to STZ; μ—STZ + L-EGCG compared to STZ + EGCG.

All antioxidant parameters (thiols, catalase, and TAC) were significantly higher in the STZ-treated group (p-values of < 0.001, 0.026, and 0.017 respectively, Figure 2a–c).

No significant differences were noted in MDA and MMP values between the pretreated group with EGCG compared to the untreated STZ group (Figure 1a, Figure 4a,b). Also, glycemia and liver parameters were not significantly different in the EGCG pretreated group, with the exception of a decrease in ALT (p-value = 0.038, Figure 3c).

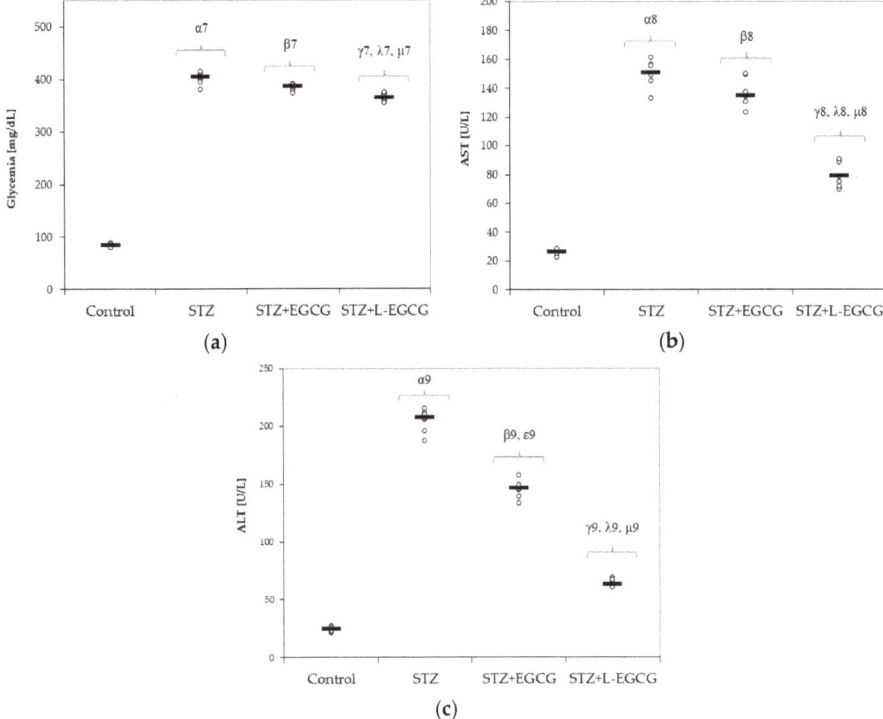

Figure 3. Distribution of (a) Glycemia, (b) AST (aspartate aminotransferase), (c) ALT (alanine aminotransferase) on all study groups (7 rats/group). STZ = streptozotocin control; STZ + EGCG = STZ and EGCG solution i.p. as pretreatment; STZ + L-EGCG = STZ and liposomal EGCG i.p. as pretreatment. The symbol–number codes correspond to the p-values < 0.05 as follows: α—STZ compared to control; β—STZ + EGCG compared to control; ε—STZ + EGCG compared to STZ; γ—STZ + L-EGCG compared to control; λ—STZ + L-EGCG compared to STZ; μ—STZ + L-EGCG compared to STZ + EGCG.

In the STZ group pretreated with L-EGCG, all oxidative stress parameters were significantly decreased and serum antioxidant capacity parameters were all increased, with better results compared to the STZ group pretreated with EGCG ($p < 0.017$, Figures 1 and 2). Also, the L-EGCG solution improved glycemic values and decreased transaminases levels better than EGCG ($p < 0.001$, Figure 3). The MMP levels were significantly lower in the L-EGCG-treated group compared to the diabetic untreated group or compared to the STZ group pretreated with EGCG (<0.001, Figure 4).

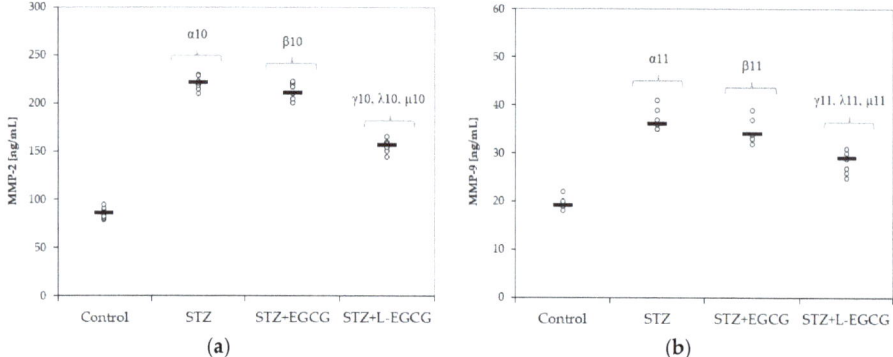

Figure 4. Distribution of matrix metalloproteinase (MMP): (**a**) MMP-2 and (**b**) MMP-9 on all study groups (7 rats/group). STZ = streptozotocin control; STZ + EGCG = STZ and EGCG solution i.p. as pretreatment; STZ + L-EGCG = STZ and liposomal EGCG i.p. as pretreatment. The symbol–number codes correspond to the p-values < 0.05 as follows: α—STZ compared to control; β—STZ + EGCG compared to control; γ—STZ + L-EGCG compared to control; λ—STZ + L-EGCG compared to STZ; μ—STZ + L-EGCG compared to STZ + EGCG.

The Kruskal–Wallis ANOVA test identified significant differences between the groups with diabetes and EGCG pretreatment for all evaluated parameters (p-values < 0.0001). The post hoc analysis identified significant differences in most of the cases with better protection for the EGCG-treated group, and significantly higher protection when liposomal EGCG solution was used (Figures 1–4).

4. Discussion

4.1. Protective Effects of EGCG on Pancreatic and Hepatic Cell Function in Diabetic Rats

In our study, EGCG reduced blood glucose levels in pretreated animals but the reduction was not statically significant (Table 1, Figure 3). Some of the antidiabetic effects of EGCG are suggested to be the suppression of appetite, adjustment of dietary fat emulsification in the gastrointestinal tract, inhibition of gastrointestinal lipolysis, and reduction of nutrient absorption enzymes [55]. The most significant hypoglycemia was obtained in liposomal EGCG-pretreated groups. This indicates a protective effect of EGCG on pancreatic cell function. Meng et al. showed that EGCG can inhibit inflammation by reducing reactive oxygen species and downregulating the production of inducible nitric oxide synthetase (iNOS) [56]. Furthermore, EGCG increases glucose tolerance [57] and decrease HbA1c levels in STZ-induced diabetes in rats, contributing to further prevention of diabetic complications [58]. Another suggested mechanism of EGCG's protective effect is the increased glucose uptake due to promoting the glucose transporter-4 (GLUT4) translocation in skeletal muscle, through activation of both phosphoinositol 3-kinase and AMP-activated protein kinase pathways [58]. EGCG also increases tyrosine phosphorylation of insulin receptors, having an insulin-like effect on H4IIE hepatoma cell lines [59].

The liver is extremely adversely affected in type 1 diabetes mellitus. In our study, we found elevated AST and ALT levels, showing liver damage, in STZ diabetic rats (Table 1, Figure 3). In STZ-induced diabetes, transaminases elevation is the consequence of the toxic effect of STZ on hepatocytes, which induces lipid peroxidation, oxidative stress enhancement, peroxisome proliferation, and mitochondrial dysfunction [60–62]. Rodriguez et al. identified increased NO levels and hepatic oxidative stress in STZ-induced diabetic rats [63]. In our study, pretreatment with EGCG decreased ALT levels, preventing hepatic damage induced by STZ. Furthermore, liposomal EGCG administration significantly reduced AST and ALT values, confirming the enhanced protective effect of L-EGCG on hepatic cells. Other studies also demonstrated the hepatic-protective effect of green tea extracts in hepatic injury reflected by decreased serum transaminase levels, and improved structural changes in histopathological examination [64]. Moreover, long-time consumption of EGCG (in healthy Wistar rats) decreases age-induced hepatic damage by lowering the ALT and AST serum levels and improving microscopic changes of the liver tissue due to the aging process [65].

4.2. Effect of EGCG on Oxidative Stress Parameters and Plasmatic Antioxidant Capacity

In this study, increased levels of MDA, NO, and TOS were observed in diabetic rats (Table 1 and Figure 1), together with low levels of antioxidant biomarkers such as thiols, catalase, and TOS (Table 1 and Figure 2). Pretreatment with EGCG and L-EGCG induced protection against STZ toxic effects, as demonstrated by reduction of oxidative stress parameters (Table 1, Figure 1) and by enhancement of antioxidant defense (Table 1, Figure 2), with best results for the liposomal form. STZ-induced diabetes in experimental models is followed by an enhanced production of reactive oxygen species (ROS) and consumption of cell antioxidant systems, as a consequence of necrotic and apoptotic degeneration of pancreatic β cells [66,67]. Hyperglycemia itself is another factor generating intracellular ROS [68]. Oxidative stress (by excessive ROS production, auto-oxidation of glycated proteins, and increased lipid peroxidation) and decreased antioxidant capacity (free radical scavengers and enzymatic systems) are also involved in the pathogenesis of diabetic complications [69–72].

Green tea component EGCG is a flavonoid with antioxidant and anti-inflammatory properties conferred by its particular structure, a flavanol core and two gallocatechol rings, which are able to bind metal ions and scavenge free oxygen radicals. As a consequence, EGCG exerts direct antioxidant effects (scavenger of ROS and cheater of metal ions), but also indirect antioxidant effects (inductor of antioxidant enzymes, such as catalase, and inhibitor of oxydases, such as NADPH—nicotinamide adenine dinucleotide phosphate, lipoxygenase, or xantin-oxydase) [73]. Anti-inflammatory effects of EGCG were also related to the increase of circulating levels of interleukin-10 (an anti-inflammatory cytokine) in nonobese diabetic mice [14]. EGCG can decrease lipid peroxidation in the liver, kidney, and brain, and reduce lymphocyte DNA damage in diabetic mice [74].

EGCG has low bioavailability which can be modified by incorporation in special drug delivery systems. Because of its highly lipophilic nature, EGCG is suitable for incorporation in liposome nanoparticles, composed of phospholipid bilayers. Minnelli et al. showed that pretreatment of adult retinal pigmented epithelium (ARPE) cells with EGCG encapsulated in magnesium liposomes increases the survival of cells exposed to hydrogen peroxide (H_2O_2), with better preserved mitochondria structure on electron microscopy examination, showing the superior antioxidant activity of L-EGCG compared with free EGCG [75]. In this regard, natural antioxidant products could be a promising therapeutic option for prevention of diabetes mellitus and its complications, conferring protection against oxidative damage by liposomal nanostructure encapsulation [69].

4.3. EGCG Effect on Matrix Metalloproteinases

In the present study, serum levels of MMP-2 and -9 increased after DM induction and were better modulated by L-EGCG (Table 1 and Figure 4). In experimental models of DM, increased MMP-2 expression and activity were linked to elevated ROS levels and oxidative stress, with consecutive pancreatic beta cell apoptosis, showing MMP-2's important role in DM pathogenesis [76]. Thus, inhibition of intracellular MMP-2 expression is an essential target for beta cell protection and DM prevention. There is also a postulated connection between MMP production and inflammatory process and proinflammatory cytokine production associated with DM. Chemokines such as MCP-1 and NF-kB can induce MMP overproduction in DM [77]. After their secretion as inactive forms, proinflammatory molecules contribute to further transformation of MMPs in active forms by different proteases that are implicated in their cleavage [38]. MMPs are also involved in regulation and duration of immune response, endothelial cell function, vascular smooth muscle migration and proliferation, Ca^{2+} signaling pathways, and vessel contraction, all of these consistently influencing vascular remodeling in DM [78,79].

Activated inflammatory cells such as leucocytes can contribute to endothelial cell dysfunction and vascular damage by direct and indirect pathways. Indirect loops comprise augmentation of MMP production by proinflammatory cytokines synthesized in activated leucocytes [70].

Activation of MMP-2 and MMP-9 is important in pathogenesis of diabetic microangiopathic complications such as diabetic retinopathy, nephropathy, and neuropathy [39]. Diabetic retinopathy, by inducing apoptosis of retinal endothelial cells and by degrading the junction proteins, is followed by increased vascular permeability [80,81]. In experimental models of DM, increased oxidative stress activates MMP-2, and antioxidant therapies inhibit the development of diabetic retinopathy by modulating retinal MMP-2 levels [32,82]. Diabetic nephropathy, one of the most severe microangiopathy in diabetes mellitus, is also characterized by MMP overexpression and accelerated ECM degradation, both being a hallmark of associated histopathologic changes [30]. MMPs' increased synthesis can also lead to neuronal injury through blood–nerve barrier (BNB) disruption, contributing to the neuropathic pain associated with diabetic neuropathy [83,84].

The multiple and complex roles exhibited by MMPs are explained by their multiple localizations. MMP-2 and MMP-9 are colocalized in vessel walls and atherosclerotic plaque, being involved in endothelial dysfunction and DM macrovascular complication and vascular remodeling [85,86]. Wang et al. reported a protective effect of EGCG after i.p. administration, by reducing the plasma levels of TNF-α, IL-6, and monocyte chemoattractant protein-1 (MCP-1) [38]. There is also evidence that EGCG can inhibit MMP-2 activation [87]. Multiple compounds of green tea can inhibit MMP-2 and -9, but the most efficient ones proved to be EGCG and epigallocatechin (EGC) [88]. Therefore, we chose the EGCG compound for our experimental study. Moreover, liposomal encapsulation brings an increased bioavailability with better results in reducing oxidative stress biomarkers and MMP plasma level. EGCG reduces MMP-2 activity by targeting the fibronectin type II repeated regions 1 and 3 of MMP-2, binds the amino acids that constitute the exosite of this enzyme, and hinders proper positioning of the substrate [89]. Due to its antioxidants effects and inhibitory action on the protein tyrosine kinases, EGCG reduces MMP-9 activity by reducing its release from the activated neutrophils [90].

From our knowledge, this is the first experimental study addressing liposomal EGCG effects in experimental DM induced by STZ in rats. Decreasing the hepatic and pancreatic damage due to STZ administration is a valuable effect of liposomal EGCG.

4.4. Potential Limitations of the Study

No measurements of EGCG and L-EGCG in the blood or pancreatic and hepatic tissue were done in this study since such quantifications were outside of our aim. Future studies could be conducted to measure the concentration of EGCG and L-EGCG in the blood and tissues. Moreover, oxidative stress parameters and MMPs could be measured in liver and pancreas tissue. Another limitation of our study is that the evaluation of endogenous insulin levels and measurement of HOMA-IR for endogenous pancreatic function were not performed.

Future studies should also investigate the effects of long-term administration of EGCG and L-EGCG on DM and its complications, as this study was focused on assessing their effects 48 h after DM induction.

5. Conclusions

L-EGCG pretreatment reduces oxidative stress biomarkers and MMP plasma levels 48 h after DM induction. Further studies are needed to detect other particularities regarding the EGCG protective mechanisms in order to improve their therapeutic efficiency. Due to the beneficial effects of EGCG nanoformulation proven by this study on oxidative stress, antioxidative defense, and MMP-2 and -9, we propose that L-EGCG could be considered as a novel adjuvant therapy in DM management.

Supplementary Materials: The following is available online at http://www.mdpi.com/2076-3921/9/2/172/s1, Table S1: *p*-values for comparisons between the study groups for all studied parameters.

Author Contributions: Conceptualization, G.D., C.M., and C.A.N.; Data curation, A.E.B., C.M., and I.C.S.; Formal analysis, M.V. and R.M.R.; Funding acquisition, G.D. and I.C.S.; Investigation, A.E.B., A.S.P., C.B., and M.V.; Methodology, P.-M.B., C.B., and C.A.N.; Project administration, A.E.B. and P.-M.B.; Resources, A.S.P., C.B., and I.C.S.; Software, P.-M.B. and M.V.; Supervision, R.M.R.; Validation, P.-M.B., A.S.P., C.M., and R.M.R.; Visualization, G.D. and C.M.; Writing—original draft, A.E.B. and I.C.S.; Writing—review & editing, A.S.P., G.D., and C.A.N. All authors have read and agreed to the published version of the manuscript.

Acknowledgments: The authors would like to thank Olivia Verișezan-Roșu for professional English language editing of the manuscript.

Conflicts of Interest: The authors declare no conflict of interest.

References

1. Park, J.H.; Bae, J.H.; Im, S.S.; Song, D.K. Green tea and type 2 diabetes. *Integr. Med. Res.* **2014**, *3*, 4–10. [CrossRef]
2. Chu, C.; Deng, J.; Man, Y.; Qu, Y. Green Tea Extracts Epigallocatechin-3-gallate for Different Treatments. *BioMed Res. Int.* **2017**, *2017*. [CrossRef] [PubMed]
3. Islam, M.A. Cardiovascular effects of green tea catechins: Progress and promise. *Recent Pat. Cardiovasc. Drug Discov.* **2012**, *7*, 88–99. [CrossRef] [PubMed]
4. Eng, Q.I.; Thanikachalam, P.V.; Ramamurthy, S. Molecular understanding of Epigallocatechin gallate (EGCG) in cardiovascular and metabolic diseases. *J. Ethnopharm.* **2018**, *210*, 296–310. [CrossRef] [PubMed]
5. Yuan, J.M. Cancer prevention by green tea: Evidence from epidemiologic studies. *Am. J. Clin. Nutr.* **2013**, *98*, 1676S–1681S. [CrossRef]
6. Suliburska, J.; Bogdanski, P.; Szulinska, M.; Stepien, M.; Pupek-Musialik, D.; Jablecka, A. Effects of green tea supplementation on elements, total antioxidants, lipids, and glucose values in the serum of obese patients. *Biol. Trace Elem. Res.* **2012**, *149*, 315–322. [CrossRef]
7. Mozaffari-Khosravi, H.; Ahadi, Z.; FallahTafti, M. The Effect of Green Tea versus Sour Tea on Insulin Resistance, Lipids Profiles and Oxidative Stress in Patients with Type 2 Diabetes Mellitus: A Randomized Clinical Trial. *Iran. J. Med. Sci.* **2014**, *39*, 424–432.
8. Turek, I.A.; Kozińska, J.; Drygas, W. Green tea as a protective factor in prophylaxis and treatment of selected cardiovascular diseases. *Kardiol. Pol.* **2012**, *70*, 848–852.
9. Larsson, S.C. Coffee, tea, and cocoa and risk of stroke. *Stroke* **2014**, *45*, 309–314. [CrossRef]
10. Li, F.J.; Ji, H.F.; Shen, L. A meta-analysis of tea drinking and risk of Parkinson's disease. *Sci. World J.* **2012**, *2012*, 923464. [CrossRef]
11. Pervin, M.; Unno, K.; Ohishi, T.; Tanabe, H.; Miyoshi, N.; Nakamura, Y. Beneficial Effects of Green Tea Catechins on Neurodegenerative Diseases. *Molecules* **2018**, *23*, 1297. [CrossRef] [PubMed]
12. Hauber, I.; Hohenberg, H.; Holstermann, B.; Hunstein, W.; Hauber, J. The main green tea polyphenol epigallocatechin-3-gallate counteracts semen-mediated enhancement of HIV infection. *Proc. Natl. Acad. Sci. USA* **2009**, *106*, 9033–9038. [CrossRef] [PubMed]
13. De Oliveira, A.; Adams, S.D.; Lee, L.H.; Murray, S.R.; Hsu, S.D.; Hammond, J.R.; Dickinson, D.; Chen, P.; Chu, T.C. Inhibition of herpes simplex virus type 1 with the modified green tea polyphenol palmitoyl-epigallocatechin gallate. *Food Chem. Toxicol.* **2013**, *52*, 207–215. [CrossRef] [PubMed]
14. Fu, Z.; Zhen, W.; Yuskavage, J.; Liu, D. Epigallocatechin gallate delays the onset of type 1 diabetes in spontaneous non-obese diabetic mice. *Br. J. Nutr.* **2011**, *105*, 1218–1225. [CrossRef]
15. Kondo, Y.; Goto, A.; Noma, H.; Iso, H.; Hayashi, K.; Noda, M. Effects of Coffee and Tea Consumption on Glucose Metabolism: A Systematic Review and Network Meta-Analysis. *Nutrients* **2019**, *11*, 48. [CrossRef]
16. Li, T.; Liu, J.; Zhang, X.; Ji, G. Antidiabetic activity of lipophilic (−)-epigallocatechin-3-gallate derivative under its role of α-glucosidase inhibition. *Biomed. Pharm.* **2007**, *61*, 91–96. [CrossRef]
17. Chiang, J.L.; Maahs, D.M.; Garvey, K.C.; Garvey, K.C.; Hood, K.K.; Laffel, L.M.; Weinzimer, S.A.; Wolfsdorf, J.I.; Schatz, D. Type 1 Diabetes in Children and Adolescents: A Position Statement by the American Diabetes Association. *Diabetes Care* **2018**, *41*, 2026–2044. [CrossRef]
18. Friederich, M.; Hansell, P.; Palm, F. Diabetes, oxidative stress, nitric oxide and mitochondria function. *Curr. Diabetes Rev.* **2009**, *5*, 120–144. [CrossRef]

19. Bulboacă, A.E.; Boarescu, P.M.; Bolboacă, S.D.; Blidaru, M.; Feștilă, D.; Dogaru, G.; Nicula, C.A. Comparative Effect of Curcumin versus Liposomal Curcumin on Systemic Pro-Inflammatory Cytokines Profile, MCP-1 and RANTES in Experimental Diabetes Mellitus. *Int. J. Nanomed.* **2019**, *14*, 8961–8972. [CrossRef]
20. Boarescu, P.-M.; Boarescu, I.; Bocșan, I.C.; Gheban, D.; Bulboacă, A.E.; Nicula, C.; Pop, R.M.; Râjnoveanu, R.-M.; Bolboacă, S.D. Antioxidant and Anti-Inflammatory Effects of Curcumin Nanoparticles on Drug-Induced Acute Myocardial Infarction in Diabetic Rats. *Antioxidants* **2019**, *8*, 504. [CrossRef]
21. Song, E.K.; Hur, H.; Han, M.-K. Epigallocatechin gallate prevents autoimmune diabetes induced by multiple low doses of streptozotocin in mice. *Arch. Pharm. Res.* **2003**, *26*, 559–563. [CrossRef] [PubMed]
22. Roghani, M.; Baluchnejadmojarad, T. Hypoglycemic and hypolipidemic effect and antioxidant activity of chronic epigallocatechin-gallate in streptozotocin-diabetic rats. *Pathophysiology* **2010**, *17*, 55–59. [CrossRef] [PubMed]
23. Granja, A.; Frias, I.; Neves, A.R.; Pinheiro, M.; Reis, S. Therapeutic Potential of Epigallocatechin GallateNanodelivery Systems. *BioMed Res. Int.* **2017**, *2017*, 5813793. [CrossRef] [PubMed]
24. Watkins, R.; Wu, L.; Zhang, C.; Davis, R.M.; Xu, B. Natural product-based nanomedicine: Recent advances and issues. *Int. J. Nanomed.* **2015**, *10*, 6055–6074.
25. Othman, A.I.; El-Sawi, M.R.; El-Missiry, M.A.; Abukhalil, M.H. Epigallocatechin-3 gallate protects against diabetic cardiomyopathy through modulating the cardiometabolic risk factors, oxidative stress, inflammation, cell death and fibrosis in streptozotocin-nicotinamide induced diabetic rats. *Biomed. Pharm.* **2017**, *94*, 362–373. [CrossRef] [PubMed]
26. Vu, T.H.; Werb, Z. Matrix metalloproteinases: Effectors of development and normal physiology. *Genes Dev.* **2000**, *14*, 2123–2133. [CrossRef]
27. Löffek, S.; Schilling, O.; Franzke, C.W. Series "matrix metalloproteinases in lung health and disease": Biological role of matrix metalloproteinases: A critical balance. *Eurrespir. J.* **2011**, *38*, 191–208. [CrossRef]
28. Peeters, S.A.; Engelen, L.; Buijs, J.; Chaturvedi, N.; Fuller, J.H.; Schalkwijk, C.G.; Stehouwer, C.D. EURODIAB Prospective Complications Study Group. Plasma levels of matrix metalloproteinase-2, -3, -10, and tissue inhibitor of metalloproteinase-1 are associated with vascular complications in patients with type 1 diabetes: The EURODIAB Prospective Complications Study. *Cardiovasc. Diabetol.* **2015**, *14*, 31.
29. Phillips, P.A.; McCarroll, J.A.; Park, S.; Wu, M.J.; Pirola, R.; Korsten, M.; Wilson, J.S.; Apte, M.V. Rat pancreatic stellate cells secrete matrix metalloproteinases: Implications for extracellular matrix turnover. *Gut* **2003**, *52*, 275–282. [CrossRef]
30. Xu, X.; Xiao, L.; Xiao, P.; Yang, S.; Chen, G.; Liu, F.; Kanwar, Y.S.; Sun, L. A glimpse of matrix metalloproteinases in diabetic nephropathy. *Curr. Med. Chem.* **2014**, *21*, 3244–3260. [CrossRef]
31. Thrailkill, K.M.; Bunn, R.C.; Moreau, C.S.; Cockrell, G.E.; Simpson, P.M.; Coleman, H.N.; Frindik, J.P.; Kemp, S.F.; Fowlkes, J.L. Matrix metalloproteinase-2 dysregulation in type 1 diabetes. *Diabetes Care* **2007**, *30*, 2321–2326. [CrossRef] [PubMed]
32. Kowluru, R.A.; Kamwar, M. Oxidative Stress and the Development of Diabetic Retinopathy: Contributory Role of Matrix Metalloproteinase-2. *Free Radicbiol. Med.* **2009**, *46*, 1677–1685. [CrossRef] [PubMed]
33. Lee, M.J.; Maliakal, P.; Chen, L.; Meng, X.; Bondoc, F.Y.; Prabhu, S.; Lambert, G.; Mohr, S.; Yang, C.S. Pharmacokinetics of tea catechins after ingestion of green tea and (−)-epigallocatechin-3-gallate by humans: Formation of different metabolites and individual variability. *Cancer Epidemiol. Biomark. Prev.* **2002**, *11*, 1025–1032.
34. Li, N.; Taylor, L.S.; Mauer, L.J. Degradation kinetics of catechins in green tea powder: Effects of temperature and relative humidity. *J. Agric. Food Chem.* **2011**, *59*, 6082–6090. [CrossRef] [PubMed]
35. Isemura, M. Catechin in Human Health and Disease. *Molecules* **2019**, *24*, 528. [CrossRef] [PubMed]
36. Tsai, Y.J.; Chen, B.H. Preparation of catechin extracts and nanoemulsions from green tea leaf waste and their inhibition effect on prostate cancer cell PC-3. *Int. J. Nanomed.* **2016**, *11*, 1907–1926.
37. Langer, R. New methods of drug delivery. *Science* **1990**, *249*, 1527–1533. [CrossRef]
38. Wang, S.; Su, R.; Nie, S.; Sun, M.; Zhang, J.; Wu, D.; Moustaid-Moussa, N. Application of nanotechnology in improving bioavailability and bioactivity of diet-derived phytochemicals. *J. Nutr. Biochem.* **2014**, *25*, 363–376. [CrossRef]
39. Mozafari, M.R.; Johnson, C.; Hatziantoniou, S.; Demetzos, C. Nanoliposomes and their applications in food nanotechnology. *J. Liposome Res.* **2008**, *18*, 309–327. [CrossRef]

40. Bulboacă, A.E.; Porfire, A.S.; Tefas, L.R.; Boarescu, P.M.; Bolboacă, S.D.; Stănescu, I.C.; Bulboacă, A.C.; Dogaru, G. Liposomal Curcumin is Better than Curcumin to Alleviate Complications in Experimental Diabetic Mellitus. *Molecules* **2019**, *24*, 846. [CrossRef]
41. Qi, S.; Wang, C.; Song, D.; Song, Y. Intraperitoneal injection of (−)-Epigallocatechin-3-gallate protects against light-induced photoreceptor degeneration in the mouse retina. *Mol. Vis.* **2017**, *23*, 171–178. [PubMed]
42. Ramachandran, B.; Jayavelu, S.; Murhekar, K.; Rajkumar, T. Repeated dose studies with pure Epigallocatechin-3-gallate demonstrated dose and route dependant hepatotoxicity with associated dyslipidemia. *Toxicol. Rep.* **2016**, *3*, 336–345. [CrossRef] [PubMed]
43. Li, C.; Peng, J.; Hu, R.; Yan, J.; Sun, Y.; Zhang, L.; Liu, W.; Jiang, H. Safety and Efficacy of Ketamine Versus Ketamine-Fentanyl-Dexmedetomidine Combination for Anesthesia and Analgesia in Rats. *Dose Response* **2019**, *17*. [CrossRef] [PubMed]
44. Porfire, A.; Tomuta, I.; Leucuta, S.E.; Achim, M. Superoxide dismutase loaded liposomes. The influence of formulation factors on enzyme encapsulation and release. *Farmacia* **2013**, *61*, 865–873.
45. Sylvester, B.; Porfire, A.; Muntean, D.M.; Vlase, L.; Luput, L.E.; Sesarman, A.; Alupei, M.C.; Banciu, M.; Achim, M.; Tomuta, I. Optimization of prednisolone loaded long circulating liposome's via application of quality by design (QbD) approach. *J. Liposome Res.* **2018**, *28*, 49–61. [CrossRef] [PubMed]
46. Postescu, I.D.; Tatomir, C.; Chereches, G.; Brie, I.; Damian, G.; Petrisor, D.; Hosu, A.M.; Miclaus, V.; Pop, A. Spectroscopic characterization of some grape extracts with potential role in tumor growth inhibition. *J. Optoelectron. Adv. Mater.* **2007**, *9*, 564–567.
47. Yagi, K. Assay for blood plasma and serum peroxides. *Methods Enzymol.* **1984**, *105*, 328–331.
48. Goel, P.; Srivastava, K.; Das, N.; Bhatnagar, V. The role of nitric oxide in portal hypertension caused by extrahepatic portal vein obstruction. *J. Indian Assocpediatrsurg.* **2010**, *15*, 117–121.
49. Bulboacă, A.E.; Porfire, A.; Bărbălată, A.; Bolboacă, S.D.; Nicula, C.; Boarescu, P.M.; Stănescu, I.; Dogaru, G. The effect of liposomal epigallocatechin gallate and metoclopramide hydrochloride co-administration on experimental migraine. *Farmacia* **2019**, *67*, 905–911. [CrossRef]
50. Erel, O. A novel automated method to measure total antioxidant response against potent free radical reactions. *Clin. Biochem.* **2004**, *37*, 112–119. [CrossRef]
51. Hu, M.L. Measurement of protein thiol groups and glutathione in plasma. *Methods Enzymol.* **1994**, *233*, 380–385. [PubMed]
52. Aebi, H. Catalase in vitro. *Methods Enzymol.* **1984**, *105*, 121–126. [PubMed]
53. Haider, R.; Annie, J. Streptozotocin-Induced Cytotoxicity, Oxidative Stress and Mitochondrial Dysfunction in Human Hepatoma HepG2 Cells. *Int. J. Mol. Sci.* **2012**, *12*, 5751–5767.
54. Weissgerber, T.L.; Milic, N.M.; Winham, S.J.; Garovic, V.D. Beyond bar and line graphs: Time for a new data presentation paradigm. *PLoS Biol.* **2015**, *13*, e1002128. [CrossRef] [PubMed]
55. Jia, J.J.; Zeng, X.S.; Song, X.Q.; Zhang, P.P.; Chen, L. Diabetes mellitus and Alzheimer's disease: The protection of epigallocatechin-3-gallate in streptozotocin injection-induced models. *Front. Pharm.* **2017**, *8*, 834. [CrossRef] [PubMed]
56. Meng, J.-M.; Cao, S.-Y.; Wei, X.-L.; Gan, R.-Y.; Wang, Y.-F.; Cai, S.-X.; Xu, X.-Y.; Zhang, P.-Z.; Li, H.-B. Effects and Mechanisms of Tea for the Prevention and Management of Diabetes Mellitus and Diabetic Complications: An Updated Review. *Antioxidants* **2019**, *8*, 170. [CrossRef]
57. Ortsäter, H.; Grankvist, N.; Wolfram, S.; Kuehn, N.; Sjöholm, A. Diet supplementation with green tea extract epigallocatechin gallate prevents progression to glucose intolerance in db/db mice. *Nutr. Metab.* **2012**, *9*, 11. [CrossRef]
58. Ueda-Wakagi, M.; Nagayasu, H.; Yamashita, Y.; Ashida, A.H. Green Tea Ameliorates Hyperglycemia by Promoting the Translocation of Glucose Transporter 4 in the Skeletal Muscle of Diabetic Rodents. *Int. J. Mol. Sci.* **2019**, *20*, 2436. [CrossRef]
59. Waltner-Law, M.E.; Wang, X.L.; Law, B.K.; Hall, R.K.; Nawano, M.; Granner, D.K. Epigallocatechin gallate, a constituent of green tea, represses hepatic glucose production. *J. Biol. Chem.* **2002**, *277*, 34933–34940. [CrossRef]
60. Kume, E.; Fujimura, H.; Matsuki, N.; Ito, M.; Aruga, C.; Toriumi, W.; Kitamura, K.; Doi, K. Hepatic changes in the acute phase of streptozotocin (SZ)-induced diabetes in mice. *Exp. Toxicol. Pathol.* **2004**, *55*, 467–480. [CrossRef]

61. Kume, E.; Aruga, C.; Takahashi, K.; Miwa, S.; Dekura, E.; Itoh, M.; Ishizuka, Y.; Fujimura, H.; Toriumi, W.; Doi, K. Morphological and gene expression analysis in mouse primary cultured hepatocytes exposed to streptozotocin. *Exp. Toxicol. Pathol.* **2005**, *56*, 245–253. [CrossRef] [PubMed]
62. Kobori, M.; Masumoto, S.; Akimoto, Y.; Takahashi, Y. Dietary quercetin alleviates diabetic symptoms and reduces streptozotocin-induced disturbance of hepatic gene expression in mice. *Mol. Nutr. Food Res.* **2009**, *53*, 859–868. [CrossRef] [PubMed]
63. Rodríguez, V.; Plavnik, L.; Tolosa de Talamoni, N. Naringin attenuates liver damage in streptozotocin-induced diabetic rats. *Biomed. Pharm.* **2018**, *105*, 95–102. [CrossRef] [PubMed]
64. Abolfathi, A.A.; Mohajeri, D.; Rezaie, A.; Nazeri, M. Protective Effects of Green Tea Extract against Hepatic Tissue Injury in Streptozotocin-Induced Diabetic Rats. *Evid.-Based Complement. Altern. Med.* **2012**, *2012*, 740671. [CrossRef]
65. Niu, Y.; Na, L.; Feng, R.; Gong, L.; Zhao, Y.; Li, Q.; Li, Y.; Sun, C. The phytochemical, EGCG, extends lifespan by reducing liver and kidney function damage and improving age-associated inflammation and oxidative stress in healthy rats. *Aging Cell* **2013**, *12*, 1041–1049. [CrossRef]
66. West, I.C. Radicals and oxidative stress in diabetes. *Diabet. Med.* **2000**, *17*, 171–180. [CrossRef]
67. Fernandes, S.M.; Cordeiro, P.M.; Watanabe, M.; Fonseca, C.D.; Vattimo, M.F. The role of oxidative stress in streptozotocin-induced diabetic nephropathy in rats. *Arch. Endocrinol. Metab.* **2016**, *60*, 443–449. [CrossRef]
68. De Almeida, D.A.T.; Braga, C.P.; Novelli, E.L.B.; Fernandes, A.A.H. Evaluation of lipid profile and oxidative stress in STZ-induced rats treated with antioxidant vitamin. *Br. Arch. Biol. Technol.* **2012**, *55*, 527–536. [CrossRef]
69. Talebanzadeh, S.; Ashrafi, M.; Kazemipour, N.; Erjaee, H.; Nazifi, S. Evaluation of the effects of saffron aqueous extract on oxidative stress in the lens of streptozotocin-induced diabetic rats. *BRAT* **2018**, *5*, 2133–2141. [CrossRef]
70. Aloud, A.A.; Veeramani, C.; Govindasamy, C.; Alsaif, M.A.; Al-Numair, K.S. Galangin, a natural flavonoid reduces mitochondrial oxidative damage in streptozotocin-induced diabetic rats. *Redox Rep.* **2018**, *23*, 29–34. [CrossRef]
71. Schmatz, R.; Belmonte, P.L.; Stefanello, N.; Mazzanti, C.; Spanevello, R.; Gutierres, J.; Bagatini, M.; Curry Martins, C.; HuseinAbdalla, F.; da Silva Serres, J.D.; et al. Effects of resveratrol on biomarkers of oxidative stress and on the activity of delta aminolevulinic acid dehydratase in liver and kidney of streptozotocin-induced diabetic rats. *Biochimie* **2012**, *94*, e374–e383. [CrossRef] [PubMed]
72. Opara, E.C. Oxidative stress, micronutrients, diabetes mellitus and its complications. *J. R. Soc. Health* **2002**, *122*, 28–34. [CrossRef] [PubMed]
73. Bernatoniene, J.; Kopustinskiene, D.M. The Role of Catechins in Cellular Responses to Oxidative Stress. *Molecules* **2018**, *23*, 965. [CrossRef] [PubMed]
74. Orsolic, N.; Sirovina, D.; Gajski, G.; Garaj-Vrhovac, V.; Jembrek, M.J.; Kosalec, I. Assessment of DNA damage and lipid peroxidation in diabetic mice: Effects of propolis and epigallocatechin gallate (EGCG). *Mutat. Res.* **2013**, *757*, 36–44. [CrossRef] [PubMed]
75. Minnelli, C.; Moretti, P.; Fulgenzi, G.; Mariani, P.; Laudadio, E.; Armeni, T.; Galeazzi, R.; Mobbili, G. A Poloxamer-407 modified liposome encapsulating epigallocatechin-3-gallate in the presence of magnesium: Characterization and protective effect against oxidative damage. *Int. J. Pharm.* **2018**, *552*, 225–234. [CrossRef] [PubMed]
76. Liu, C.; Wan, X.; Ye, T.; Fang, F.; Chen, X.; Chen, Y.; Dong, Y. Matrix Metalloproteinase 2 Contributes to Pancreatic Beta Cell Injury Induced by Oxidative Stress. *PLoS ONE* **2014**, *9*, e110227. [CrossRef]
77. Macarie, R.D.; Vadana, M.; Ciortan, L.; Tucureanu, M.M.; Ciobanu, A.; Vinereanu, D.; Manduteanu, I.; Simionescu, M.; Butoi, E. The expression of MMP-1 and MMP-9 is up-regulated by smooth muscle cells after their cross-talk with macrophages in high glucose conditions. *J. Cell Mol. Med.* **2018**, *22*, 4366–4376. [CrossRef]
78. Smigiel, K.S.; Parks, W.C. Matrix Metalloproteinases and Leukocyte Activation. *Prog. Mol. Biol. Transl. Sci.* **2017**, *147*, 167–195.
79. Cui, N.; Hu, M.; Khalil, R.A. Biochemical and Biological Attributes of Matrix Metalloproteinases. *Prog. Mol. Biol. Transl. Sci.* **2017**, *147*, 1–73.
80. Mohammad, G. Role of matrix metalloproteinase-2 and -9 in the development of diabetic retinopathy. *J. Ocul. Biol. Dis. Inform.* **2012**, *5*, 1–8. [CrossRef]

81. Drankowska, J.; Kos, M.; Kościuk, A.; Marzęda, P.; Boguszewska-Czubara, A.; Tylus, M.; Święch-Zubilewicz, A. MMP targeting in the battle for vision: Recent developments and future prospects in the treatment of diabetic retinopathy. *Life Sci.* **2019**, *229*, 149–156. [CrossRef] [PubMed]
82. Kowluru, R.A.; Kanwar, M.; Chan, P.S.; Zhang, J.P. AREDS-based micronutrients inhibit retinopathy and retinal metabolic abnormalities in diabetic rats. *Arch. Ophthalmol.* **2008**, *126*, 1266–1272. [CrossRef] [PubMed]
83. Hughes, P.M.; Wells, G.M.; Perry, V.H.; Brown, M.C.; Miller, K.M. Comparison of matrix metalloproteinase expression during Wallerian degeneration in the central and peripheral nervous systems. *Neuroscience* **2002**, *113*, 273–287. [CrossRef]
84. Kuhad, A.; Singh, P.; Chopra, K. Matrix metalloproteinases: Potential therapeutic target for diabetic neuropathic pain. *Expert Opin. Ther. Targets* **2015**, *19*, 177–185. [CrossRef]
85. Raffetto, J.D.; Khalil, R.A. Matrix metalloproteinases and their inhibitors in vascular remodeling and vascular disease. *Biochem. Pharmacol.* **2008**, *75*, 346–359. [CrossRef]
86. Kiugel, M.; Hellberg, S.; Käkelä, M.; Liljenbäck, H.; Saanijoki, T.; Li, X.-G.; Tuomela, J.; Knuuti, J.; Saraste, A.; Roivainen, A. Evaluation of [68Ga]Ga-DOTA-TCTP-1 for the Detection of Metalloproteinase 2/9 Expression in Mouse Atherosclerotic Plaques. *Molecules* **2018**, *23*, 3168. [CrossRef]
87. Djerir, D.; Iddir, M.; Bourgault, S.; Lamy, S.; Annabi, B. Biophysical evidence for differential gallated green tea catechins binding to membrane type-1 matrix metalloproteinase and its interactors. *Biophys. Chem.* **2018**, *234*, 34–41. [CrossRef]
88. Demeule, M.; Brossard, M.; Pagé, M.; Gingras, D.; Béliveau, R. Matrix metalloproteinase inhibition by green tea catechins. *Biochim. Biophys. Acta* **2000**, *1478*, 51–60. [CrossRef]
89. Jha, S.; Kanaujia, S.P.; Limaye, A.M. Direct inhibition of matrix metalloproteinase-2 (MMP-2) by (−)-epigallocatechin-3-gallate: A possible role for the fibronectin type II repeats. *Gene* **2016**, *593*, 126–130. [CrossRef]
90. Kim-Park, W.K.; Allam, E.S.; Palasuk, J.; Kowolik, M.; Park, K.K.; Windsor, L.J. Green tea catechin inhibits the activity and neutrophil release of Matrix Metalloproteinase-9. *J. Tradit. Complement. Med.* **2016**, *6*, 343–346. [CrossRef]

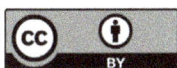

© 2020 by the authors. Licensee MDPI, Basel, Switzerland. This article is an open access article distributed under the terms and conditions of the Creative Commons Attribution (CC BY) license (http://creativecommons.org/licenses/by/4.0/).

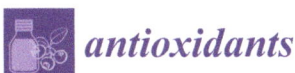

Article

A Novel Pectic Polysaccharide of Jujube Pomace: Structural Analysis and Intracellular Antioxidant Activities

Ximeng Lin [1], Keshan Liu [1], Sheng Yin [2], Yimin Qin [3], Peili Shen [3,*] and Qiang Peng [1,*]

1. College of Food Science and Engineering, Northwest A&F University, Yangling 712100, China; ximenglin423@nwsuaf.edu.cn (X.L.); Liukeshan@nwafu.edu.cn (K.L.)
2. Beijing Engineering and Technology Research Center of Food Additives, Beijing Technology & Business University (BTBU), Beijing 100048, China; yinsheng@btbu.edu.cn
3. State Key Laboratory of Bioactive Seaweed Substances, Ministry of Agriculture Key Laboratory of Seaweed Fertilizers, Qingdao Brightmoon Seaweed Group Co Ltd., Qingdao 266400, China; yiminqin1965@126.com
* Correspondence: spl@bmsg.com (P.S.); pengqiang@nwsuaf.edu.cn (Q.P.)

Received: 29 December 2019; Accepted: 30 January 2020; Published: 2 February 2020

Abstract: After extraction from jujube pomace and purification by two columns (DEAE-Sepharose Fast Flow and Sepharcyl S-300), the structure of SAZMP4 was investigated by HPGPC, GC, FI-IR, GC-MS, NMR, SEM, and AFM. Analysis determined that SAZMP4 (Mw = 28.94 kDa) was a pectic polysaccharide mainly containing 1,4-linked GalA (93.48%) with side chains of 1,2,4-linked Rha and 1,3,5-linked Ara and terminals of 1-linked Rha and 1-linked Ara, which might be the homogalacturonan (HG) type with side chains of the RG-I type, corresponding to the results of NMR. In AFM and SEM images, self-assembly and aggregation of SAZMP4 were respectively observed indicating its structural features. The antioxidant activity of SAZMP4 against H_2O_2-induced oxidative stress in Caco-2 cells was determined by activity of superoxide dismutase (SOD) and glutathione peroxidase (GSH-Px) as well as malondialdehyde (MDA) and reactive oxygen species (ROS) levels, indicating SAZMP4 can be a natural antioxidant. Also, a better water retention capacity and thermal stability of SAZMP4 was observed based on DSC analysis, which could be applied in food industry as an additive.

Keywords: polysaccharide; jujube pomace; structural analysis; antioxidant activity

1. Introduction

Pectin is a natural macromolecular compound, generally considered as a complex polysaccharide containing α-1,4-linked galacturonic acid, which might be partly methyl esterified and have side chains of various neutral sugars, such as rhamnose, arabinose, galactose, and so on [1]. It widely exists in the cell wall and the middle lamella structure of all higher plants [2]. Because of pectin's gelatification, thickening, and stabilization, it is widely applied in food, medical, chemical, and other industries [3]. China, the original country of jujube, has cultivated jujube since around 7000 years ago. Since jujube fruits are rich in sugar, and the abundant intracellular and cell wall polysaccharides are more soluble in alkaline solution, it is better to use alkaline solution for extraction to take full advantage of the pomace [4]. According to previous research, jujube polysaccharides have different biological activities, such as antioxidant activity [5], immunoregulatory activity [6], hepatoprotective effects [7], anti-hyperlipidemia effects [8], and antitumor activity [9]. Obviously, biological activities of polysaccharides are associated with their structural characteristics. Many researchers have determined the composition, the average molecular weight, and the type of linkages of polysaccharides can affect the biological activities of polysaccharides [10–12]. Thus, there exists an importance to determine the structural characterizations of pectic polysaccharide.

It is widely acknowledged that free radicals are indispensable in metabolic processes. However, oxidative stress is an important factor in these diseases. Reactive oxygen species (ROS), chemically active substances mainly including peroxide, superoxide, hydroxyl radicals, and singlet oxygen [13], plays a necessary role in physiological regulation and message passing in moderate amount. Normally, there exists an antioxidant system containing antioxidants and antioxidant enzymes that controls the metabolic balance of free radicals. However, as a result of some unnormal factors and conditions like ischemia, hypoxia, chemicals, ionizing radiation, chemotherapy drugs, and ultraviolet radiation, abundant free radicals will be produced and break the metabolic balance. Under this circumstance, oxidative stress will occur. Also, excessive free radical accumulation can injure the components of cells, such as DNA and proteins, leading to the development and progression of diseases such as diabetes, cancer, and cardiovascular diseases [14,15]. Thus, it is imperative to improve antioxidant activity in order to prevent and control these diseases.

In this study, the structure of a pectic polysaccharide extracted from jujube pomace was characterized by chemical and instrumental methods, and the antioxidant activity was investigated by the Caco-2 cells model.

2. Materials and Methods

2.1. Materials and Reagents

The dry fruits (*Ziziphus jujuba* cv. Muzao) were provided by the Loess Plateau Experimental Orchard from Yulin in Shaanxi province, China. The chromatographic columns (DEAE-Sepharose Fast Flow and Sepharcyl S-300) were purchased from GE Healthcare Life Sciences (Piscataway, NJ, USA). The standards arabinose, fucose, galactose, glucose, mannose, rhamnose, and xylose were from Solarbio Life Sciences Co. (Beijing, China). The standards glucuronic acid and galacturonic acid were purchased from Aladdin Biochemical Technology Co., (Shanghai, China). All other chemicals were analytical grade.

2.2. Extraction and Purification of SAZMP4

Jujube pomace was obtained by removing the water-insoluble polysaccharide jujube powder. Alkaline extraction (0.1 M NaOH, 25 °C, 1 h) was applied to jujube pomace for obtaining crude polysaccharide. Then, an anion-exchange column of DEAE-Sepharose Fast Flow (2.6 × 100 cm), using 0.3 M NaCl as mobile phase at room temperature with a flow rate of 1.2 mL/min, and a gel-permeation chromatography column of Sepharcyl S-300 (2.6 × 100 cm), using ultrapure water as mobile phase at room temperature with a flow rate of 0.8 mL/min, were used to purify the crude polysaccharide in order to derive the purified polysaccharide, SAZMP4 [16].

2.3. Structural analysis of SAZMP4

2.3.1. Physical and Chemical Analysis

The phenol-sulfuric acid method [17], the Bradford method [18], and the Folin–Ciocalteu reagent method [19] were used to measure the content of total sugar, protein, and total phenolics.

The UV-Vis spectrum was recorded by a UV7 spectrophotometer (METTLER, TOLEDO, Zurich, Switzerland) in the 200–400 nm region to detect the protein and nuclear acids [20], and the FI-IR spectrum was recorded with a Fourier transform infrared spectrometer (FI-IR, Vetex70, Bruker Co., Ettlingen, Germany) in the 4000–400 cm^{-1} region by KBr pellets to determine the primary functional groups [21].

High-performance gel-permeation chromatography (HPGPC) equipped with an Agilent 1200 series high-performance liquid chromatography system, a Waters 2414 refractive index detector, and a TSK gel G5000PWXL column (300 × 7.8 mm, Tosoh, Japan) were used to determine the homogeneity and average molecular weight of the purified polysaccharide [22]. The retention time was used to calculate the average molecular weight of SAZMP4.

Gas chromatography (GC, GC-2014, Shimadzu Co., Kyoto, Japan) with a capillary column of DB-17 (30 m × 0.25 mm × 0.25 μm, Agilent, Santa Clara, CA, US) was used to indicate the monosaccharide composition of SAZMP4 [23], and the mixed standard monosaccharides were used for the monosaccharide identification and quantification.

A differential scanning calorimeter (DSC, Q2000, Waters, Milford, MA, USA) was used to analyze the thermal properties of SAZMP4 [24]. The dried and powdered polysaccharide (3 mg) was put into a standard aluminum crucible and sealed immediately. The program raised the temperature from 40 °C to 300 °C at a rate of 10 °C/min in a dynamic inert nitrogen atmosphere (50 mL/min). Simultaneously, an empty standard aluminum crucible was used as a reference.

2.3.2. Methylation Analysis

After the uronic acid reduction by Taylor and Conrad [25], SAZMP4 was methylated by a method reported previously [26]. The disappearance of the absorption band of O-H around 3400 cm^{-1} in the FI-IR spectrum indicated complete methylation of the sample. Then, the sample was hydrolyzed by trifluoroacetic acid, restored with sodium borohydride, acetylated by acetic anhydride, and dissolved in chloroform. A GCMS-QP2010A instrument (Shimadzu Co., Kyoto, Japan) equipped with a Rtx-50 capillary column (30 m × 0.25 mm × 0.25 μm) and an ion trap MS detector was used to determine the derivatives.

2.3.3. NMR Analysis

The dried SAZMP4 was dissolved (D_2O) and lyophilized three times. Fifty milligrams of deuterium-exchanged SAZMP4 was dissolved in 0.5 mL D_2O. NMR spectra of ^1H and ^{13}C were recorded with a Brucker AVANCE III 500 MHz nuclear magnetic resonance spectrometer (NMR) using standard pulse sequences at 25 °C [27].

2.4. Molecular Morphological Analysis

A field emission scanning electron microscope (SEM, S-4800, Hitachi, Tokyo, Japan) was used to record the surface morphological properties of SAZMP4 [28]. Before observation, SAZMP4 was covered with a gold layer.

An atomic force microscope (AFM, Multimode-8, Bruker Co., Billerica, MA, USA) was used to document the properties of the molecular morphology of the polysaccharide. Ten microliters of the polysaccharide solution (1 μg/mL) was dropped onto a mica carrier and then dried at room temperature, using tapping mode on the AFM for record [29].

2.5. Antioxidant Activity of SAZMP4

2.5.1. Cell Culture

Human colorectal adenocarcinoma cells (Caco-2) were obtained from Shanghai Institute of Cell Biology (Shanghai, China). The cells were cultured in high-glucose Dulbecco's modified Eagle's medium (H-DEME, Hyclone, Logan, UT, USA) with 10% fetal bovine serum (FBS, Biological Industries Beit Haemek, Kibbutz, Israel), 100 units/mL penicillin, and 100 μg/mL streptomycin and in a humidified atmosphere of 5% CO_2 at 37 °C. Between 3 and 15 passages of the cells were used in this study.

2.5.2. Cell Viability Analysis

Cell Counting Kit-8 (CCK-8, EnoGene Co., Shanghai, China) was used to evaluate the cell viability. In brief, Caco-2 cells were cultured in 96-well plates with a density of 5×10^3 cells/mL and incubated for 24 h in a 37 °C incubator with a humidified 5% CO_2 atmosphere. After that, the cells were treated with different concentrations of SAZMP4 (50, 100, 200, 400, and 800 μg/mL) for 24 h. Then, 10 μL of

CCK-8 solution was added, and the cells were incubated in the same environment for 1 h. The cell viability was determined by a multifunctional enzyme marker (victorX3, PerkinElmer Co., Waltham, Massachusetts, US) at a wavelength of 450 nm and was expressed as a relative percentage to the blank control group.

2.5.3. Treatment Procedure

For treatment, the cells (5×10^3 cells/mL) were cultured in 96-well plates and incubated at 37 °C for 24 h. Then, the cells were treated with different concentrates of SAZMP4 (25, 50, 100, and 200 μg/mL) for 24 h. After removing the medium, the cells were exposed to 200 μM of H_2O_2 for 2 h. The cell viability, superoxide dismutase (SOD), glutathione peroxidase (GSH-Px), ROS, and malondialdehyde (MDA) levels were determined by relevant commercial kits.

2.5.4. Measurement of SOD and GSH-Px

Cell lysates treated without or with different concentrations of SAZMP4 were collected for antioxidant enzymes (SOD and GSH-Px) analysis. The activities of SOD were measured by the relevant commercial kits (Beyotime, Biotechnology, Shanghai, China) using the xanthine oxidase method for determination. The activity of SOD was defined as the corresponding SOD content when the SOD inhabitation rate in each milliliter of reaction liquid reached 50%.

The activities of GSH-Px were measured by the relative commercial kits (Beyotime, Biotechnology, Shanghai, China). The activities of GSH-Px were determined by the consumption of GSH in enzymatic reactions.

2.5.5. Intracellular ROS and MDA Levels

The intracellular ROS was determined by a Reactive Oxygen Species Assay Kit (Beyotime, Biotechnology, Shanghai, China), investigated by fluorophore 2,7-dichlorofluorescein diacetate (DCFH-DA). After incubating the cells in a black 96-well plate for 24 h and removing the medium, the cells were washed with phosphate-buffered saline (PBS, 100 μL). After that, the cells were cultured with DCFH-DA at a concentration of 10 μM at 37 °C for 30 min. The results were determined by a multimode microplate reader (PerkinElmer, Waltham, MA, USA) and expressed as fold changes in fluorescence intensity versus control.

The MDA levels were indicated by corresponding detection kits (Jiancheng Bioengineering Institute, Nanjing, China) following the manufacturer's instructions.

2.6. Data Analysis

All test data were expressed as mean ± SD from no fewer than three determinations and analyzed with variance (ANOVA) following multiple tests. SPSS version 22.0 was used for all statistical analyses, and $p < 0.05$ was considered to be significant.

3. Results

3.1. Separation and Purification of SAZMP4

SAZMP4 was extracted from jujube pomace by alkaline solution and purified by the column of DEAE-Sepharose Fast Flow with mobile phase of 0.3 M NaCl and the column of Sepharcyl S-300 with ultrapure water. The yield of crude polysaccharide was 5.3% relative to jujube pomace, and the yield of SAZMP4 was 5.10% relative to crude polysaccharide. Other jujube researchers [5,7,9] obtained similar results to this study.

3.2. Preliminary Characterizations of SAZMP4

According to the phenol-sulfuric acid assay, SAZMP4 was 96.52% sugar. It had a low protein content of 0.78%, coinciding with UV–Vis analysis that the polysaccharide contained no protein (<3%)

based on the no absorption peaks at 280 nm. Also, no absorption peaks at 260 nm in the spectrum indicated no nucleic acid in SAZMP4. The total phenol content was not detected in SAZMP4. These results were similar to other acidic jujube polysaccharides from Z. *Jujuba* [30].

In the FI-IR spectrum (Figure 1), the peaks of the intramolecular or intermolecular stretching vibration of O-H was around 3400 cm^{-1} and the stretching vibration of C–H was around 2940 cm^{-1}, indicating the SAZMP4 was a polysaccharide. The peaks at approximately 1620 cm^{-1} were attributed to the stretching vibration of carboxyl, which implied that SAZMP4 might contain uronic acid [31]. The absorptions at 1420 and 1325 cm^{-1} belonged to the bending vibration of C–H. Also, the signals at 1200–800 cm^{-1} of the fingerprint area of carbohydrates indicated that the bands at 1093 and 1012 cm^{-1} were the bending vibration of C–O in the pyranose form. In addition, the weak absorption bands at 941 and 838 cm^{-1} were probably attributed to α-glycosidic bonds, further supported by the out-of-plane bending vibration of C–H at around 630 cm^{-1}, which implied the presence of α-glycosidic bonds in SAZMP4 [32].

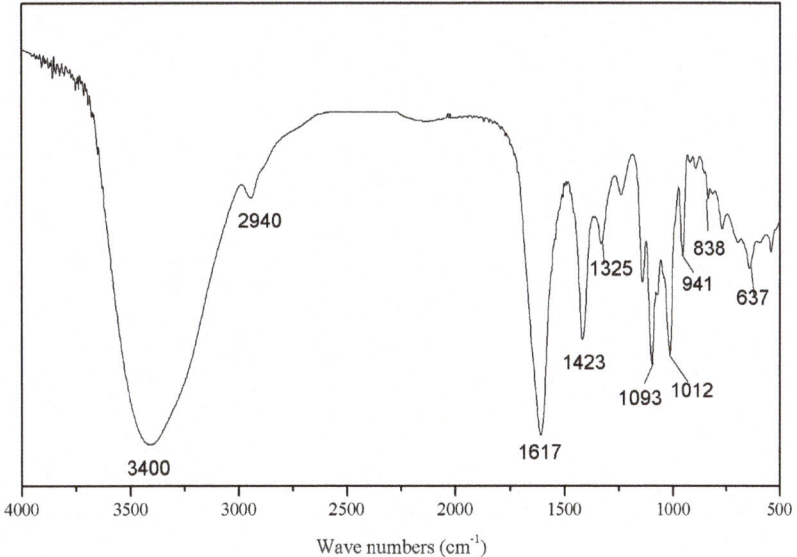

Figure 1. FI-IR spectrum of SAZMP4.

According to the equation, the average molecular weight of SAZMP4 was calculated to be 28.94 kDa with the retention time of 19.91 min. Also, the single and symmetric elution peak from the HPGPC indicated SAZMP4 was a homogeneous fraction.

GC analysis, as shown in Table 1, determined that the monosaccharide composition of SAZMP4 mainly contained galacturonic acid at a molar rate of 93.48%, which coincided with the feature of pectin. This result was similar with other pectic polysaccharides [30,33,34], but the galacturonic acid content of SAZMP4 was higher than them.

Table 1. Monosaccharide analysis data of SAZMP4.

Peak No.	Retention Time (min)	Monosaccharide	Molar Radio
1	11.645	Rhamnose	1
2	12.289	Arabinose	0.9
3	12.921	Xylose	0.05
4	22.800	Mannose	0.07
5	38.020	Galacturonic acid	28.9

The thermodynamic properties of SAZMP4 were examined by DSC from 40 to 300 °C. In the DSC thermogram of SAZMP4 (Figure 2), an endothermic peak and an exothermic peak were observed, and the parameters of them were labeled, such as melting temperature (T_m), melting enthalpy (ΔH_m), degradation temperature (T_d), and degradation enthalpy (ΔH_d). T_m and ΔH_m were determined by the composition and structural characterizations of polysaccharides. A polysaccharide with lower molecular weight and less uronic acid content has worse capacity to sustain water, so the T_m and ΔH_m were lower [35]. The high T_m and ΔH_m indicated the better capacity of SAZMP4 to sustain water, coinciding with results of HPGPC and GC analyses. The second peak was caused by the degradation of the polysaccharide in the process [36]. Apparently, T_d was primarily impacted by the composition of the polysaccharides, while the ΔH_d of polysaccharides was mainly affected by its galacturonic acid content. The T_d implied that SAZMP4 was stable below 240 °C, related to the better thermal stability, which might be applied in the food industry.

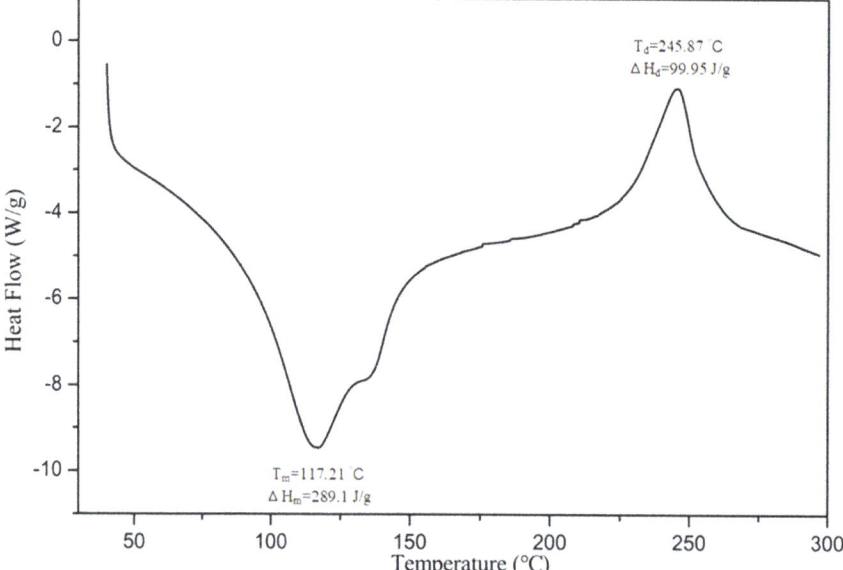

Figure 2. DSC thermogram of SAZMP4.

3.3. Methylation Analysis

For the determination of linkage types between sugar residues with GC-MS, SAZMP4 was firstly subjected to uronic acid reduction in order to avoid β-condensation reaction during methylation, which might cause structural changes to sugar chains [37]. According to the retention time of sugar residues and the standard data of CCRC Spectral Database, the results of the methylation analysis are exhibited in Table 2. SAZMP4 mainly included five types of glycosidic linkages: 1-linked Rha*p*, 1-linked Ara*f*, 1,2,4-liked Rha*p*, 1,3,5-linked Ara*f*, and 1,4-linked Gal*p* with a molar ratio of 0.4: 0.38: 0.62: 0.58: 28.7. This conformed to the GC analysis, which indicated that the structures of sugar chains were not destroyed in the methylation process. Besides, GC analysis showed SAZMP4 contained only galacturonic acid, and no galactose exited in it. Thus, the linkage type of galacturonic acid was 1,4-linked GalA*p*. Obviously, SAZMP4 was a pectic polysaccharide containing 1,4-linked galacturonic acid with side chains of 1,2,4-liked Rha*p* and 1,3,5-linked Ara*f* as well as terminals of 1-linked Rha*p* and 1-linked Ara*f*, which indicated that SAZMP4 might be homogalacturonan (HG) with side chains of rhamnogalacturonan (RG) type I [38].

Table 2. Methylation analysis data of SAZMP4.

Peak No.	Retention Time (min)	Methylated Sugars	Linkage Patterns	Molar Radio
1	20.355	2,3,4-Me$_3$-Rha$p$	1-linked Rha$p$	0.5
2	26.563	2,3,5-Me$_3$-Ara$f$	1-linked Ara$f$	0.47
3	31.915	2-Me-Ara$f$	1,3,5-linked Ara$f$	0.46
4	34.707	3-Me-Rha$p$	1,2,4-linked Rha$p$	0.52
5	35.092	2,3,6-Me$_3$-Gal$p$	1,4-linked Gal$p$	28.8

3.4. NMR Analysis

The ^{1}H (Figure 3A) and ^{13}C NMR (Figure 3B) spectra of SAZMP4 were displayed, and the chemical shifts in the spectra were classified based on previous research [39]. In the ^{1}H spectrum, the weak peak of δ 1.84 belonged to H-6 of 1,2,4-linked Rha$p$ or 1-linked Rha$p$, and the other strong signs of δ 4.34, 4.06, 3.92, and 3.60 were respectively attributed to H-5, H-4, H-3, and H-2 of 1,4-linked GalAp. The strong signs of δ 160.45, 99.07, 71.44, 69.67, 68.28, and 62.70 belonged to the C-6, C-1, C-4, C-5, C-3, and C-2 of 1,4-linked GalAp in the ^{13}C spectrum, respectively.

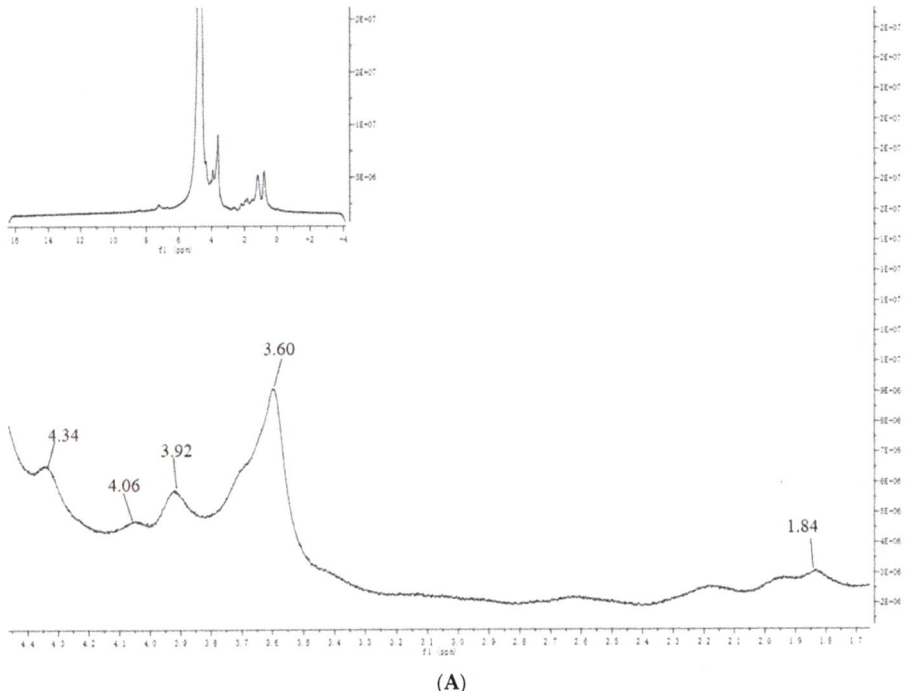

(**A**)

Figure 3. *Cont.*

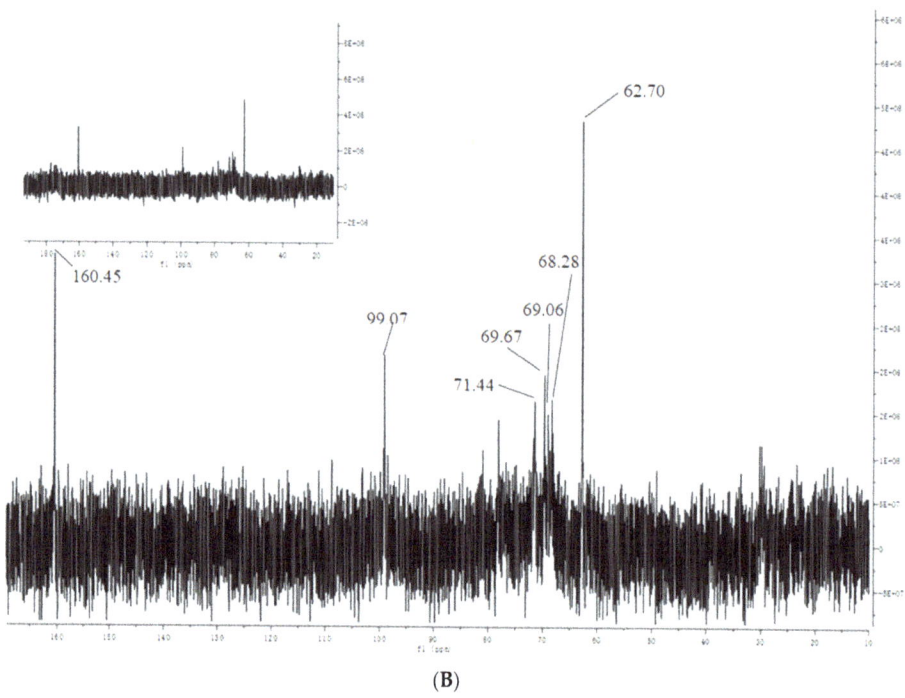

Figure 3. The NMR spectra of SAZMP4 in D_2O: ^1H spectrum (**A**); ^{13}C spectrum (**B**).

3.5. Molecular Morphological Properties

It is widely acknowledged that SEM can be used to observe the surface morphology of polysaccharides, and the SEM images can exhibit the molecular morphological properties of polysaccharide. At low magnification (400-fold and 3000-fold, Figure 4A,B), SAZMP4 was observed to have a smooth surface and debris shape, while it showed a smooth surface and a thin but large lamellar shape in the image of high magnification (8000-fold and 20,000-fold, Figure 4C,D). These results were different to those of previous research [40] possibly because of the different preparation and purification methods and the structural differences of polysaccharides.

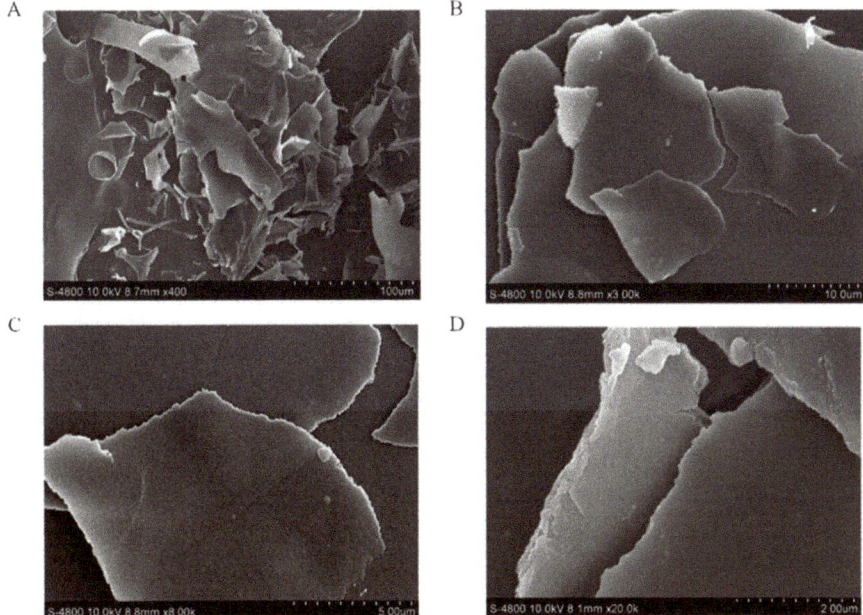

Figure 4. The SEM images of SAZMP4 (**A**: × 400, **B**: × 3000, **C**: × 8000, **D**: × 20,000).

AFM is another tool that can not only provide two-dimensional images but also observe three-dimensional surface images of polysaccharides directly in the natural conditions. Generally speaking, sugar chains with different compositions always have the tendency to form into a conformation with the lowest free energy. According to the AFM images (Figure 5B), SAZMP4 was observed to have an irregular bulk structure, indicating the molecular aggregation caused by intermolecular and intramolecular interactions of hydroxyl groups on polysaccharide chains, and these results coincided with the results of SEM analysis. The height analysis in the planar image (Figure 5E,F) revealed the aggregation extent of SAZMP4. A branched, ring-like, helical or an interconnected network structure in the AFM image (Figure 5A,B) implied molecular self-assembly of SAZMP4, which undergoes a spontaneous process from disorder to order based on the weak, noncovalent interaction of hydrogen bonds and van der Waals forces as well as the hydrophobic effect [41]. These results indicated that SAZMP4 might aggregate at first and then self-assemble to form a long chain; this is why the molecular morphology of SAZMP4 appeared the way it did in SEM and AFM images. In addition, SAZMP4 was also observed to have a core structure with branches probably related to the α-1,4 glycosidic bonds, which might be galacturonic acid, coinciding with the methylation analysis [42].

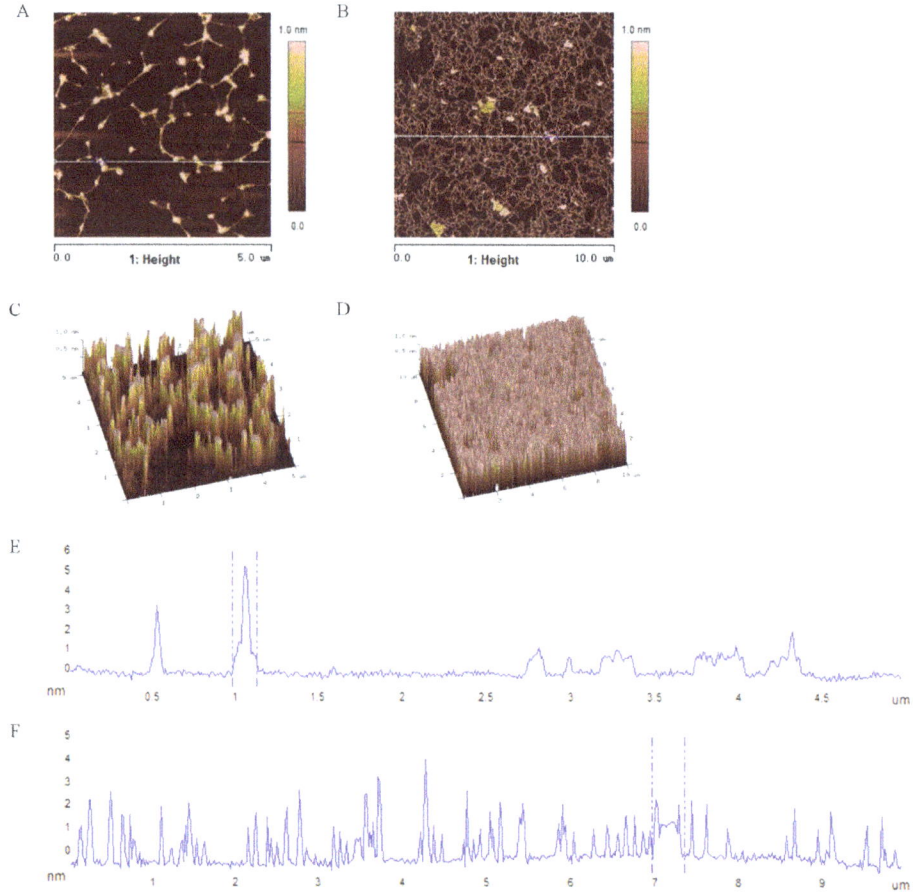

Figure 5. The AFM planar image (**A**) and (**B**); three-dimensional image of AFM (**C**) and (**D**); the height analysis of the planar image at the line (**E**) and (**F**).

3.6. Antioxidant Activity of SAZMP4

3.6.1. The Cytotoxicity of SAZMP4 to Caco-2 Cells

The cytotoxic effects of different concentrations of SAMZP4 on Caco-2 cells were evaluated by the CCK-8 commercial kit. As shown in Figure 6A, SAZMP4 of 50 and 100 μg/mL presented no significant effects on cell viability compared to the control group, while SAZMP4 at high concentrations (200, 400, and 800 μg/mL) caused a significant dose-dependent decrease of cell viability. Hence, the following experiments were carried out with 25, 50, and 100 μg/mL of SAZMP4 for treatment in order to reduce the interference with the polysaccharide.

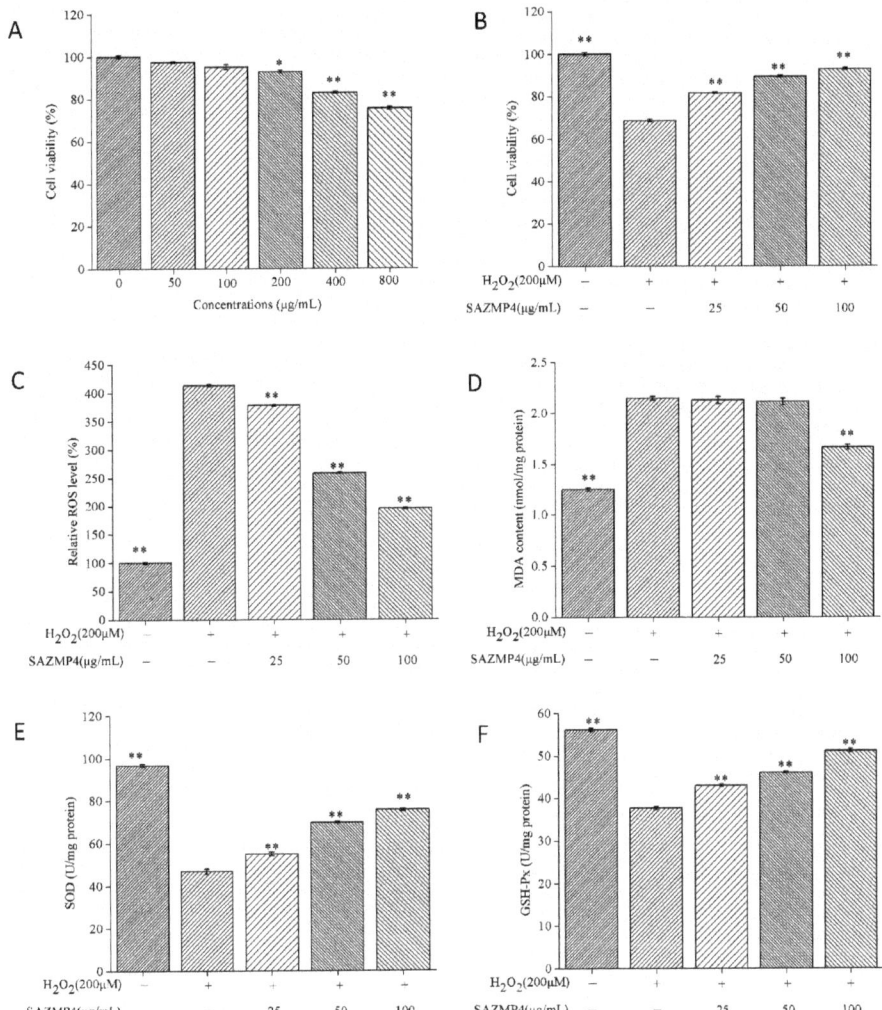

Figure 6. Cell viability of Caco-2 with different concentrations of SAZMP4 (**A**). Cell viability of Caco-2 with 200 μM H_2O_2 and different concentrations of SAZMP4 (**B**). Intracellular level of ROS in Caco-2 cells (**C**). Intracellular level of MDA in Caco-2 cells (**D**). Activity of SOD in Caco-2 cells (**E**). Activity of GSH-Px in Caco-2 cells (**F**). The data are expressed as the mean ± SD (n = 5 wells per group). (*) $p < 0.05$ and (**) $p < 0.01$ versus the control group.

3.6.2. Protective Effect against H_2O_2-induced Toxicity

After treating with different concentrations of SAZMP4 for 24 h, the cells were exposed to 200 μM H_2O_2 for 2 h. The results are exhibited in Figure 6B. The cell viability of the group only exposed to H_2O_2 declined to 68.6%, indicating the cells were in the state of oxidative stress. Pretreatment of SAZMP4 for 24 h enabled the cells to resist the toxic effects of H_2O_2, causing the viability to be greater than 81.6%. However, these results were not precise to indicate SAZMP4 had antioxidant activity. Thus, the determinations of ROS and MDA levels and SOD and GSH-Px activities were inevitable.

3.6.3. ROS and MDA Levels in Caco-2 Cells

The ROS and MDA levels in Caco-2 cells after pretreatment of SAZMP4 and treatment of 200 µM H_2O_2 are exhibited in Figure 6C. There was a significant increase in the ROS level in the group without pretreatment of SAZMP4 compared to the control group. Pretreated groups had significant decreases of ROS levels and exhibited a dose-dependent response. Also, similar results were exhibited in the changes of MDA levels (Figure 6D). At 100 µg/mL, SAZMP4 presented significant decreases compared to the group only exposed to 200 µM H_2O_2. Apparently, these results suggested that SAZMP4 could help the cells resist the toxicity of H_2O_2.

3.6.4. The Activity of SOD and GSH-Px in Caco-2 Cells

Figure 6E,F, respectively, showed the activity of SOD and GSH-Px in Caco-2 cells. Compared to the control group, the activity of SOD and GSH-Px significantly declined in the no pretreatment group. With pretreatment of SAZMP4, the activity of SOD and GSH-Px had a significant increase comparing to the 200 µM H_2O_2-treated group and showed a dose-dependent relationship. Obviously, these results indicated that SAZMP4 might protect the cells from oxidant injury of H_2O_2 by activating the antioxidant enzymes (SOD and GSH-Px).

4. Discussion

Mitochondria, bearing the responsibilities of the generation of cell energy (adenosine triphosphate, ATP), the main source of ROS, and the apoptosis of cells, is the core and hub of the entire cell and its vital activities. Also, it can participate in cell signaling. All these physiological functions of mitochondria are mainly needed to regulate energy metabolism and ROS production. In normal cells, there exists a balance between oxidation and antioxidation. However, metabolic disorders of ROS in mitochondria cause oxidative stress, leading to cell apoptosis and some diseases such as cancer, cardiovascular diseases (hypertension, diabetes), and neurodegenerative diseases (Parkinson's disease). One of the ways to cause oxidative stress is lack of antioxidants. When cells are in the state of oxidative stress, they cannot scavenge the free radicals generated by mitochondria. As previous research reported [43–47], the antioxidant activity of polysaccharides is associated with their composition of sugar chains, branched chains, molecular weight, substituents, and conformation. The higher the molecular weight and the higher the content of uronic acid the polysaccharide has, the stronger its antioxidant ability. In this study, the structural analysis of SAZMP4 determined that it mainly contained galacturonic acid with higher molecular weight and branched chains. Hence, SAZMP4 could become a natural antioxidant because it could be the electronic acceptor and scavenge free radicals.

As polysaccharides can only be digested in the intestinal tract, this study used Caco-2 as the cell model and H_2O_2 as the irritant to induce cellular oxidative stress [47]. The antioxidant system in the human body has the ability to recover and regulate itself. When the body is in a state of oxidative stress, the relevant antioxidant system will produce corresponding antioxidants to control the injury of oxidative stress. SOD is an important kind of enzyme in the antioxidant system that can catalyze superoxide anions to translate into H_2O_2. GSH-Px is another kind of enzyme in the human body. It can scavenge H_2O_2 and block the lipid peroxidation radical chain reaction to protect cell membranes and other biological tissues from oxidant injury. Compared to the blank group, the cell viability of the model group had an obvious reduction indicating the success of this oxidative stress model. The stronger activity of antioxidant enzymes (SOD and GSH-Px) and the reduction of MDA and ROS levels compared to the model group indicated SAZMP4 had antioxidant effects and could improve the antioxidant ability of the cells. However, the antioxidant mechanism of polysaccharides has not clearly determined yet. The signaling pathway of Nrf2-keap2-ARE is the primary antioxidant signaling pathway in the body [48]. Nrf2 is the most important transcription factor in this signaling pathway. Active Nrf2 dissociates with keap1 and enters the nucleus to interact with antioxidant response elements (AREs) to start the transcription of antioxidant enzyme genes. At present, many antioxidants from natural plants have been determined to play an antioxidant role by promoting the dissociation of keap1-Nrf2 and activation of Nrf2, such as curcumin and phenyl ethyl caffeic acid [49]. Since polysaccharides are macromolecules, they cannot get into the membrane. Thus, it is possible that polysaccharides are decomposed into small molecules by intestinal flora at first and then enter the cells to active Nrf2. Moreover, antioxidant polysaccharides also can serve as electronic acceptors by their hydroxyl and carboxyl groups and scavenge free radicals by their special structure to play an antioxidant role in the body. Hence, polysaccharides with more uronic acid and a higher molecular weight can have a stronger antioxidant activity.

In recent years, because of the toxicity and carcinogenesis of synthetic antioxidants, people are more interested in natural antioxidants. Thus, SAZMP4 could be used as a natural antioxidant for food and medicine industries to produce some products for the prevention and control of diseases. In this study, we only investigated the structure and intercellular antioxidant activity of SAZMP4. There is no denying that further research in mice or humans is needed in order to determine the structure–activity relationship based on this study.

5. Conclusions

In conclusion, SAZMP4 (Mw = 28.94 kDa) is a novel pectic polysaccharide, mainly containing 1,4-linked GalA with side chains of 1,2,4-linked Rha and 1,3,5-linked Ara and terminals of 1-linked Rha and 1-linked Ara, and it has a tendency to aggregate and self-assemble. SAZMP4 can be a natural antioxidant and can be applied in the medicine industry. In addition, SAZMP4 has a better water retention capacity and thermal stability, indicating the potential capacity to be used as an additive in the food industry. This is a systematic work investigating the structure and antioxidant activity of a novel pectic polysaccharide, and it can provide a theoretical basis in further research.

Author Contributions: Conceptualization, X.L. and K.L.; methodology, X.L.; software, X.L.; validation, S.Y., P.S. and Q.P.; formal analysis, X.L.; investigation, K.L.; resources, Q.P.; data curation, X.L.; writing—original draft preparation, X.L.; writing—review and editing, X.L. and Y.Q.; visualization, K.L.; supervision, Q.P.; project administration, P.S.; funding acquisition, P.S. All authors have read and agreed to the published version of the manuscript.

Funding: This research was financially supported by the Beijing Engineering and Technology Research Center of Food Additives, Beijing Technology & Business University (BTBU) and Open Foundation of Ministry of Agriculture Key Laboratory of Seaweed Fertilizers (MAKLSF1807).

Conflicts of Interest: The authors declare no conflict of interest.

Abbreviations

SAZMP4: purified polysaccharide from crude polysaccharide with sodium hydroxide solution (0.3 M); HPGPC, high-performance gel permeation chromatography; GC, gas chromatography; FI-IR, Fourier transform infrared spectroscopy; NMR, nuclear magnetic resonance; SEM, scanning electron microscopy; AFM, atomic force microscopy; DSC, differential scanning calorimeter; RG, rhamnogalacturonan; SOD, superoxide dismutase; GSH-Px, glutathione peroxidase; MDA, malondialdehyde; ROS, reactive oxygen species.

References

1. Noreen, A.; Nazli, Z.I.H.; Akram, J.; Rasul, I.; Mansha, A.; Yaqoob, N.; Iqbal, R.; Tabasum, S.; Zuber, M.; Zia, K.M. Pectins functionalized biomaterials; a new viable approach for biomedical applications: A review. *Int. J. Biol. Macromol.* **2017**, *101*, 254–272. [CrossRef] [PubMed]
2. Qiu, N.; Tian, Y.; Qiao, S.; Deng, H. Apple Pectin Behavior Separated by Ultrafiltration. *Agri. Sci. China* **2009**, *8*, 1193–1202. [CrossRef]
3. John, I.; Muthukumar, K.; Arunagiri, A. A review on the potential of citrus waste for D-Limonene, pectin, and bioethanol production. *Int. J. Green Energy.* **2017**, *14*, 599–612. [CrossRef]
4. Sun, Y.; Hou, S.; Song, S.; Zhang, B.; Ai, C.; Chen, X.; Liu, N. Impact of acidic, water and alkaline extraction on structural features, antioxidant activities of *Laminaria japonica* polysaccharides. *Int. J. Biol. Macromol.* **2018**, *112*, 985–995. [CrossRef] [PubMed]

5. Li, J.; Liu, Y.; Fan, L.; Ai, L.; Shan, L. Antioxidant activities of polysaccharides from the fruiting bodies of *Zizyphus Jujuba* cv. Jinsixiaozao. *Carbohydr. Polym.* **2011**, *84*, 390–394. [CrossRef]
6. Chen, J.; Du, C.Y.; Lam, K.Y.; Zhang, W.L.; Lam, C.T.; Yan, A.L.; Yao, P.; Lau, D.T.; Dong, T.T.; Tsim, K.W. The standardized extract of ziziphus jujuba fruit (Jujube) regulates pro-inflammatory cytokine expression in cultured murine macrophages: suppression of lipopolysaccharide-stimulated NF-kB activity. *Phytother. Res.* **2014**, *28*, 1527–1532. [CrossRef] [PubMed]
7. Yue, Y.; Wu, S.; Zhang, H.; Zhang, X.; Niu, Y.; Cao, X.; Huang, F.; Ding, H. Characterization and hepatoprotective effect of polysaccharides from *Ziziphus jujuba* Mill. var. spinosa (Bunge) Hu ex HF Chou sarcocarp. *Food Chem. Toxicol.* **2014**, *74*, 76–84. [CrossRef]
8. Zhao, Y.; Yang, X.; Ren, D.; Wang, D.; Xuan, Y. Preventive effects of jujube polysaccharides on fructose-induced insulin resistance and dyslipidemia in mice. *Food Funct.* **2014**, *5*, 1771–1778. [CrossRef]
9. Wang, Y.; Liu, X.; Zhang, J.; Liu, G.; Liu, Y.; Wang, K.; Yang, K.; Cheng, H.; Zhao, Z. Structural characterization and in vitro antitumor activity of polysaccharides from *Zizyphus jujuba* cv. Muzao. *RSC Adv.* **2015**, *5*, 7860–7867. [CrossRef]
10. Huang, H.; Chen, F.; Long, R.; Huang, G. The antioxidant activities in vivo of bitter gourd polysaccharide. *Int. J. of Biol. Macromol.* **2020**, *145*, 141–144. [CrossRef]
11. Chen, S.; Huang, H.; Huang, G. Extraction, derivatization and antioxidant activity of cucumber polysaccharide. *Int. J. of Biol. Macromol.* **2019**, *140*, 1047–1053. [CrossRef] [PubMed]
12. Su, Y.; Li, L. Structural characterization and antioxidant activity of polysaccharide from four auriculariales. *Carbohydr. Polym.* **2020**, *229*, 115407. [CrossRef] [PubMed]
13. Wang, M.; Zhu, P.; Zhao, S.; Nie, C.; Wang, N.; Du, X.; Zhou, Y. Characterization, antioxidant activity and immunomodulatory activity of polysaccharides from the swollen culms of Zizania latifolia. *Int. J. of Biol. Macromol.* **2017**, *95*, 809–817. [CrossRef] [PubMed]
14. Harman, D. Aging: A theory based on free radical and radiation chemistry. *Lawrence Berkeley Natl. Lab.* **1955**, *11*, 298–300. [CrossRef]
15. Sugamura, K.; Keaney, J.F. Reactive oxygen species in cardiovascular disease. *Free. Radic. Biol. Med.* **2011**, *51*, 978–992. [CrossRef]
16. Lin, X.; Ji, X.; Wang, M.; Yin, S.; Peng, Q. An alkali-extracted polysaccharide from Zizyphus jujuba cv. Muzao: Structural characterizations and antioxidant activities. *Int. J. of Biol. Macromol.* **2019**, *136*, 607–615. [CrossRef]
17. Dubois, M.; Gilles, K.A.; Harmilton, J.K.; Rebers, P.A.; Smith, F. Colorimetric method for determination of sugars and related substances. *Anal. Chem.* **1956**, *28*, 350–356. [CrossRef]
18. Bradford, M.M. A rapid and sensitive method for the quantitation of microgram quantities of protein utilizing the principle of protein binding. *Anal. Biochem.* **1976**, *72*, 248–254. [CrossRef]
19. Singleton, V.L.; Rossi, J.A. Colorimetry of total phenolics with phosphomolybdic-phosphotungstic acid reagents. *Am. J. of Enol. Vitic.* **1965**, *16*, 144–158.
20. Seedevi, P.; Moovendhan, M.; Sudharsan, S.; Sivasankar, P.; Sivakumar, L.; Vairamani, S.; Shanmugam, A. Isolation and chemical characteristics of rhamnose enriched polysaccharide from Grateloupia lithophila. *Carbohydr. Polym.* **2018**, *195*, 486–494. [CrossRef]
21. Ren, J.; Hou, C.; Shi, C.; Lin, Z.; Liao, W.; Yuan, E. A polysaccharide isolated and purified from Platycladus orientalis (L.) Franco leaves, characterization, bioactivity and its regulation on macrophage polarization. *Carbohydr. Polym.* **2019**, *213*, 276–285. [CrossRef] [PubMed]
22. Wang, X.; Lu, X. Characterization of pectic polysaccharides extracted from apple pomace by hot-compressed water. *Carbohydr. Polym.* **2014**, *102*, 174–184. [CrossRef] [PubMed]
23. Wang, X.; Zhang, L.; Wu, J.; Xu, W.; Wang, X.; Lu, X. Improvement of simultaneous determination of neutral monosaccharides and uronic acids by gas chromatography. *Food Chem.* **2017**, *220*, 198–207. [CrossRef] [PubMed]
24. Li, Q.; Li, J.; Li, H.; Xu, R.; Yuan, Y.; Cao, J. Physicochemical properties and functional bioactivities of different bonding state polysaccharides extracted from tomato fruit. *Carbohydr. Polym.* **2019**, *219*, 181–190. [CrossRef] [PubMed]
25. Taylor, R.L.; Conrad, H.E. Stoichiometric depolymerization of polyuronides and glycosaminoglycuronans to monosaccharides following reduction of their carbodiimide-activated carboxyl groups. *Biochem.* **1972**, *11*, 1383–1388. [CrossRef]

26. Needs, P.W.; Selvendran, R.R. Avoiding oxidative-degradation during dodium-hydroxide methyl iodlde-mediated carbohydrate methylation in dimethyl-sulfoxide. *Carbohydr. Polym.* **1993**, *245*, 1–10. [CrossRef]
27. Chaves, P.F.P.; Iacomini, M.; Cordeiro, L.M.C. Chemical characterization of fructooligosaccharides, inulin and structurally diverse polysaccharides from chamomile tea. *Carbohydr. Polym.* **2019**, *214*, 269–275. [CrossRef]
28. Yan, J.K.; Ding, Z.C.; Gao, X.; Wang, Y.Y.; Yang, Y.; Wu, D.; Zhang, H.N. Comparative study of physicochemical properties and bioactivity of Hericium erinaceus polysaccharides at different solvent extractions. *Carbohydr. Polym.* **2018**, *193*, 373–382. [CrossRef]
29. Wang, L.; Liu, H.M.; Qin, G.Y. Structure characterization and antioxidant activity of polysaccharides from Chinese quince seed meal. *Food Chem.* **2017**, *234*, 314–322. [CrossRef]
30. Zou, M.; Chen, Y.; Sun-Waterhouse, D.; Zhang, Y.; Li, F. Immunomodulatory acidic polysaccharides from Zizyphus jujuba cv. Huizao: Insights into their chemical characteristics and modes of action. *Food Chem.* **2018**, *258*, 35–42. [CrossRef]
31. Huang, F.; Liu, H.; Zhang, R.; Dong, L.; Liu, L.; Ma, Y.; Jia, X.; Wang, G.; Zhang, M. Physicochemical properties and prebiotic activities of polysaccharides from longan pulp based on different extraction techniques. *Carbohydr. Polym.* **2019**, *206*, 344–351. [CrossRef] [PubMed]
32. Zhang, L.; Hu, Y.; Duan, X.; Tang, T.; Shen, Y.; Hu, B.; Liu, A.; Chen, H.; Li, C.; Liu, Y. Characterization and antioxidant activities of polysaccharides from thirteen boletus mushrooms. *Int. J. of Biol. Macromol.* **2018**, *113*, 1–7. [CrossRef] [PubMed]
33. Zhang, L.; Liu, X.; Wang, Y.; Liu, G.; Zhang, Z.; Zhao, Z.; Cheng, H. In vitro antioxidative and immunological activities of polysaccharides from Zizyphus Jujuba cv. Muzao. *Int. J. of Biol. Macromol.* **2017**, *95*, 1119–1125. [CrossRef] [PubMed]
34. Ji, X.; Yan, Y.; Hou, C.; Shi, M.; Liu, Y. Structural characterization of a galacturonic acid-rich polysaccharide from Ziziphus Jujuba cv. Muzao. *Int. J. of Biol. Macromol.* **2019**. [CrossRef]
35. Iijima, M.; Nakamura, K.; Hatakeyama, T.; Hatakeyama, H. Phase transition of pectin with sorbed water. *Carbohydr. Polym.* **2000**, *41*, 101–106. [CrossRef]
36. Godeck, R.; Kunzek, H.; Kabbert, R. Thermal analysis of plant cell wall materials depending on the chemical structure and pre-treatment prior to drying. *Eur. Food Res. Technol.* **2001**, *213*, 395–404. [CrossRef]
37. Bjorndal, H.; Hellerqv, C.; Lindberg, B.; Svensson, S. Gas-liquid chromatography and mass spectrometry in methylation analysis of polysaccharides. *Angew. Chem. -Int. Ed.* **1970**, *9*, 610–618. [CrossRef]
38. Ridley, B.L.; O'Neill, M.A.; Mohnen, D. Pectins: structure, biosynthesis, and oligogalacturonide-related signaling. *Phytochem.* **2001**, *57*, 927–967. [CrossRef]
39. Agrawal, P.K. NMR spectroscopy in the structural elucidation of oligosaccharides and glycoside. *Phytochem.* **1992**, *31*, 3307–3330. [CrossRef]
40. Zhang, X.; Chen, H.; Zhang, N.; Chen, S.; Tian, J.; Zhang, Y.; Wang, Z. Extrusion treatment for improved physicochemical and antioxidant properties of high-molecular weight polysaccharides isolated from coarse tea. *Food Res. Int.* **2013**, *53*, 726–731. [CrossRef]
41. Myrick, J.M.; Vendra, V.K.; Krishnan, S. Self-assembled polysaccharide nanostructures for controlled-release applications. *Nanotechnol. Rev.* **2014**, *3*, 319–346. [CrossRef]
42. Ochiai, A.; Itoh, T.; Kawamata, A.; Hashimoto, W.; Murata, K. Plant cell wall degradation by saprophytic Bacillus subtilis strains: gene clusters responsible for rhamnogalacturonan depolymerization. *Appl. Environ. Microbiol.* **2007**, *73*, 3803–3813. [CrossRef] [PubMed]
43. He, P.; Zhang, A.; Zhang, F.; Linhardt, R.J.; Sun, P. Structure and bioactivity of a polysaccharide containing uronic acid from Polyporus umbellatus sclerotia. *Carbohydr. Polym.* **2016**, *152*, 222–230. [CrossRef] [PubMed]
44. Zhao, Z.; Li, J.; Wu, X.; Dai, H.; Gao, X.; Liu, M.; Tu, P. Structures and immunological activities of two pectic polysaccharides from the fruits of Ziziphus jujuba Mill. cv. jinsixiaozao Hort. *Food Res. Int.* **2006**, *39*, 917–923. [CrossRef]
45. Misaki, M.K.A.; Sasaki, T.; Tanaka, M.; Miyaji, H. Studies on interrelation of structure and antitumor effects of polysaccharides: Antitumor action of periodate-modified, branched $(1 \rightarrow 3)$- β-d-glucan of auricularia auricula-judae, and other polysaccharides containing $(1 \rightarrow 3)$-glycosidic linkages. *Carbohydr. Res.* **1981**, *92*, 115–129. [CrossRef]
46. Ahn, S.; Halake, K.; Lee, J. Antioxidant and ion-induced gelation functions of pectins enabled by polyphenol conjugation. *Int. J. of Biol. Macromol.* **2017**, *101*, 776–782. [CrossRef]

47. Klosterhoff, R.R.; Bark, J.M.; Glanzel, N.M.; Iacomini, M.; Martinez, G.R.; Winnischofer, S.M.B.; Cordeiro, L.M.C. Structure and intracellular antioxidant activity of pectic polysaccharide from acerola (Malpighia emarginata). *Int. J. of Biol. Macromol.* **2018**, *106*, 473–480. [CrossRef]
48. Yu, X.; Kensler, T. Nrf2 as a target for cancer chemoprevention. *Mutat. Res.* **2005**, *591*, 93–102. [CrossRef]
49. Ramyaa, P.; Krishnnaswamy, R.; Padma, V.V. Quercetin modulates OTA-induced oxidative stress and redox signaling in HepG2 cells-up regulation of Nrf2 expression and down regulation of NF- NF-κB and COX-2. *Biochim. et Biophys. Acta-Gen. Subj.* **2014**, *1840*, 681–692. [CrossRef]

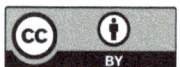

© 2020 by the authors. Licensee MDPI, Basel, Switzerland. This article is an open access article distributed under the terms and conditions of the Creative Commons Attribution (CC BY) license (http://creativecommons.org/licenses/by/4.0/).

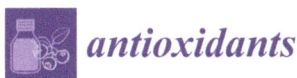

Article

Induction of Antioxidant Protein HO-1 Through Nrf2-ARE Signaling Due to Pteryxin in *Peucedanum Japonicum* Thunb in RAW264.7 Macrophage Cells

Junsei Taira [1],* and Takayuki Ogi [2]

1 Department Bioresources Engendering, Okinawa College, National Institute of Technology, Okinawa 905-2192, Japan
2 Department of Environment and Natural Resources, Okinawa Industrial Technology Center, Okinawa 904-2234, Japan; ogitkyuk@pref.okinawa.lg.jp
* Correspondence: taira@okinawa-ct.ac.jp; Tel.: +81-980-55-4207

Received: 11 November 2019; Accepted: 1 December 2019; Published: 5 December 2019

Abstract: This study focused on exploring the nuclear factor-erythroid-2-related factor (Nrf2) active compound to avoid oxidative stress related to various diseases, such as obesity and diabetes mellitus. The activity of the Nrf2-ARE (antioxidant response element) signaling was evaluated by a reporter assay involving over five hundred various edible medicinal herbs, and the highest Nrf2 activity was found in the ethanol extract of *Peucedanum japonicum* leaves. The active compound in the extract was isolated by high performance liquid chromatography (HPLC), and the chemical structure was identical to pteryxin based on ^{1}H, ^{13}C-NMR spectra and liquid chromatography/time-of-fright mass spectrometer (LC/TOF/MS). From the pteryxin, the transcription factor Nrf2 was accumulated in the nucleus and resulted in the expression of the antioxidant protein, heme oxygenase-1 (HO-1). In addition, the Nrf2 activity involving HO-1 expression due to coumarin derivatives was evaluated together with pteryxin. This suggested that the electrophilicity, due to the α,β-carbonyl and/or substituted acyl groups in the molecule, modulates the cysteine residue in Keap1 via the Michel reaction, at which point the Nrf2 is dissociated from the Keap1. These results suggest that pteryxin will be a useful agent for developing functional foods.

Keywords: coumarin; pteryxin; HO-1; Nrf2; oxidative stress; *Peucedanum japonicum* Thunb; RAW264.7 cells

1. Introduction

Some *Peucedanum* species belonging to the *Apiaceae* family contain therapeutic properties and are used in traditional medicine against various conditions, including sore throats, coughs, colds, and headaches [1]. A species of *Peucedanum japonicum* Thunb has been used as a folk medicine in Japan, Taiwan, and China, and the antioxidant and antityrosinase active compounds were found in the leaf extract of the *Peucedanum* species [2,3]. Recent studies have demonstrated that the ethanol (EtOH) extract of *P. japonicum* has an anti-obesity effect and that it contains coumarin-related compounds that the affect diabetes and obesity, both of which are bioaccessible to the systemic tissues [4–9].

Oxidative stress, with the excess production of reactive oxygen species (ROS), is related to an increased risk of developing several diseases, including obesity and diabetes mellitus. The ROS and reactive nitrogen species (RNS), due to the oxidative stress in the cells, induce antioxidant enzymes such as SOD, glutathione peroxidase, and thioredoxin (Trx) as the first line of defense. The Nrf2 (Nuclear factor-erythroid-2-related factor)-ARE (antioxidant response element) signaling responds to the cell damage with the excess production of ROS and RNS or electrophiles. The Nrf2 dissociates from the Kelch-like ECH-associated protein 1 (Keap1) by electrophiles and the oxidative stress, which regulates the expression of the ARE region containing phase II detoxifying/antioxidant enzymes, such as glutathione S-transferase, NAD(P)H quinone oxidoreductase-1, Trx, and heme oxygenase-1 (HO-1) [10]. The Nrf2 plays a significant role in the regulation of adipocyte differentiation, obesity, and insulin resistance [11]. Certain dietary chemopreventive agents target the Keap1 by oxidizing or chemically modifying its specific cysteine thiols, which can induce ARE-mediated genes expression [12,13]. In our previous studies, it was demonstrated that marine natural products modulate the HO-1 protein expression through Nrf2 activation in both normal cells and cancer cells [14,15].

This study assessed the Nrf2 activity in various edible medicinal plants, and the highest Nrf2 activity was found in the EtOH extract of *P. japonicum* leaves. In addition, this study shows that pteryxin was the active compound in the extract, which was enhanced by the HO-1 protein expression through the Nrf2-ARE signaling.

2. Materials and Methods

2.1. Materials

Coumarin and 3,4-dihydrocoumarin were purchased from the FUJI Firm Wako Pure Chemical Corporation (Osaka, Japan) and pyranocoumarin was obtained from Sigma-Aldrich Co. LLC (St. Louis, USA). The products of the antibodies, such as anti-Nrf2 (Santa Cruz Biotechnology, Inc., TX, USA), anti-HO-1 (StressMarq Biosciences, Inc., Victoria, Canada), and anti-β-actin (FUJI Firm Wako Pure Chemical Corporation) were used for detecting the protein expressions. The cytotoxicity was determined using 3-(4,5-dimethyl-2-thiazlyl)-2,5-diphenyltetrazolium bromide (MTT, FUJI Firm Wako Pure Chemical Corporation).

2.2. Isolation of Pteryxin

Pteryxin was isolated from the dried-leaf powder of *P. japonicum*. The dried-leaf powder of *P. japonicum* (20 g) was extracted by 50% EtOH (210 mL) using a Dionex ASE 350 accelerated solvent extractor (Thermo Fisher Scientific, Inc., Waltham, MA, USA). The extract was loaded on a Diaion HP20 column (100 × 20 mm I.D., Mitsubishi Rayon Aqua Solutions Co. Ltd., Tokyo, Japan), then the sample was sequentially eluted, each with 100 mL of 50% and absolute EtOH. The EtOH fraction was evaporated in vacuo, and the residue (325 mg) was separated by centrifugal partition chromatography (Easy-PREPccc, 318 mL of coil column, Kutuwa Sangyo, Hiroshima, Japan) in the two-phase solvent system of n-hexane/chloroform/70% methanol (9:1:10 in *v/v/v*). Its lower layer (mobile phase) was separated at 3.0 mL/min and 1110 rpm. The collected fractions (31.8 mg) were purified on a reversed-phase chromatographic column (XBridge C18 column, 150 × 19 mm, I.D., 5 µm particle size, Waters Corp., MA, USA) at the flow rate of 12.0 mL/min by the elution of formic acid/H_2O/acetonitrile (0.1/55/45 in *v/v/v*) using an HPLC apparatus (PU-980 HPLC Pump, JASCO Corp., Tokyo, Japan), then the yield (0.029%) of 5.8 mg pteryxin was purified.

2.3. Analysis of Pteryxin

The structure of pteryxin was determined by its ^{1}H and ^{13}C-NMR spectra (Avance III HD Ascend 400 MHz spectrometer, Bruker Billerica, MA, USA), and its molecular formula was determined by Q-TOF LC/MS (Agilent 6530 Accurate-Mass Q-TOF LC/MS system Agilent Technologies, CA, USA) on a reversed-phase chromatographic column (ACQUITY UPLC BEH C18, 50 × 2.1 mm I.D., 1.7 µM particle size, Waters Corp., MA, USA) at 40 °C. The mobile phase consisting of a 0.1% formic acid aqueous solution / 0.1% formic acid containing acetonitrile (1:1) was carried out at the flow rate of 0.4 mL/min by a linear gradient to 0.1% formic acid aqueous solution/0.1% formic acid containing acetonitrile (1:19) at 3 min. The high-resolution mass spectra (HRMS) was measured under the following conditions: a positive ion mode; a desolvation temperature, 350 °C; a desolvation pressure, 40 psig; and a desolvation gas flow, 8 L/min.

2.4. Cell Culture

RAW264.7 cells (mouse macrophages) were obtained from American Type Culture Collection (VA, USA). Cells were cultured in DMEM medium (including 10 % FBS, 100 U/mL penicillin and 100 µg/mL streptomycin) at 37 °C in a 5% CO_2 atmosphere.

2.5. Cell Survaival

The cell viability treatment, with or without a test sample in a well, was examined by an MTT assay, as previously reported [16]. After the culture, MTT (0.05%) was added to each well and incubated for 3 h. The formazan reduced from an MTT was extracted with DMSO (100 µL) and determined as an index of the surviving cells at 570 nm using a microplate reader (BIO-RAD Model 550, BIO-RAD, CA, USA).

2.6. Activity of Nrf2-ARE Signaling

The activity of Nrf2-ARE signal treatment, with or without a test sample, was examined by a reporter assay, as previously reported (14,15). The RAW264.7 cells, with or without the test sample, were pre-cultured on a 12-well microplate (5×10^5 cells/well) for 24 h, and then the pGL4.37 [luc/ARE/Hygro] plasmid and VIOFECTINE (as the transfection reagent) were co-transfected in cells. After 24 h, the cells were washed twice in PBS and lysed in 100 µL lysis buffer. The luciferase activity of the lysate cells (50 µL) was assayed using a luciferase substrate, then the chemiluminescence (CL) in cells was measured by a microplate reader (GLOMAX MULTI Detection system, Promega, WI, USA). The protein concentration of the cells was determined using a BCA protein assay kit (Thermo Fisher Scientific, Inc., MA, USA).

2.7. Nuclear Extraction and Determination of Nrf2

The Nrf2 translocation in nucleus was examined as previously reported (14). Cells (1.0×10^6 cells/mL) with or without the compound (50 and 100 µM) were incubated for 24 h. After 24 h, the cells were treated with trypsin. The nucleus of the cells was extracted using an extraction kit (NE-PER Nuclear and Cytoplasmic Extraction Reagent, Thermo Fisher Scientific K.K, Yokohama, Japan). Nrf2 protein was detected using anti-Nrf2 by a Western blot analysis, and the Nrf2 protein expression was expressed as % of the untreated sample cells (control).

2.8. Protein Expression by Western Blot Analysis

The assessed cells were treated with the lysis buffer. The cellular lysates were centrifuged at 13,800 g for 5 min. The cellular extracts were separated on SDS-polyacrylamide gels (4–12% SDS-polyacrylamide, Invitrogen, CA, USA) and transferred to a nitrocellulose membrane (iBlot Gel Transfer Mini, Invitrogen) using an iBlot Gel Transfer Device (Invitrogen). The protein was detected with the antibodies, such as Nrf2 and HO-1, and the protein expression was determined by densitometry analysis.

3. Results

3.1. Determination of Pteryxin

The chemical structure of (+)-pteryxin ($[\alpha]_D^{24} = 10.9°$ (c 0.13, EtOH)) was determined by the following ^{1}H and ^{13}C NMR spectra. The ^{1}H NMR (400 MHz, CDCl$_3$, δ_H 7.26): 7.59 (1H, d, J = 9.5 Hz, H-4), 7.35 (1H, d, J = 8.6 Hz, H-5), 6.80 (1H, d, J = 8.6 Hz, H-6), 6.63 (1H, d, J = 5.0 Hz, H-4'), 6.22 (1H, d, J = 9.5 Hz, H-3), 6.03 (1H, qq, J = 7.2, 1.5 Hz, H-3"), 5.35 (1H, d, J = 5.0 Hz, H-3'), 2.09 (3H, s, OCOCH$_3$), 2.00 (3H, dq, J = 7.2, 1.5 Hz, H-4"), 1.86 (3H, dq, J = 4.5, 1.5 Hz, H-5"), 1.46 (3H, s, 2'-CH$_3$), 1.43 (3H, s, 2'-CH$_3$). ^{13}C NMR (100 MHz, CDCl$_3$, δ_C 77.0): δ_C 169.8 (OCOCH$_3$), 166.9 (C-1"), 159.7 (C-2), 156.6 (C-7), 154.0 (C-9), 143.1 (C-4), 137.9 (C-3"), 129.2 (C-5), 127.4 (C-2"), 114.4 (C-6), 113.3 (C-3), 112.5 (C-10),

107.3 (C-8), 77.3 (C-2′), 70.5 (C-3′), 60.1 (C-4′), 25.3 (2′-CH$_3$), 22.2 (2′-CH$_3$), 20.7 (OCOCH$_3$), 20.4 (C-5″), 15.6 (C-4′).

In addition, the molecular formula was established as C$_{21}$H$_{22}$O$_7$ on the basis of HRMS (m/z 387.1448 [M+H]$^+$, calcd. 387.1438, and m/z 409.1262 [M+Na]$^+$, calcd. 409.1258). The chemical structure of pteryxin is shown in Figure 1. Pteryxin is an angular-type khellacton coumarin substituted acyl groups. In this study, the Nrf2 activity of the major types of coumarins, such as angular type pyranocoumarin, simple coumarin, and its dihydotype coumarin (3,4-dihydrocoumarin), were assessed together with the pteryxin (Figure 1).

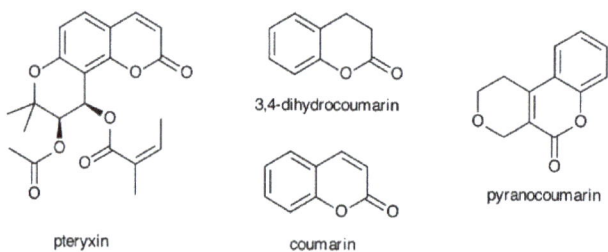

Figure 1. Chemical structures of pteryxin and the derivatives used in this study.

3.2. Nrf2-ARE Signaling

P. japonicum leaves were extracted with ethanol, and the cytotoxicity of the extract was evaluated by an MTT assay. As shown in Figure 2a, the cytotoxicity of the extract was not detected in the range of the test concentrations. The various concentrations (100, 200 and 400 µg/mL) of the extract were evaluated for the activity of the Nrf2-ARE signaling in RAW264.7 cells (Figure 2b). The extract was significantly activated in a dose-dependent manner, suggesting that the Nrf2 activator is contained in the extract (Figure 2b).

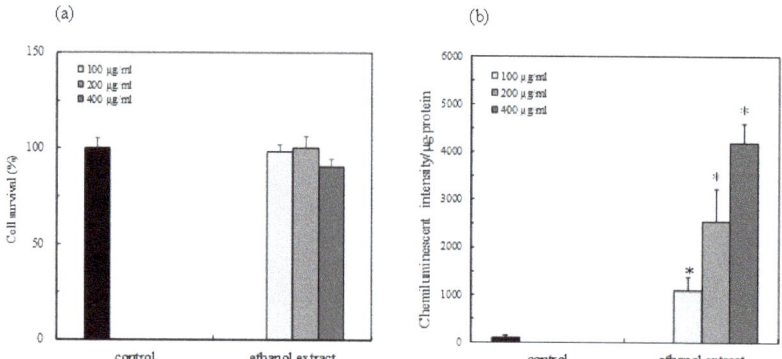

Figure 2. Activation of the Nrf2 (Nuclear factor-erythroid-2-related factor)-ARE (antioxidant response element) signaling in the presence of the ethanol extract of *Peucedanum japonicum* Thunb leaves in RAW264.7 macrophage cells. (**a**) Cell viability with treated samples at the test concentrations was examined by an MTT assay. The cell viability was expressed as % of the control cells without sample. The Nrf2-ARE signaling activity of the EtOH extract of the *P. japonicum* leaves was evaluated by the reporter assay as described in the text. (**b**) The effect of the various concentrations (100–400 µg/mL) of the EtOH extract of *P. japonicum* leaves in RAW264.7 cells. The activity (%) was indicated as % of induction for the control cells without a sample. Data were expressed as mean ± SD, and the significant difference was analyzed by the student's *t*-test. * $p < 0.01$ indicated as a significant difference from the control.

Pteryxin was isolated from the ethanol extract of *P. japonicum* leaves. As shown in Figure 3a, the cytotoxicity of pteryxin was not detected in the range of the test concentrations. When pteryxin was placed in the Nrf2-ARE signaling cell system, the Nrf2 activity was significantly induced in the concentration range of 25–100 µM, indicating that pteryxin is one of the active compounds in the *P. japonicum* leaves (Figure 3b).

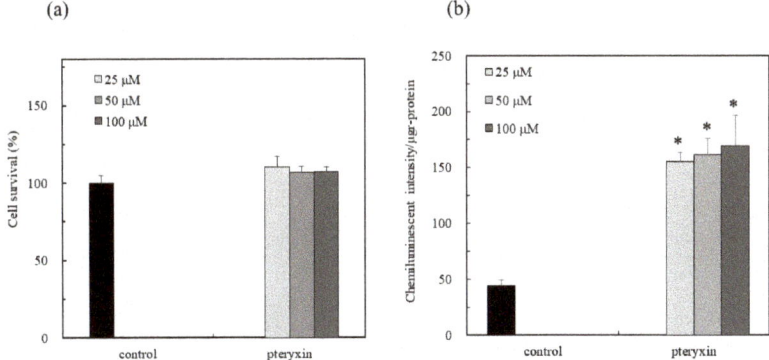

Figure 3. Nrf2-ARE signaling activity due to pteryxin in RAW264.7 macrophage cells. The Nrf2-ARE signaling activity in the presence of pteryxin (25–100 µM) was evaluated by the reporter assay, as described in the text. (**a**) Cell viability with treated samples at the test concentrations was examined by an MTT assay. The cell viability was expressed as % of control cells without a sample. (**b**) The effect of the various concentrations (25–100 µM) of pteryxin in RAW264.7 cells. The activity was indicated as induction (%) for control cells without sample. Data were expressed as mean ± SD, and the significant difference was analyzed by the student's *t*-test. * $p < 0.01$ indicated a significant difference from the control.

3.3. Nrf2 Expression in Cytoplasm and Nuclei

The expression of cytoplasmic Nrf2 in the presence of a compound was determined by Western blot analysis. The Nrf2 was accumulated in the cytoplasm in a dose-dependent manner, and the accumulation of the transcription factor Nrf2 was also detected in the nucleus, suggesting that the cytoplasmic Nrf2 translocated into the nucleus through the Nrf2-ARE signaling (Figure 4a,b). Consequently, the transcription factor Nrf2 would be activated on the ARE regions, resulting in the expression of the HO-1 protein.

3.4. HO-1 Expression

The expression of the antioxidant protein HO-1 in the presence of the target compound was determined by Western blot analysis. The protein expression increased in the concentration range of 25–100 µM (Figure 5a,b). Consequently, the Nrf2 in the nucleus was enhanced by the HO-1 protein expression (Figure 4). This result indicates that the pteryxin plays a significant role in delaying the oxidative stress in a biological system.

3.5. Nrf2-ARE Signaling Activity and HO-1 Protein Expression by Coumarin Derivatives

The Nrf2-ARE signaling activity of pteryxin was compared to the other types of coumarins, such as simple coumarin, 3,4-dihydrocoumarin, and pyranocoumarin. The Nrf2 activity of these compounds was determined by the reporter assay (Figure 6a). As a result, the Nrf2 activity was detected by the α,β–carbonyl coumarins, except for 3,4-dihydrocoumarin, which suggested that the electrophyllicity in the molecule contributes to the cysteine thiol oxidation of Keap1 and leads to the activation of the Nrf2-ARE signaling. Particularly, the activity of pteryxin, which was the highest of the evaluated coumarin derivatives, indicated that the structure of khellacton is suitable for the electrophyllicity.

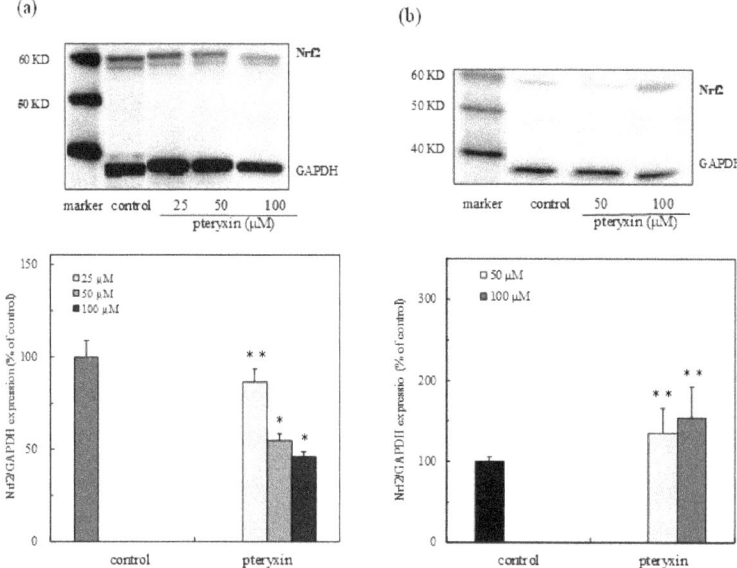

Figure 4. Expression of the transcription factor Nrf2 protein due to pteryxin in RAW 264.7 macrophage cells. The Nrf2 protein expression in the presence of a compound was detected by western blot analysis and determined by densitometry. (**a**) Cytoplasmic Nrf2 protein expression and (**b**) nuclear Nrf2 protein expression in the presence of a compound. Data were expressed as mean ± SD, and the significant difference was analyzed by the student's t-test. * $p < 0.01$ and ** $p < 0.05$ indicated a significant difference from the control.

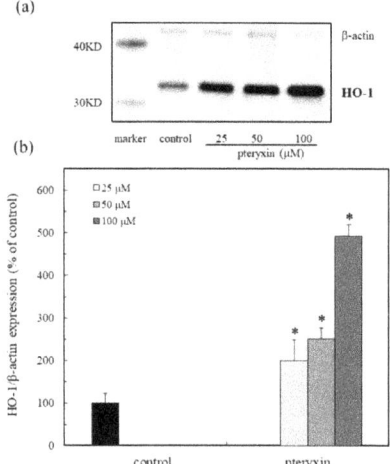

Figure 5. HO-1 (heme oxygenase-1) expression due to pteryxin in RAW 264.7 macrophage cells. The HO-1 protein expression due to pteryxin (25–100 μM) on the Nrf2-ARE signaling in the cells was examined. (**a**) Western blot analysis of the HO-1 protein in the presence of a compound. (**b**) Densitometry analysis of the expression of the HO-1 protein. Data were expressed as mean ± SD, and the significant difference was analyzed by the student's t-test. * $p < 0.01$ indicated a significant difference from the control.

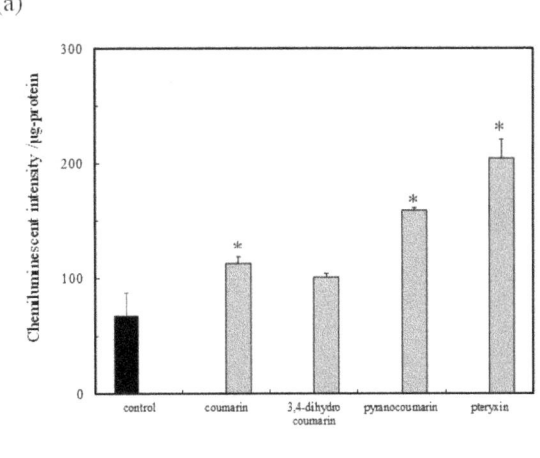

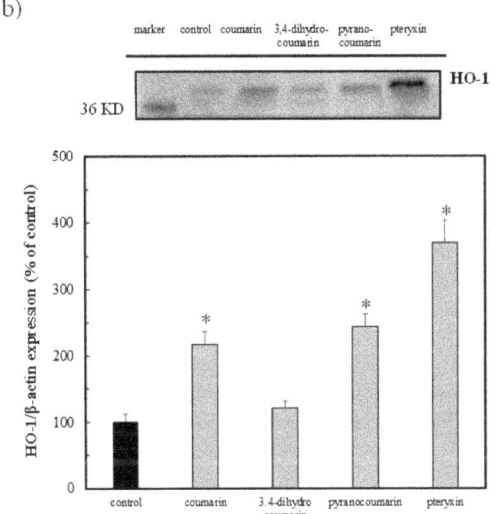

Figure 6. Activation of Nrf2-ARE signaling and the HO-1 protein expression due to coumarin derivatives in the RAW 264.7 macrophage cells. (**a**) The activation of Nrf2-ARE signaling due to the coumarin derivatives (50 µM) was assessed by the reporter assay. (**b**) The HO-1 protein expression due to the various coumarins (50 µM) was detected by Western blot analysis. The expression of the HO-1 protein was determined by a densitometry analysis. Data were expressed as mean ± SD, and the significant difference was analyzed by the student's t-test. * $p < 0.01$ indicated a significant difference from the control.

The HO-1 protein expression, due to the structurally different coumarins, was assessed together with pteryxin. The pteryxin and pyranocoumarin, in common with an angular-type skeleton, presented a high expression, which had a similar result to that of the Nrf2 activity (Figure 6b). Particularly, the pteryxin, which consisted of khellacton-substituted acyl groups, had the highest Nrf2 activity involving the HO-1 protein expression. These results suggest that the difference in the Nrf2 activity due to the compounds may be dependent on the individual potential electrophyllicity.

4. Discussion

Peucedanum species are used as a traditional medicine for sore throats, coughs, colds, and headaches [1]. Recent studies have demonstrated that the extract of *P. japonicum* Thunb plays a role in suppressing obesity. Particularly, some coumarins in the *Peucedanum* species have been examined based on their anti-diabetes and anti-obesity activities [4,7,8]. In addition, several anti-obesity components, including pteryxin and the other coumarin derivatives, were found in *P. japonicum* Thunb, and they were mainly exerted by inhibition of lipogenesis in the adypocytes.

A more recent study indicated that the oxidative stress in the hypothalamus induces insulin resistance and obesity. The Nrf2 activity then suppressed the hypothalamic oxidative stress, subsequently improving the resistance of insulin and leptin related to obesity [17]. This study demonstrated that the leaf extract of *P. japonicum* Thunb has the physiological function of activating the Nrf2-ARE signaling to avoid cell damage by the excess production of the reactive oxygen species (ROS) under oxidative stress (Figure 2). In addition, the pteryxin, as one of the main Nrf2 activators in the extract, dissociated the Nrf2 from Keap1, and then the Nrf2 translocated into the nucleus, activated the ARE region containing the promoter and enhancer regions-mediated antioxidant enzyme, HO-1 (Figures 3–5). Some α,β carbonyls in the molecule will be potential electrophiles that react with the nucleophile protein, Keap1 [18]. When the cysteine residue in the Keap1 is oxidized by an electrophile, the Nrf2 part from Keap1 binds to the ARE region in the DNA sequences. Our results, together with previous knowledge, suggest that the coumarins that are effective against diabetes mellitus and obesity may also act in conjunction with the Nrf2 activity [8].

Coumarins are a large class of plant secondary compounds with a benzopyrone skeleton; they are distributed across four major sub-types: simple coumarins, furanocoumarins, pyran-substituted coumarins, and pyranocoumarins. The pteryxin is an angular-type pyranocoumarin (khellacton coumarin) substituted acyl group (Figure 1). In this study, the Nrf2 activity of the structurally different coumarins—angular-type pyranocoumarin, simple coumarin, and 3,4-dihydrocoumari—were examined together with the pteryxin, and the activation of the Nrf2 activity was detected by the α,β carbonyl coumarins, except for 3,4-dihydrocoumarin (Figure 6a). The HO-1 expression was also similar to the result of the Nrf2 signaling activity (Figure 6b). A previous study demonstrated that the α,β carbonyl in 1,2-naphtoquintione is an electrophile that resulted in the nucleophile protein, Keap1, which is added to the carbon β by Michael addition [18]. A similar result was obtained, except for 3,4-dihydrocoumarin, which suggested that the α,β carbonyl in the molecule plays a significant role as an electrophile for the Nrf2 activator. Also, pteryxin and pyranocoumarin indicated a high Nrf2 activity, which suggested that the angular skeleton will be an effective structure for an Nrf2 activator. In addition, the pteryxin, consisting of khellacton-substituted acyl groups, indicated the highest Nrf2 activity involving HO-1 expression, suggesting that the acyl groups may also contribute to the electrophyllicity in the molecule.

Choi et al. reported the anti-adipogenic and anti-diabetic effects of cis-3,4-diisovalerylkhellactone isolated from *P. japonicum* Thunb [8]. This khellacton coumarin substituted acyl group has a structure similar to that of pteryxin, which may have potential Nrf2 activity. In a previous study, the effect anti-obesity effect due to pteryxin was elucidated through animal testing [14]. The Nrf2 plays a significant role in the regulation of obesity and insulin resistance [11]. The Nrf2 activity suppressed the hypothalamic oxidative stress, resulting in the improvement of the resistance of insulin and leptin related to obesity [17]. Thus, the Nrf2 active function will play a key role in prohibiting obesity and diabetes mellitus. In addition, pteryxin will be a useful agent for functional foods, preventing the metabolic syndrome based on insulin resistance.

5. Conclusions

In this study, the highest Nrf2 activity was found in EtOH extract of *P. japonicum* leaves, and its Nrf2 active compound was identical to that of pteryxin. The accumulation of the Nrf2 in the nucleus due to pteryxin induced the expression of the antioxidant protein, HO-1. In addition, the Nrf2 active function, due to pteryxin, was suggested to hold electrophillicity due to the α,β-carbonyl and/or substituted acyl groups in the molecule modulating the dissociation of Nrf2 from the Keap 1.

Author Contributions: All authors participated in the design of the study. T.O. isolated pteryxin used in this study; J.T. organized this study including experiment, interpreted the data, and wrote the manuscript.

Funding: Works described here were supported by Grants from Okinawa Industrial Technology Center (OITC) and Okinawa Science and Technology Promotion Center (OSTC).

Acknowledgments: We acknowledge graduate students in our laboratory, Okinawa College for their technical support.

Conflicts of Interest: The authors declare no conflict of interest.

References

1. Sarkhail, P. Traditional uses, phytochemistry and pharmacological properties of the genus. *J. Ethnopharmacol.* **2014**, *156*, 235–270. [CrossRef] [PubMed]
2. Hisamoto, M.; Kikuzaki, H.; Ohigashi, H.; Nakatani, N. Antioxidant compounds from the leaves of *Peucedanum japonicum* Thunb. *J. Agric. Food Chem.* **2003**, *51*, 5255–5261. [CrossRef] [PubMed]
3. Hisamoto, M.; Kikuzaki, H.; Ohigashi, H.; Nakatani, N. Constituents of the leaves of *Peucedanum japonicum* Thunb. and their biological activity. *J. Agric. Food Chem.* **2004**, *52*, 445–450. [CrossRef] [PubMed]
4. Nukitrangsan, N.; Okabe, T.; Toda, T.; Inafuku, M.; Iwasaki, H.; Oku, H. Anti-obesity activity of *Peucedanum japonicum* Thunb extract in obese diabetic animal model C57BL/6JHam Slc-ob/ob Mice. *Int. J. Life Sci. Med. Res.* **2012**, *2*, 28–34. [CrossRef]
5. Nugara, R.N.; Inafuku, M.; Iwasaki, H.; Oku, H. Partially purified *Peucedanum japonicum* Thunb extracts exert anti-obesity effects in vitro. *Nutrition* **2014**, *30*, 575–583. [CrossRef] [PubMed]
6. Nugara, R.N.; Inafuku, M.; Takara, K.; Iwasaki, H.; Oku, H. Pteryxin: A coumarin in *Peucedanum japonicum* Thunb leaves exerts antiobesity activity through modulation of adipogenic gene network. *Nutrition* **2014**, *30*, 1177–1184. [CrossRef]
7. Okabe, T.; Toda, T.; Nukitrangsan, N.; Inafuku, M.; Iwasaki, H.; Oku, H. *Peucedanum japonicum* Thunb inhibits high-fat diet induced obesity in mice. *Phytother. Res.* **2011**, *25*, 870–877. [CrossRef]
8. Choi, R.Y.; Nam, S.J.; Ham, J.R.; Lee, H.I.; Yee, S.T.; Kang, K.Y.; Lee, M.K. Anti-adipogenic and anti-diabetic effects of cis-3, 4-diisovalerylkhellactone isolated from *Peucedanum japonicum* Thunb leaves in vitro. *Bioorganic Med. Chem. Lett.* **2016**, *26*, 4655–4660. [CrossRef] [PubMed]
9. Taira, N.; Nugara, R.N.; Inafuku, M.; Takara, K.; Ogi, T.; Ichiba, Y.; Iwasaki, H.; Okabe, T.; Oku, H.J. In vivo and in vitro anti-obesity activities of dihydropyranocoumarins derivatives from *Peucedanum japonicum* Thunb. *J. Funct. Foods.* **2017**, *29*, 19–28. [CrossRef]
10. Kaspar, J.W.; Niture, S.K.; Jaiswal, A.K. Nrf2:INrf2 (Keap1) signaling in oxidative stress. *Free Radic. Biol. Med.* **2009**, *47*, 1304–1309. [CrossRef] [PubMed]
11. Seo, H.-A.; Lee, I.-K. The Role of Nrf2: Adipocyte differentiation, obesity, and insulin resistance. *Oxid. Med. Cell. Longev.* **2013**, 1–7. [CrossRef] [PubMed]
12. Chen, C.; Kong, A.N. Dietary chemopreventive compounds and ARE/EpRE signaling. *Free Radic. Biol. Med.* **2004**, *36*, 1505–1516. [CrossRef] [PubMed]
13. Surh, Y.-J.; Kundu, J.K.; Na, H.-K. Nrf2 as a master redox switch in turning on the cellular signaling involved in the induction of cytoprotective genes by some chemopreventive phytochemicals. *Planta Med.* **2008**, *74*, 1526–1539. [CrossRef] [PubMed]
14. Taira, J.; Sonamoto, M.; Uehara, M. Dual biological functions of a cytoprotective effect and apoptosis induction by bioavailable marine carotenoid fucoxanthinol through modulation of the Nrf2 activation in RAW264.7 macrophage cells. *Mar. Drugs* **2017**, *15*, 305. [CrossRef] [PubMed]
15. Taira, J.; Miyazato, H.; Ueda, K. Marine peroxy sesquiterpenoids induce apoptosis by modulation of Nrf2-ARE signaling in HCT116 colon cancer cells. *Mar. Drugs* **2018**, *16*, 347. [CrossRef] [PubMed]
16. Taira, J.; Nanbu, H.; Ueda, K. Nitric oxide-scavenging compounds in *Agrimonia pilosa* Ledeb on LPS-induced RAW264.7 macrophages. *Food Chem.* **2009**, *115*, 1221–1227. [CrossRef]

17. Yagishita, Y.; Uruno, A.; Fukutomi, T.; Sugiyama, F.; Takahashi, S.; Yamamoto, M. Nrf2 improves leptin and insulin resistance provoked by hypothalamic oxidative stress. *Cell Rep.* **2017**, *18*, 2030–2044. [CrossRef] [PubMed]
18. Takayama, N.; Iwamoto, N.; Sumi, D.; Shinkai, Y.; Tanaka-Kagawa, T.; Jinno, H.; Kumagai, Y. Peroxiredoxin 6 is a molecular target for 1, 2-naphthoquinone, an atmospheric electrophile in human pulmonary epithelial A549 cells. *J. Toxicol. Sci.* **2011**, *36*, 817–821. [CrossRef] [PubMed]

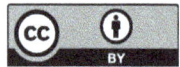

© 2019 by the authors. Licensee MDPI, Basel, Switzerland. This article is an open access article distributed under the terms and conditions of the Creative Commons Attribution (CC BY) license (http://creativecommons.org/licenses/by/4.0/).

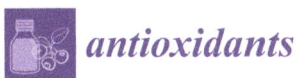

Article

Protective Effect of Tomato-Oleoresin Supplementation on Oxidative Injury Recoveries Cardiac Function by Improving β-Adrenergic Response in a Diet-Obesity Induced Model

Artur Junio Togneri Ferron [1,*], Giancarlo Aldini [2], Fabiane Valentini Francisqueti-Ferron [1], Carol Cristina Vágula de Almeida Silva [1], Silmeia Garcia Zanati Bazan [1], Jéssica Leite Garcia [1], Dijon Henrique Salomé de Campos [1], Luciana Ghiraldeli [1], Koody Andre Hassemi Kitawara [1], Alessandra Altomare [2], Camila Renata Correa [1], Fernando Moreto [1] and Ana Lucia A. Ferreira [1]

1. Medical School, Sao Paulo State University (Unesp), Botucatu 18618-687, Brazil
2. Department of Pharmaceutical Sciences, University of Milan, 20133 Milan, Italy
* Correspondence: artur.ferron@gmail.com; Tel.: +55-14-3880-1722

Received: 30 June 2019; Accepted: 17 August 2019; Published: 2 September 2019

Abstract: The system redox imbalance is one of the pathways related to obesity-related cardiac dysfunction. Lycopene is considered one of the best antioxidants. The aim of this study was to test if the tomato-oleoresin would be able to recovery cardiac function by improving β-adrenergic response due its antioxidant effect. A total of 40 animals were randomly divided into two experimental groups to receive either the control diet (Control, $n = 20$) or a high sugar-fat diet (HSF, $n = 20$) for 20 weeks. Once cardiac dysfunction was detected by echocardiogram in the HSF group, animals were re- divided to begin the treatment with Tomato-oleoresin or vehicle, performing four groups: Control ($n = 6$); (Control + Ly, $n = 6$); HSF ($n = 6$) and (HSF + Ly, $n = 6$). Tomato oleoresin (10 mg lycopene/kg body weight (BW) per day) was given orally every morning for a 10-week period. The analysis included nutritional and plasma biochemical parameters, systolic blood pressure, oxidative parameters in plasma, heart, and cardiac analyses in vivo and in vitro. A comparison among the groups was performed by two-way analysis of variance (ANOVA). Results: The HSF diet was able to induce obesity, insulin-resistance, cardiac dysfunction, and oxidative damage. However, the tomato-oleoresin supplementation improved insulin-resistance, cardiac remodeling, and dysfunction by improving the β-adrenergic response. It is possible to conclude that tomato-oleoresin is able to reduce the oxidative damage by improving the system's β-adrenergic response, thus recovering cardiac function.

Keywords: high sugar-fat diet; obesity; β-adrenergic system; cardiac dysfunction; lycopene; tomato-oleoresin

1. Introduction

Clinical studies show that the excessive body fat leads to many cardiac abnormalities, among them, morphologic and functional changes [1,2]. Animal studies have demonstrated myocardial dysfunction in obese rodents fed with hypercaloric diets [3–7]. Although it is evident that many cardiac changes and/or impairments in performance occur due to adipose tissue accumulation [3,8], the responsible mechanisms by which these changes are not clarified. The system redox unbalance, characterized by a high production of reactive species and inefficient antioxidant activity, is one of the pathways associated with the obesity-related cardiac dysfunction [9].

The β-adrenergic system is one of the most important mechanisms responsible for myocardial contraction and relaxation [10–12]. However, chronic expositions to reactive species are associated with sustained adrenergic stimulation, resulting in arrhythmias and heart failure [13]. Considering the redox system's role in the pathogenesis of obesity and cardiac disorders, the use of antioxidants as therapeutic strategies has been tested [14,15].

Lycopene is a carotenoid present in tomato and red fruits and considered a potent antioxidant [16–18]. The tomato, and tomato product consumption are one of the Mediterranean diet's characteristics, which is associated with health benefits [18]. However, there is a lack of studies regarding lycopene dose ingestion in countries with a Mediterranean diet. Moreover, the few studies which bring information about lycopene consumption have a big variability [19] among the results (for example: in Italy the average intake is 7.4 mg per day while in Spain is 1.6mg per day [18]). The effect of lycopene on cardiovascular disease has been evaluated in clinical [20,21] and experimental studies [22]. Although obesity and oxidative stress are able to lead to cardiac dysfunction, no studies have evaluated the cardiac modulation by lycopene due the antioxidant effect. So, this study aimed to test if the tomato-oleoresin would be able to recovery the cardiac function by improving β-adrenergic response due its antioxidant effect.

2. Materials and Methods

2.1. Animals and Experimental Protocol

In the present study, male Wistar rats (±187 g) were initially divided into two experimental groups to receive control diet (Control, $n = 20$) or high sugar-fat diet (HSF, $n = 20$) for 20 weeks. The diets and water were provided ad libitum. The diet composition has been described in our previous studies [15,23]. All the animals were housed in an environmental controlled room (22 °C ± 3 °C, 12 h light-dark cycle and relative humidity of 60 ± 5%). All of the experiments were performed in accordance with the National Institute of Health's Guide for the Care and Use of Laboratory Animals and the procedures were approved by the Animal Ethics Committee of Botucatu Medical School (1196/2016).

At week 20 of this study, the cardiac dysfunction was detected by echocardiogram in the HSF group. Thus, the animals were casually divided to begin the treatment with tomato-oleoresin or vehicle, performing four groups: Control ($n = 6$); Control supplemented with lycopene- tomato oleoresin (Control + Ly, $n = 6$); HSF ($n = 6$) and HSF supplemented with lycopene- tomato oleoresin (HSF + Ly, $n = 6$). Tomato oleoresin was mixed with corn oil correspondent to 10 mg lycopene/kg of body weight (BW) per day and given orally every day, in the morning, for a 10-week period [24,25]. To avoid differences in the energy provided, all the groups received the same corn oil amount (about 2 ml/kg BW per day). The supplementation time and dose were chosen based in previous studies from our research group and others from the literature [24–26].

2.2. Tomato-Oleoresin Preparation

The tomato-oleoresin (Lyc-O-Mato 6% dewaxed; LycoRed Natural Products Industries, Beersheba, Israel) was mixed with corn oil and kept in the dark, at 4 °C, until the moment to be used [27]. The tomato oleoresin-corn oil mixture stayed for 20 min in a water-bath at 54 °C before the animals receive. The total amount of lycopene in each solution was 5mg/ml. Lycopene stability was confirmed by diode-array spectra at 450 nm, as previously described [28].

2.3. Nutritional Evaluation

Nutritional evaluation included: feed consumption (FC)-daily consumed amount in grams of chow feed; final body weight (BW); caloric intake (CI), calculating according to the following formula for the control group: caloric intake (kcal/day) = feed consumption (g) × dietary energy (3.59 kcal/g). For the HSF group, the caloric intake was calculated as following: water volume consumed (mL) × 0.25 (equivalent to 25% fructose) × 4 (calories per gram of carbohydrate) + caloric intake providing by the chow (feed consumption (g) × dietary energy (4.35 kcal/g).

Feed efficiency (FE) is defined as the ability to convert the caloric intake to body weight. It was calculated according to the formula: FE (%) = BW gain (g)/total caloric intake (kcal) × 100 [15,23]. The adiposity index, considered an obesity marker, was calculated as follow: adiposity index = (total body fat (BF)/final body weight) × 100. BF was evaluated considering the sum of the individual fat pad weights: BF = epididymal fat + retroperitoneal fat + visceral fat.

2.4. Metabolic and Hormonal Analysis

The plasma used for the biochemical analysis was collected after 12 h of fasting. The glucose levels were evaluated by a glucometer (Accu-Chek Performa; Roche Diagnostics, Indianapolis, IN, USA). The insulin levels were analyzed by ELISA assay with commercial kits (Millipore) [23]. The HOMA-IR (homeostatic model of insulin resistance), considered an insulin resistance index, was calculated by the following formula: HOMA-IR = [fasting glucose (mmol/L) × fasting insulin (μU/mL)]/22.5 [15].

2.5. Systolic Blood Pressure (SBP)

SBP was evaluated by a non-invasive tail-cuff method with a NarcoBioSystems® Electro-Sphygmomanometer (International Biomedical, Austin, TX, USA) with the conscious rats. For this, the animals were heat during 4–5min in a wooden box (50 × 40 cm), with two incandescent lamps and temperature between 38–40 °C, to induce arterial vasodilation in the tail. Then, the rats were transferred to an iron cylindrical support specially made to allow the total exposure of the animal's tail [29]. After this procedure, a cuff with a pneumatic pulse sensor was attached to the tail and inflated to 200 mmHg pressure and successively deflated. Blood pressure values were documented on a Gould RS 3200 polygraph (Gould Instrumental Valley View, Cleveland, OH, USA). The final SBP of each animal considered the average of three pressure readings.

2.6. Lycopene Bioavailability Evaluation

The presence of lycopene was determined in plasma and cardiac tissue homogenate. To extract the carotenoids, samples were incubated with internal standard (equinenone), chloroform/methanol $CHCl_3/CH_3OH$ (3 mL, 2:1, v/v) and 500 mL of saline 8.5 g/L. Then the samples were centrifuged at 2000× g for 10 min and the supernatant was collected and hexane was added. The chloroform and hexane layers were evaporated under nitrogen and the residue was resuspended in 150 mL of ethanol and sonicated for 30 s. 50 μL of this aliquot was injected into the HPLC. The HPLC system was a Waters Alliance 2695 (Waters, Wilmington, MA, USA) and consisted of pump and chromatography bound to a 2996 programmable photodiode array detector, a C30 carotenoid column (5 μm, 150 × 4.6 mm, YMC-Yamamura Chemical Research, Wilmington, NC, USA), and Empower software (Empower 3, chromatographic data software Milford, MA, USA). The HPLC system programmable photodiode array detector was set at 450 nm for carotenoids. The mobile phase consisted of ethanol/methanol/methyl-tert-butyl ether/water (83:15:2, $v/v/v$, 15 g/L with ammonium acetate in water, solvent A) and methanol/methyl-tert-butyl ether/water (8:90:2, $v/v/v$, 10 g/L with ammonium acetate in water, solvent B). The gradient procedure, at a flow rate of 1 mL/min (16 °C), was as follows: (1) 100% solvent A was used for 2 min followed by a 6 min linear gradient to 70% solvent A; (2) a 3 min hold followed by a 10 min linear gradient to 45% solvent A; (3) a 2 min hold, then a 10 min linear gradient to 5% solvent A; (4) a 4 min hold, then a 2 min linear gradient back to 100% solvent A. For the quantification of the chromatograms, a comparison was made between the area ratio of the substance and area of the internal standard obtained in the analysis [30].

2.7. Cardiac Malondialdehyde (MDA) Levels

MDA is the main lipid peroxidation marker. It is considered an oxidative stress index [31] and associated with cardiovascular diseases [32]. Thus, MDA levels were used to evaluate the cardiac lipid oxidation as follow:

Cardiac tissue (±150 mg) was homogenized (ULTRA-TURRAX®T25 basic IKA® Werke Staufen/Germany) with 1.0 mL of cold phosphate buffered saline (PBS) pH 7.4, and centrifuged at 800 g at 4 °C for 10 min. Then, 100 µL from the supernatant was mixed with 700 µL of 1% orthophosphoric acid and 200 µL of thiobarbituric acid (42 mM). After this, the samples were kept at 100 °C for 60 min in a water bath, and immediately cooled on ice. In a 2 mL tube, 200 µL was mixed with 200 µL sodium hydroxide/methanol (1:12 v/v). After vortex, the samples were centrifuged for 3 min at 13,000 g. 200 µL from the supernatant was transferred to a glass vial and 50µL was injected into the column. The HPLC used was a Shimadzu LC-10AD system (Kyoto, Japan) with a C18 Luna column (5 µm, 150 × 4.60 mm, Phenomenex Inc., Torrance, CA, USA), and a Shimadzu RF-535 fluorescence detector (excitation 525 nm, emission 551 nm), and 0.5mL/min phosphate buffer flow (KH2PO4 1mM, pH 6.8) [25]. The MDA levels considered the peak area determination in the chromatograms relative to the standard curve of known concentrations.

2.8. Circulating Advanced Oxidation Protein Products

Advanced oxidation protein products (AOPPs) are oxidized plasma proteins resulting from the exposure to oxidation products and are transported by albumin in the circulation [33]. The literature reports that high AOPP circulating levels contribute to cardiac diseases [34].

AOPP determination was based on spectrophotometric detection according to Kalousova et al. [35]. Plasma samples (200 µL) were diluted 1:5 with PBS. It was also used 200 µL of chloramin T (0–100 µmol/L) for calibration curve and the blank was only PBS (200 µL). All the samples were put on a microtiter plate and mixed with 10 µL of KI 1.16 M and 20 µL of acetic acid. The absorbance was measured immediately at 340 nm (spectrophotometer Multiskan Ascent, Labsystems, Vantaa, Finland). The final AOPP concentration is expressed in chloramine units (µmol/L).

2.9. Circulating Carboxymethyl Lysine

Advanced glycation end products (AGEs) are a group of several molecules generated by both non-enzymatic glycation and protein, lipids and nucleic acids oxidation, able to modify tissue function and mechanical properties [36]. In vivo, CML is the main AGE associated with cardiac pathologies [37]. The plasmatic carboxymethyl lysine (CML) levels were evaluated using an ELISA commercial kit (OxiSelect™ CML, Cell Biolabs Inc., San Diego, CA, USA) following the manufacturer's instructions.

2.10. Echocardiographic Study

The analyze was performed in the live animals by transthoracic echocardiography, with a Vivid S6 system equipped with multifrequency ultrasonic transducer 5.0 to 11.5 MHz (General Electric Medical Systems, Tirat Carmel, Israel). The animals were lightly anesthetized by intraperitoneal injection with a mixture of ketamine (50 mg/kg) and xylazine (1 mg/kg), put in left decubitus position and only one examiner made all the exams. The heart image structural measurements were obtained in one-dimensional mode (M-mode) guided by the images in two-dimensional mode with the transducer in the parasternal position, minor axis. Left ventricular (LV) evaluation was performed with the cursor M-mode just below the mitral valve plane at the level of the papillary muscles. The aorta and left atrium images were obtained by positioning the M-mode course to plan the aortic valve level [23].

The following cardiac structures were evaluated: diastolic diameter (LVDD); systolic (LVSD) LV; left ventricle diastolic thickness posterior wall (LVPWD); aorta diameter (AD); left atrium (LA). The LV diastolic function was assessed by the transmitral flow early peak velocity (E). The LV systolic function was evaluated by ejection fraction and posterior wall shortening velocity (PWSV). The joint assessment of diastolic and systolic LV function was performed using the Tei index (sum of isovolumetric contraction and IRT time, divided by the left ventricular ejection time). The study was complemented by tissue Doppler evaluation, considering early diastolic (E'), and late (A') of the mitral annulus (arithmetic average travel speeds of lateral and septal walls), and the ratio by the waves E and E' (E/E').

2.11. Myocardial Function by Isolated Papillary Muscle Study

Besides echocardiographic analysis, myocardial function was also assessed by LV isolated papillary muscles. This procedure has been used by several authors [6,7,29]. Conventional mechanical parameters at $Lmax$ were calculated from isometric contraction: maximum developed tension normalized per cross-sectional area (DT [g/mm^2]), resting tension normalized per cross-sectional area (RT [g/mm^2]), positive (+dT/dt [g/mm^2/s]) and negative (−dT/dt [g/mm^2/s]) tension derivative normalized per cross-sectional area of papillary muscle (CSA).

2.12. β-Adrenergic System Study

β-adrenergic receptors (βAR) are important to regulate cardiac function in both normal and pathologic conditions [11]. The receptors activity was assessed by the dose-response relationship between the isoproterenol and conventional mechanical parameters of papillary muscle at $Lmax$. After baseline values determination, the isoproterenol was added to the vat in the presence of 1.0 mM [Ca^{2+}] to increase progressively the concentrations for 10^{-8}, 10^{-7} and 10^{-6} mol/L.

The stabilization of contractile response occurs nearly 3–5min after adding each isoproterenol dose. Data were sampled and expressed as the stimulation mean percent (%) [29]. At the end of the study, length (mm), weight (mg), and CSA (mm^2) [38] were measured for papillary muscle characterization. The CSA was calculated from papillary muscle length and weight, assuming uniformity and a specific gravity of 1.0. The muscle length at $Lmax$ was measured with a cathetometer (Gartner Scientific Corporation, Chicago, IL, USA), and the muscle between the two clips was blotted dry and weighed.

2.13. Statistical Analysis

The results are expressed in mean ± standard deviation (SD). Two-way analysis of variance (ANOVA) for independent samples was used to determine the differences among the groups. In order to evaluate the positive and negative inotropic effects on myocardial function, it was used a repeated-measures two-way ANOVA. Once detected significant differences ($p < 0.05$), the Tukey post hoc test for multiple comparisons were carried out. All the statistical analyses were performed using SigmaStat for Windows (Version 3.5, San Jose, CA, USA).

3. Results

The lycopene bioavailability is presented in the Table 1. It is possible to verify the presence of lycopene in both groups, which were supplemented (Control + Ly and HSF + Ly).

The HSF group presented increased caloric intake (kcal/d), final body weight (g), adiposity index, glucose levels, HOMA-IR and systolic blood pressure values compared to the control group. The HSF + Ly showed the same changes observed in HSF group when compared to control + Ly, except for HOMA-IR. Tomato-oleoresin suppressed the insulin resistance in HSF + Ly compared to HSF (Figure 1). No effect was observed of tomato-oleoresin on the other parameters.

Table 1. Lycopene Bioavailability.

Lycopene Concentration	Groups			
	Control	Control + Ly	HSF	HSF + Ly
Plasma (µg/mL)	ND	3.61 ± 0.68	ND	3.59 ± 2.31
Heart (µg/g of tissue)	ND	4.83 ± 2.37	ND	2.41 ± 0.36

Data are expressed in mean ± standard deviation ($n = 4$ animals/group). ND: Not detectable.

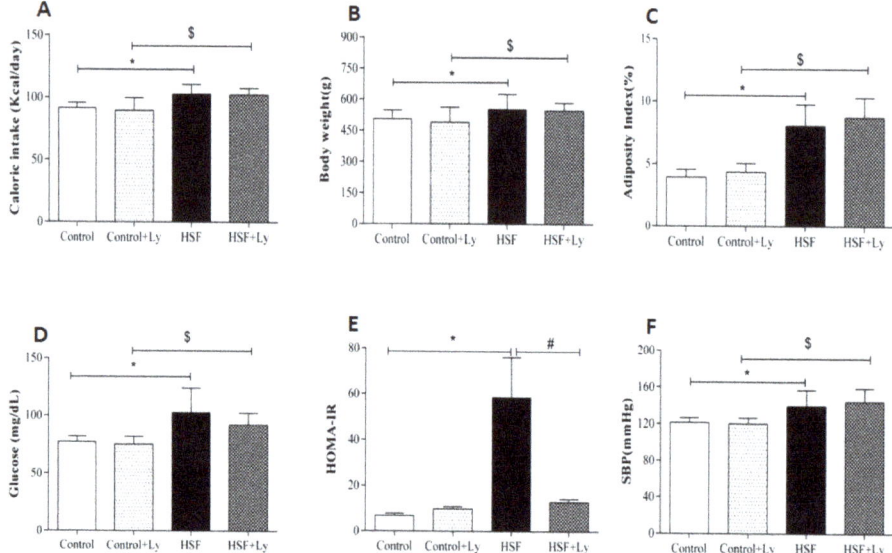

Figure 1. Nutritional and cardio- metabolic parameters. **A**—caloric intake (kcal/day); **B**—adiposity index (%); **C**—final body weight (g); **D**—glucose (mg/dL); **E**—HOMA-IR; **F**—systolic blood pressure (mmHg). Data are expressed in mean ± standard deviation (n = 6 animals/group). Comparison by Two-way ANOVA with Tukey post-hoc ($p < 0.05$): * HSF vs Control; # HSF vs HSF + Ly; $ HSF + Ly vs Control + Ly.

The HSF group presented cardiac remodeling (increased LVDS, LVPWD and reduced LVDD), and deterioration of both systolic (decreased ejection fraction, Tei-a and Tei-b) and diastolic (increased E/E' and decreased Tei-a and Tei-b) functions compared to control group. Regarding the tomato-oleoresin supplementation effect, HSF + Ly group showed improvement in some remodeling, systolic and diastolic parameters compared to HSF (Table 2).

Table 2. Echocardiographic study.

Variables	Groups				Effect		
	Control	Control + Ly	HSF	HSF + Ly	Diet	Ly	Interaction
LVDD (mm)	7.15 ± 0.11	7.02 ± 0.11	6.70 ± 0.12 *	6.92 ± 0.11	0.019	0.665	0.123
LVDS (mm)	2.83 ± 0.10	2.74 ± 0.10	3.17 ± 0.11 *	2.91 ± 0.10	0.016	0.098	0.417
LVPWD (mm)	1.63 ± 0.04	1.53 ± 0.04	1.73 ± 0.04 *	1.62 ± 0.04 #	0.031	0.014	0.932
AD (mm)	3.91 ± 0.06	3.86 ± 0.06	3.89 ± 0.07	3.88 ± 0.06	0.999	0.682	0.740
LA (mm)	4.86 ± 0.11	4.85 ± 0.11	5.02 ± 0.11	4.88 ± 0.11	0.388	0.483	0.536
HR (bpm)	254 ± 14	265 ± 14	262 ± 15	262 ± 14	0.871	0.716	0.713
E (cm/s)	73.6 ± 2.1	73.2 ± 2.18	76.1 ± 2.1	75.1 ± 2.3	0.351	0.742	0.895
PWSV (cm/s)	58.6 ± 1.3	61.1 ± 1.3	56.1 ± 1.3	59.8 ± 1.4	0.181	0.028	0.622
Dec. time (ms)	47.2 ± 1.3	42.1 ± 1.3	50.6 ± 1.3	42.7 ± 1.4	0.128	<0.001	0.322
Tei-a (ms)	116.1 ± 2.5	116.8 ± 2.5	99.1 ± 2.5 *	111.7 ± 2.6 #	<0.001	0.012	0.024
Tei-b (ms)	86.6 ± 2.9	92.6 ± 2.9	77.7 ± 2.9 *	85.5 ± 3.1 #	0.012	0.028	0.761
EF (%)	0.93 ± 0.008	0.93 ± 0.008	0.88 ± 0.008 *	0.93 ± 0.008 #	<0.001	0.006	0.008
E/E'	13.3 ± 0.4	12.7 ± 0.4	15.3 ± 0.4 *	13.9 ± 0.50 #	0.002	0.049	0.439

Data are expressed in mean ± standard deviation (n = 6 animals/group). Comparison by Two-way ANOVA with Tukey post-hoc ($p < 0.05$): * HSF vs Control; # HSF vs HSF+Ly. LVDD, left ventricular diastolic diameter; LVSD, left ventricular systolic diameter; LVPWD, diastolic thickness posterior wall of the left ventricle; AD, aorta diameter; LA, left atrium diameter during ventricular systole; HR, heart rate; E, E-wave peak transmitral early diastolic inflow velocity; PWSV, posterior wall shortening velocity; Dec. time, deceleration time; Transmitral flow, Tei-a and Tei-b; EF, ejection fraction; E/E'.

The myocardial papillary muscle study at baseline condition with 2.5 mM Ca^{2+} is presented in the Table 3. HSF group showed functional impairment in the maximum developed tension (DT) compared to control group. Tomato-oleoresin supplementation was effective to recovery the DT capacity in HSF + Ly group compared to HSF (Table 3).

Table 3. Isolated papillary muscle at baseline condition (2.5 mM Ca^{2+}).

Variables	Groups				Effect		
	Control	Control + Ly	HSF	HSF + Ly	Diet	Ly	Interaction
DT(g/mm^2)	5.96 ± 1.25	6.29 ± 1.65	4.41 ± 1.11 *	6.05 ± 1.19 #	0.066	0.046	0.173
RT(g/mm^2)	0.65 ± 0.11	0.61 ± 0.11	0.63 ± 0.08	0.57 ± 0.11	0.512	0.202	0.844
+dT/dt(g/mm^2/s)	61.9 ± 10.1	63.5 ± 18.4	60.8 ± 11.7	65.5 ± 19.7	0.934	0.573	0.773
−dT/dt(g/mm^2/s)	16.8 ± 2.4	17.5 ± 2.9	15.5 ± 3.3	16.1 ± 2.9	0.193	0.569	0.933
CSA(mm^2)	1.11 ± 0.12	1.10 ± 0.23	1.25 ± 0.27	1.17 ± 0.3	0.181	0.801	0.912

Data are expressed in mean ± standard deviation (n = 6 animals/group). Comparison by Two-way ANOVA with Tukey post-hoc (p < 0.05): * HSF vs Control; # HSF vs HSF+Ly. DT, Maximum developed tension normalized per cross-sectional area of the papillary muscle; RT, Resting tension normalized per cross-sectional area of the papillary muscle; peak of the positive, +dT/dt and negative, −dT/dt tension derivatives normalized per cross-sectional area of the papillary muscle; CSA, cross-sectional area.

Figure 2 shows the β-adrenergic stimulation on the papillary muscle function. The isoproterenol stimulation demonstrated that the HSF group presented functional impairment in DT (10^{-6} M) and −dT/dt (10^{-7} and 10^{-6} M) compared to control group. Tomato-oleoresin supplementation was effective to recover the −dT/dt (10^{-7} and 10^{-6} M) capacity in HSF + Ly group compared to HSF.

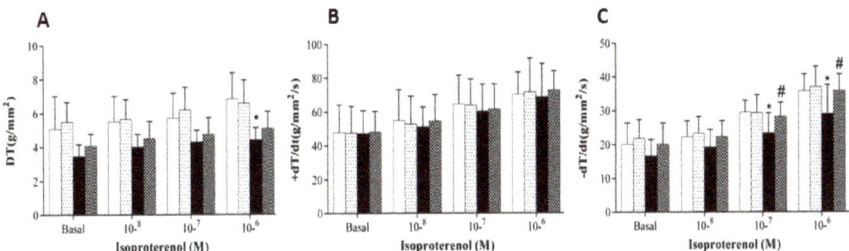

Figure 2. β-adrenergic stimulation in papillary muscles. Data are expressed in mean ± standard deviation (n = 6 animals/group). Baseline calcium concentration (1.0 mM) is presented as 100%. A, Maximum developed tension normalized per cross-sectional area [DT, g/mm^2]. B, positive [+dT/dt, g/mm^2/s] and C, negative [−dT/dt, g/mm^2/s] tension derivative normalized per cross-sectional area of the papillary muscle. Two-way ANOVA repeated-measures with Tukey post-hoc was used to compare the groups (p < 0.05); * HSF vs Control; # HSF vs HSF + Ly.

Figure 3 shows the oxidative stress parameters in plasma and cardiac tissue. All the parameters increased in HSF group compared to control group. By contrast, it is possible to note that CML, AOPP and cardiac MDA plasma levels reduced in HSF + Ly group in respect to HSF to demonstrate a positive effect of tomato-oleoresin.

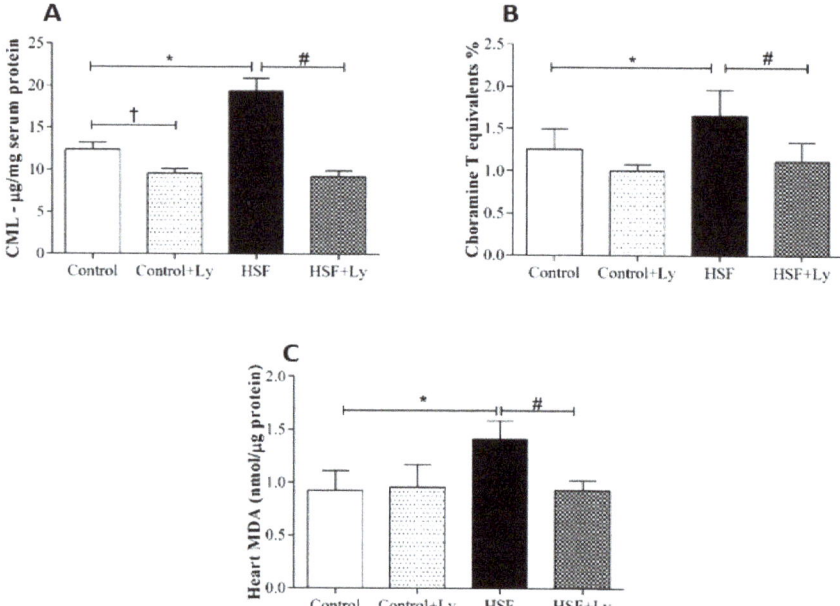

Figure 3. Plasma and cardiac tissue redox state parameters. **A**—Carboxymethyl lysine (CML-pg/mg protein); **B**—Cholaramine T equivalents %; **C**—Malondyhaldeide (MDA-nmol/µg protein). Data are expressed in mean ± standard deviation (n = 6 animals/group). Comparison by Two-way ANOVA with Tukey post-hoc ($p < 0.05$), * HSF vs Control; # HSF vs HSF + Ly.

4. Discussion

This study aimed to test if the tomato-oleoresin would be able to recovery the cardiac function by improving β-adrenergic response due its antioxidant effect. The results show that the HSF groups presented with obesity, characterized by the higher values of body weight and adiposity index, and metabolic syndrome, with insulin resistance, dyslipidemia, and hypertension, all diseases usually associated with obesity [39]. These findings confirm that the diet model used in this study was efficient to lead obesity and related disorders, corroborating the literature [6,7,15,23]. Regarding the lycopene effect on obesity and related disorders, it was observed a positive action only on insulin resistance in the HSF + Ly group, represented by the reduction in HOMA-IR. The literature attributes the tomato-oleoresin benefic effects on diabetes to the lycopene antioxidant potential [40]. Another explanation for this amelioration is the anti-inflammatory effect of tomato-oleoresin. Since insulin resistance and type 2 diabetes are conditions closely related with inflammation and studies already showed that tomato-oleoresin ameliorates the inflammation, this property may explain the beneficial effect on glucose metabolism [41]. The antioxidant and anti-inflammatory effect of lycopene can also be explained by considering its well-established ability, through electrophilic metabolites, to activate Nrf2 pathway thus inducing phase II detoxifying/antioxidant enzymes and inhibiting NF-κB activation [42–44].

Obesity is also associated with cardiac abnormalities, among them morphological, hemodynamic and functional alterations [1,8,23]. Considering the lycopene absence effect on obesity and hypertension in the HSF + Ly group, should both HSF groups present cardiac damage. However, the echocardiographic analysis showed cardiac remodeling and impairment in ventricular systolic and diastolic function only in HSF group after 30 weeks. In opposition, the HSF group supplemented with tomato-oleoresin showed a cardiac remodeling and function recovery.

Several mechanisms could explain the obesity-induced cardiac dysfunction, among them is the β-adrenergic system responsiveness. The myocardial β-adrenergic mechanism is the main responsible by regulating the cardiac performance, especially by intracellular Ca^{2+} handling [6,7]. Although functional studies using isolated papillary muscle have showed that obesity is able to lead to impairment in cardiac contractile [3,5,7], a small number of studies have evaluated the β-adrenergic response in high sugar-fat diet obesity-induced experimental models [29,45–49]. Our results demonstrated that the isoproterenol stimulation leaded to negative responses in both systolic (DT) and diastolic ($-dT/dt$) response in the HSF group while the HSF + Ly group showed an improvement in the β-adrenergic response. However, it is still unclear how the high sugar-fat diet obesity-induced leads to a reduction in the β-adrenergic response.

One hypothesis for the β-adrenergic response impairment is the chronic exposition to reactive oxygen species (ROS) promoted by obesity [9,50]. The literature reports that the direct contact with ROS exerts the same action of isoproterenol on β-adrenergic response, increasing the calcium transient amplitude, therefore, exerting a modulator role in the myocardial contractility [13]. However, this continues exposition to ROS may result in deleterious effects and contribute the development of cardiac arrhythmias and failure [9]. Considering the lycopene antioxidant effect, the amelioration in the β-adrenergic responsiveness of the HSF + Ly group can be attributed to this carotenoid property [14].

Another hypothesis is that the redox system imbalance in obesity conditions may lead to damage to lipids and proteins, generating such biomarkers as MDA, CML and AOPP, which were evaluated in this study [33,51–53]. These oxidative products can damage directly the cardiac tissue by altering its geometry and functionality, or indirectly by the carbonylation of proteins involved in the myocardial contractility regulatory response, as the β-adrenergic pathway [13,54,55]. While the HSF group presented higher levels of MDA, CML and AOPP and cardiac function deterioration, the tomato-oleoresin antioxidant effect is confirmed by reduced levels of these markers and cardiac function recovery in the HSF + Ly group.

5. Conclusions

In summary, this study found that the HSF diet induced obesity-related cardiac dysfunction and the tomato-oleoresin was able to attenuate this condition. Therefore, it is possible to conclude that tomato-oleoresin is able to reduce oxidative damage, thereby improving the system's β-adrenergic response and recovering cardiac function.

Author Contributions: Conceptualization, A.J.T.F., F.V.F.-F., G.A., F.M. and A.L.A.F.; methodology, A.J.T.F., F.V.F.-F., J.L.G., L.G., S.G.Z.B., K.A.H.K., C.C.V.d.A.S.; D.H.S.d.C. and A.A.; data curation, A.J.T.F., F.V.F.-F., S.G.Z.B., and A.A.; writing—original draft preparation, A.J.T.F.; F.V.F.-F.; C.R.C.; A.L.A.F.; writing—review and editing, F.V.F.-F., G.A., F.M. and A.L.A.F.; supervision, A.L.A.F.; project administration, A.J.T.F.

Funding: This work was funded by Conselho Nacional de Desenvolvimento Científico e Tecnológico CNPq (424209/2016-0) and Fundação de Amparo à Pesquisa do Estado de São Paulo FAPESP and Universidade Estadual Paulista "Julio de Mesquita Filho".

Conflicts of Interest: The authors declare no conflict of interest.

References

1. Alpert, M.A.; Lambert, C.R.; Panayiotou, H.; Terry, B.E.; Cohen, M.V.; Massey, C.V.; Hashimi, M.W.; Mukerji, V. Relation of duration of morbid obesity to left ventricular mass, systolic function, and diastolic filling, and effect of weight loss. *Am. J. Cardiol.* **1995**, *76*, 1194–1197. [CrossRef]
2. Scaglione, R.; Dichiara, M.A.; Indovina, A.; Lipari, R.; Ganguzza, A.; Parrinello, G.; Capuana, G.; Merlino, G.; Licata, G. Left ventricular diastolic and systolic function in normotensive obese subjects: Influence of degree and duration of obesity. *Eur. Heart J.* **1992**, *13*, 738–742. [CrossRef] [PubMed]
3. Relling, D.P.; Esberg, L.B.; Fang, C.X.; Johnson, W.T.; Murphy, E.J.; Carlson, E.C.; Saari, J.T.; Ren, J. High-fat diet-induced juvenile obesity leads to cardiomyocyte dysfunction and upregulation of Foxo3a transcription factor independent of lipotoxicity and apoptosis. *J. Hypertens.* **2006**, *24*, 549–561. [CrossRef] [PubMed]

4. du Toit, E.F.; Nabben, M.; Lochner, A. A potential role for angiotensin II in obesity induced cardiac hypertrophy and ischaemic/reperfusion injury. *Basic Res. Cardiol.* **2005**, *100*, 346–354. [CrossRef] [PubMed]
5. Ren, J.; Zhu, B.-H.; Relling, D.P.; Esberg, L.B.; Ceylan-Isik, A.F. High-fat diet-induced obesity leads to resistance to leptin-induced cardiomyocyte contractile response. *Obesity* **2008**, *16*, 2417–2423. [CrossRef] [PubMed]
6. Leopoldo, A.S.; Sugizaki, M.M.; Lima-Leopoldo, A.P.; do Nascimento, A.F.; Luvizotto, R.D.A.M.; de Campos, D.H.S.; Okoshi, K.; Pai-Silva, M.D.; Padovani, C.R.; Cicogna, A.C. Cardiac remodeling in a rat model of diet-induced obesity. *Can. J. Cardiol.* **2010**, *26*, 423–429. [CrossRef]
7. Leopoldo, A.S.; Lima-Leopoldo, A.P.; Sugizaki, M.M.; Nascimento, A.F.D.; de Campos, D.H.S.; Luvizotto, R.D.A.M.; Castardeli, E.; Alves, C.A.B.; Brum, P.C.; Cicogna, A.C. Involvement of L-type calcium channel and serca2a in myocardial dysfunction induced by obesity. *J. Cell. Physiol.* **2011**, *226*, 2934–2942. [CrossRef]
8. Panchal, S.K.; Poudyal, H.; Iyer, A.; Nazer, R.; Alam, A.; Diwan, V.; Kauter, K.; Sernia, C.; Campbell, F.; Ward, L.; et al. High-carbohydrate, high-fat diet-induced metabolic syndrome and cardiovascular remodeling in rats. *J. Cardiovasc. Pharmacol.* **2011**, *57*, 611–624. [CrossRef]
9. Tsutsui, H.; Kinugawa, S.; Matsushima, S. Oxidative Stress and Heart Failure. *Am. J. Physiol. Heart Circ. Physiol.* **2011**, *301*, H2181–H2190. [CrossRef]
10. Opie, L. *The Heart. Physiology from Cell to Circulation*; Lippincott Williams & Wilkins: Philadelphia, PA, USA, 1998.
11. Bers, D.M. Cardiac excitation-contraction coupling. *Nature* **2002**, *415*, 198–415. [CrossRef]
12. Carvajal, K.; Balderas-Villalobos, J.; Bello-Sanchez, M.D.; Phillips-Farfán, B.; Molina-Munoz, T.; Aldana-Quintero, H.; Gómez-Viquez, N.L. Ca^{2+} mishandling and cardiac dysfunction in obesity and insulin resistance: Role of oxidative stress. *Cell Calcium* **2014**, *56*, 408–415. [CrossRef] [PubMed]
13. Andersson, D.C.; Fauconnier, J.; Yamada, T.; Lacampagne, A.; Zhang, S.J.; Katz, A.; Westerblad, H. Mitochondrial production of reactive oxygen species contributes to the β-adrenergic stimulation of mouse cardiomycetes. *J. Physiol.* **2011**, *589*, 1791–1801. [CrossRef] [PubMed]
14. Pereira, B.L.; Reis, P.P.; Severino, F.E.; Felix, T.F.; Braz, M.G.; Nogueira, F.R.; Silva, R.A.C.; Cardoso, A.C.; Lourenço, M.A.M.; Figueiredo, A.M.; et al. Tomato (*Lycopersicon esculentum*) or lycopene supplementation attenuates ventricular remodeling after myocardial infarction through different mechanistic pathways. *J. Nutr. Biochem.* **2017**, *46*, 117–124. [CrossRef] [PubMed]
15. Francisqueti, F.; Minatel, I.; Ferron, A.; Bazan, S.; Silva, V.; Garcia, J.; De Campos, D.; Ferreira, A.; Moreto, F.; Cicogna, A.; et al. Effect of Gamma-Oryzanol as Therapeutic Agent to Prevent Cardiorenal Metabolic Syndrome in Animals Submitted to High Sugar-Fat Diet. *Nutrients* **2017**, *9*, 1299. [CrossRef] [PubMed]
16. Di Mascio, P.; Kaiser, S.; Sies, H. Lycopene as the most efficient biological carotenoid singlet oxygen quencher. *Arch. Biochem. Biophys.* **1989**, *274*, 532–538. [CrossRef]
17. Stahl, W.; Sies, H. Antioxidant activity of carotenoids. *Mol. Asp. Med.* **2003**, *24*, 345–351. [CrossRef]
18. Story, E.N.; Kopec, R.E.; Schwartz, S.J.; Harris, G.K. An Update on the Health Effects of Tomato Lycopene. *Annu. Rev. Food Sci. Technol.* **2010**, *1*, 189–210. [CrossRef]
19. Porrini, M.; Riso, P. What are Typical Lycopene Intakes? *J. Nutr.* **2005**, *135*, 2042–2045. [CrossRef]
20. Araujo, F.B.; Barbosa, D.S.; Hsin, C.Y.; Maranhao, R.C.; Abdalla, D.S.P. Evaluation of oxidative stress in patients with hyperlipidemia. *Atherosclerosis* **1995**, *117*, 61–71. [CrossRef]
21. Engelhard, Y.N.; Gazer, B.; Paran, E. Natural antioxidants from tomato extract reduce blood pressure in patients with grade-1 hypertension: A double-blind, placebo-controlled pilot study. *Am. Heart J.* **2006**, *151*. [CrossRef]
22. Bansal, P.; Gupta, S.K.; Ojha, S.K.; Nandave, M.; Mittal, R.; Kumari, S.; Arya, D.S. Cardioprotective effect of lycopene in the experimental model of myocardial ischemia-reperfusion injury. *Mol. Cell. Biochem.* **2006**, *289*, 1–9. [CrossRef] [PubMed]
23. Ferron, A.; Francisqueti, F.; Minatel, I.; Silva, C.; Bazan, S.; Kitawara, K.; Garcia, J.; Corrêa, C.; Moreto, F.; Ferreira, A. Association between Cardiac Remodeling and Metabolic Alteration in an Experimental Model of Obesity Induced by Western Diet. *Nutrients* **2018**, *10*, 1675. [CrossRef] [PubMed]

24. Luvizotto, R.D.A.M.; Nascimento, A.F.; Imaizumi, E.; Pierine, D.T.; Conde, S.J.; Correa, C.R.; Yeum, K.-J.; Ferreira, A.L.A. Lycopene supplementation modulates plasma concentrations and epididymal adipose tissue mRNA of leptin, resistin and IL-6 in diet-induced obese rats. *Br. J. Nutr.* **2013**, *110*, 1803–1809. [CrossRef] [PubMed]
25. Pierine, D.T.; Navarro, M.E.L.; Minatel, I.O.; Luvizotto, R.A.M.; Nascimento, A.F.; Ferreira, A.L.A.; Yeum, K.-J.; Corrêa, C.R. Lycopene supplementation reduces TNF-α via RAGE in the kidney of obese rats. *Nutr. Diabetes* **2014**, *4*, e142. [CrossRef] [PubMed]
26. Rao, A.V.; Shen, H. Effect of low dose lycopene intake on lycopene bioavailability and oxidative stress. *Nutr. Res.* **2002**, *22*, 1125–1131. [CrossRef]
27. Anjos Ferreira, A.L.; Russell, R.M.; Rocha, N.; Placido Ladeira, M.S.; Favero Salvadori, D.M.; Oliveira Nascimento, M.C.M.; Matsui, M.; Carvalho, F.A.; Tang, G.; Matsubara, L.S.; et al. Effect of lycopene on doxorubicin-induced cardiotoxicity: An echocardiographic, histological and morphometrical assessment. *Basic Clin. Pharmacol. Toxicol.* **2007**, *101*, 16–24. [CrossRef] [PubMed]
28. Luvizotto, R.; Nascimento, A.; Miranda, N.; Wang, X.-D.; Ferreira, A. Lycopene-rich tomato oleoresin modulates plasma adiponectin concentration and mRNA levels of adiponectin, SIRT1, and FoxO1 in adipose tissue of obese rats. *Hum. Exp. Toxicol.* **2015**, *34*, 612–619. [CrossRef] [PubMed]
29. Ferron, A.J.T.; Jacobsen, B.B.; Grippa, P.; Ana, S. Cardiac Dysfunction Induced by Obesity Is Not Related to β -Adrenergic System Impairment at the Receptor-Signalling Pathway. *PLoS ONE* **2015**, *10*. [CrossRef] [PubMed]
30. Ferreira, A.L.A.; Salvadori, D.M.F.; Nascimento, M.C.M.O.; Rocha, N.S.; Correa, C.R.; Pereira, E.J.; Matsubara, L.S.; Matsubara, B.B.; Ladeira, M.S.P. Tomato-oleoresin supplement prevents doxorubicin-induced cardiac myocyte oxidative DNA damage in rats. *Mutat. Res. Genet. Toxicol. Environ. Mutagen.* **2007**, *631*, 26–35. [CrossRef]
31. Yagi, K. Simple Assay for the Level of Total Lipid Peroxides in Serum or Plasma. *Free Radic. Antioxid. Protoc.* **1998**, *108*, 101–106.
32. Lee, R.; Margaritis, M.; Channon, K.M.; Antoniades, C. Evaluating oxidative stress in human cardiovascular disease: Methodological aspects and considerations. *Curr. Med. Chem.* **2012**, *19*, 2504–2520. [CrossRef] [PubMed]
33. Feng, W.; Zhang, K.; Liu, Y.; Chen, J.; Cai, Q.; He, W.; Zhang, Y.; Wang, M.-H.; Wang, J.; Huang, H. Advanced oxidation protein products aggravate cardiac remodeling via cardiomyocyte apoptosis in chronic kidney disease. *Am. J. Physiol. Circ. Physiol.* **2017**, *314*, H475–H483. [CrossRef] [PubMed]
34. Zuwala-Jagiello, J.; Murawska-Cialowicz, E.; Pazgan-Simon, M. Increased Circulating Advanced Oxidation Protein Products and High-Sensitive Troponin T in Cirrhotic Patients with Chronic Hepatitis C: A Preliminary Report. *Biomed. Res. Int.* **2015**, *2015*. [CrossRef] [PubMed]
35. Kalousová, M.; Škrha, J.; Zima, T. Advanced glycation end-products and advanced oxidation protein products in patients with insulin dependent diabetes melli.us. *Med. J. Bakirkoy* **2011**, *7*, 130–135.
36. Hegab, Z.; Gibbons, S.; Neyses, L.; Mamas, M.A. Role of advanced glycation end products in cardiovascular disease. *World J. Cardiol.* **2012**, *4*, 90. [CrossRef] [PubMed]
37. Fishman, S.L.; Sonmez, H.; Basman, C.; Singh, V.; Poretsky, L. The role of advanced glycation end-products in the development of coronary artery disease in patients with and without diabetes mellitus: A review. *Mol. Med.* **2018**, *24*, 59. [CrossRef] [PubMed]
38. Lima-Leopoldo, A.P.; Leopoldo, A.S.; Sugizaki, M.M.; Bruno, A.; Nascimento, A.F.; Luvizotto, R.A.; de Oliveira Júnior, S.A.; Castardeli, E.; Padovani, C.R.; Cicogna, A.C. Myocardial Dysfunction and Abnormalities in Intracellular Calcium Handling in Obese Rats. *Arq. Bras. Cardiol.* **2011**, *97*, 232–240. [CrossRef] [PubMed]
39. Maioli, T.U.; Gonçalves, J.L.; Miranda, M.C.G.; Martins, V.D.; Horta, L.S.; Moreira, T.G.; Godard, A.L.B.; Santiago, A.F.; Faria, A.M.C. High sugar and butter (HSB) diet induces obesity and metabolic syndrome with decrease in regulatory T cells in adipose tissue of mice. *Inflamm. Res.* **2016**, *65*, 169–178. [CrossRef] [PubMed]
40. Assis, R.; Arcaro, C.; Gutierres, V.; Oliveira, J.; Costa, P.; Baviera, A.; Brunetti, I. Combined effects of curcumin and lycopene or bixin in yoghurt on inhibition of LDL oxidation and increases in HDL and paraoxonase levels in streptozotocin-diabetic rats. *Int. J. Mol. Sci.* **2017**, *18*, 332. [CrossRef] [PubMed]
41. Zeng, Z.; He, W.; Jia, Z.; Hao, S. Lycopene Improves Insulin Sensitivity through Inhibition of STAT3/Srebp-1c-Mediated Lipid Accumulation and Inflammation in Mice fed a High-Fat Diet. *Exp. Clin. Endocrinol. Diabetes* **2017**, *125*, 610–617. [CrossRef]

42. Kawata, A.; Murakami, Y.; Suzuki, S.; Fujisawa, S. Anti-inflammatory activity of β-carotene, lycopene and tri-n-butylborane, a scavenger of reactive oxygen species. *In Vivo* **2018**, *32*, 255–264. [PubMed]
43. Yang, P.M.; Chen, H.Z.; Huang, Y.T.; Hsieh, C.W.; Wung, B.S. Lycopene inhibits NF-κB activation and adhesion molecule expression through Nrf2-mediated heme oxygenase-1 in endothelial cells. *Int. J. Mol. Med.* **2017**, *39*, 1533–1540. [CrossRef] [PubMed]
44. Barros, M.P.; Rodrigo, M.J.; Zacarias, L. Dietary Carotenoid Roles in Redox Homeostasis and Human Health. *J. Agric. Food Chem.* **2018**, *66*, 5733–5740. [CrossRef] [PubMed]
45. Carroll, J.F.; Kyser, C.K.; Martin, M.M. beta-Adrenoceptor density and adenylyl cyclase activity in obese rabbit hearts. *Int. J. Obes. Relat. Metab. Disord.* **2002**, *26*, 627–632. [CrossRef] [PubMed]
46. Carroll, J.F.; Jones, A.E.; Hester, R.L.; Reinhart, G.A.; Cockrell, K.; Mizelle, H.L. Reduced cardiac contractile responsiveness to isoproterenol in obese rabbits. *Hypertension* **1997**, *30*, 1376–1381. [CrossRef] [PubMed]
47. Lima-Leopoldo, A.P.; Sugizaki, M.M.; Leopoldo, A.S.; Carvalho, R.F.; Nogueira, C.R.; Nascimento, A.F.; Martinez, P.F.; Luvizotto, R.A.M.; Padovani, C.R.; Cicogna, A.C. Obesity induces upregulation of genes involved in myocardial Ca^{2+} handling. *Braz. J. Med. Biol. Res.* **2008**, *41*. [CrossRef] [PubMed]
48. Dincer, U.D. Cardiac β-adrenoceptor expression is markedly depressed in Ossabaw swine model of cardiometabolic risk. *Int. J. Gen. Med.* **2011**, *4*, 493–499. [CrossRef] [PubMed]
49. Pinotti, M.F.; Silva, M.D.P.; Sugizaki, M.M.; Novelli, Y.S.D.; Sant'ana, L.S.; Aragon, F.F.; Padovani, C.R.; Novelli, E.L.B.; Cicogna, A.C. Artigo Original Influências de Dietas Ricas em Ácidos Graxos Saturados e Insaturados sobre o Miocárdio de Ratos. *Arq. Bras. Cardiol.* **2007**, *88*, 346–353. [CrossRef]
50. de Lucia, C.; Eguchi, A.; Koch, W.J. New insights in cardiac β-Adrenergic signaling during heart failure and aging. *Front. Pharmacol.* **2018**, *9*, 904. [CrossRef]
51. Wu, I.; Shiesh, Â.S.; Kuo, P.; Lin, X. High Oxidative Stress Is Correlated with Frailty in Elderly Chinese. *J. Am. Geriatr. Soc.* **2009**, *57*, 1666–1671. [CrossRef]
52. Zhang, G.X.; Kimura, S.; Nishiyama, A.; Shokoji, T.; Rahman, M.; Yao, L.; Nagai, Y.; Fujisawa, Y.; Miyatake, A.; Abe, Y. Cardiac oxidative stress in acute and chronic isoproterenol-infused rats. *Cardiovasc. Res.* **2005**, *65*, 230–238. [CrossRef] [PubMed]
53. Ojha, S.; Goyal, S.; Sharma, C.; Arora, S.; Kumari, S.; Arya, D.S. Cardioprotective effect of lycopene against isoproterenol-induced myocardial infarction in rats. *Hum. Exp. Toxicol.* **2013**, *32*, 492–503. [CrossRef] [PubMed]
54. Yilmaz, S.; Atessahin, A.; Sahna, E.; Karahan, I.; Ozer, S. Protective effect of lycopene on adriamycin-induced cardiotoxicity and nephrotoxicity. *Toxicology* **2006**, *218*, 164–171. [CrossRef] [PubMed]
55. Folden, D.V.; Gupta, A.; Sharma, A.C.; Li, S.Y.; Saari, J.T.; Ren, J. Malondialdehyde inhibits cardiac contractile function in ventricular myocytes via a p38 mitogen-activated protein kinase-dependent mechanism. *Br. J. Pharmacol.* **2003**, *139*, 1310–1316. [CrossRef] [PubMed]

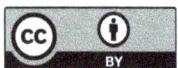 © 2019 by the authors. Licensee MDPI, Basel, Switzerland. This article is an open access article distributed under the terms and conditions of the Creative Commons Attribution (CC BY) license (http://creativecommons.org/licenses/by/4.0/).

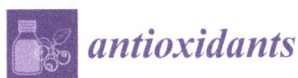

Review
Dietary Antioxidants and Parkinson's Disease

Han-A Park * and Amy C. Ellis

Department of Human Nutrition and Hospitality Management, College of Human Environmental Sciences, The University of Alabama, Tuscaloosa, AL 35487, USA; aellis@ches.ua.edu
* Correspondence: hpark36@ches.ua.edu; Tel.: +1-205-348-8051

Received: 26 May 2020; Accepted: 26 June 2020; Published: 1 July 2020

Abstract: Parkinson's disease (PD) is a neurodegenerative disorder caused by the depletion of dopaminergic neurons in the basal ganglia, the movement center of the brain. Approximately 60,000 people are diagnosed with PD in the United States each year. Although the direct cause of PD can vary, accumulation of oxidative stress-induced neuronal damage due to increased production of reactive oxygen species (ROS) or impaired intracellular antioxidant defenses invariably occurs at the cellular levels. Pharmaceuticals such as dopaminergic prodrugs and agonists can alleviate some of the symptoms of PD. Currently, however, there is no treatment to halt the progression of PD pathology. Due to the nature of PD, a long and progressive neurodegenerative process, strategies to prevent or delay PD pathology may be well suited to lifestyle changes like dietary modification with antioxidant-rich foods to improve intracellular redox homeostasis. In this review, we discuss cellular and genetic factors that increase oxidative stress in PD. We also discuss neuroprotective roles of dietary antioxidants including vitamin C, vitamin E, carotenoids, selenium, and polyphenols along with their potential mechanisms to alleviate PD pathology.

Keywords: antioxidant; mitochondria; neurodegeneration; nutrient; apoptosis

1. Introduction

Parkinson's disease (PD) is a neurodegenerative disorder characterized by inadequate levels of dopamine that is caused by loss of dopaminergic neurons in the substantia nigra pars compacta (SNpc) of the basal ganglia. Dopamine also acts in other regions of the brain like the striatum, a substructure of the forebrain that regulates the motor system. Patients with PD exhibit motor symptoms including tremor, bradykinesia, rigidity, and speech difficulties, and also frequently suffer from nonmotor symptoms including depression and insomnia [1,2]. The incidence of sporadic PD is influenced by many factors including lifestyle, environment, age, and pre-existing conditions. Oxidative stress generated by many of these factors has been addressed as a major contributor to the development and progression of neurodegeneration at the cellular levels (Figure 1) [3–5]. In particular, mitochondrial dysfunction is a key finding in reactive oxygen species (ROS)-induced PD pathology [4–7]. Complex I, also known as NADH oxidoreductase of the electron transport chain (ETC) transfers electrons from NADH to ubiquinone and so plays a key role in oxidative phosphorylation. Complex I is vulnerable to oxidative damage, and its inhibition is also strongly associated with the generation of ROS such as superoxide and hydrogen peroxide presenting a positive feedback loop [8–10]. Currently, neurotoxins that target complex I like 1-methyl-4-phenyl-1,2,3,6-tetrahydropyridine (MPTP) and rotenone are used to induce parkinsonism in both in vitro and in vivo models for research, and treatment with these drugs is known to induce oxidative stress [11,12]. In addition, imbalances in dopamine metabolism contribute to ROS generation, thus damaging dopaminergic neurons. Under normal physiological conditions, dopamine is synthesized from the amino acids tyrosine and tyramine. Hydroxylation and decarboxylation of tyrosine produce dopamine, and dopamine is further converted to norepinephrine and epinephrine or undergoes degradation. However, dopamine can also undergo metabolism by monoamine oxidase

(MAO) producing the highly reactive metabolite 3,4-dihydroxyphenylacetaldehyde (DOPAL) [13], and dopamine itself can undergo oxidation. Accumulation of DOPAL and oxidized dopamine increases the production of ROS damaging mitochondria [14–18].

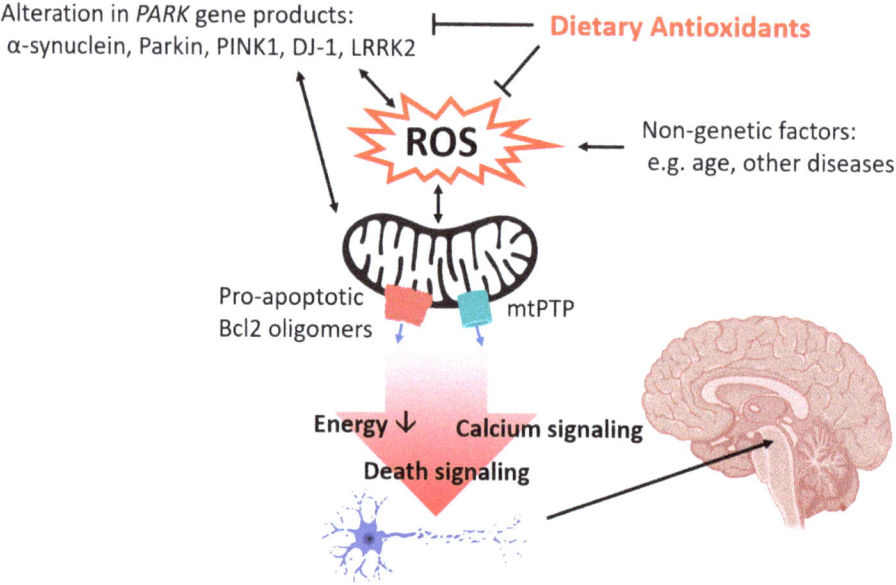

Figure 1. Summary of the protective roles of dietary antioxidants in Parkinson's disease (PD). Both genetic and nongenetic factors contribute to the accumulation of oxidative stress by enhancing ROS production and impairing cellular antioxidant defense systems. Oxidative stress damages intracellular organelles, most notably the mitochondria, impairing neuronal energy metabolism and thus hindering the energy-demanding process in the brain including neurotransmission and neuritogenesis. Mitochondrial dysfunction primes apoptosis, calcium release, and opening of mtPTP which leads to the death of neurons, including the specific dopaminergic population of the SNpc which produces the signs and symptoms of PD. Illustration by BioRender.

2. Oxidative Stress and *PARK* Genes

Approximately 5-10% of PD cases are associated with abnormalities of *PARK* genes [19–21]. The mutation of *PARK* genes increases oxidative stress in neurons by enhancing the production of ROS or impairing intracellular antioxidant defense systems. ROS predisposes *PARK* genes to abnormal protein production and vice versa (Figure 1). α-synuclein is a protein encoded by the *SNCA (PARK1)* gene. Although α-synuclein supports synaptogenesis and synaptic plasticity during normal physiology [22,23], α-synuclein aggregation-associated neuronal damage is a common finding in PD affected tissue. Application of oligomeric α-synuclein increases ROS production and lipid peroxidation [24,25]. α-synuclein is translocated to mitochondria and directly interacts with mitochondrial proteins including ATP synthase to lower mitochondrial inner membrane potential, thus altering neuronal energy metabolism and opening mitochondrial death channels [24,26]. Increased oxidative stress induced by treatment with hydrogen peroxide or depletion of antioxidant enzymes enhances post-translational modification and aggregation of α-synuclein and worsens the progression of PD [27–29].

Parkin, the ubiquitin E3 ligase encoded by the *PARK2* gene, regulates mitochondrial quality control. Mutations of *PARK2* are the most common cause of early-onset PD. Approximately 77% of early-onset familial PD in patients younger than 30 years old have Parkin mutations [30]. Parkin works in conjunction with the myocytes lacking PTEN-induced kinase 1 (PINK1), a key enzyme responsible for carrying out autophagy, encoded by the *PARK6* gene. PINK1-mediated phosphorylation of ubiquitin activates Parkin, and this enhances the removal of unwanted mitochondria [31]. Additionally, Parkin-mediated ubiquitination also targets mitofusin and miro, key components of mitochondrial fusion and mitochondrial transport, respectively [32,33]. The deletion of Parkin or PINK1 impairs mitophagy, and failure to remove dysfunctional mitochondria increases ROS production [34]. *PARK2* knockout transgenic mice treated with chronic ethanol, a stimulator of ROS, show abnormally high superoxide accumulation and glutathione depletion [35]. Application of the mitophagy inducer, autophagy and beclin 1 regulator 1 (AMBRA1), restores mitophagy in PINK1 knockout mice and suppresses ROS production [36]. Overall, the Parkin/PINK1 system plays a critical role in regulating intracellular ROS by mitochondrial quality control, removing inefficient and damaged mitochondria.

Protein deglycase DJ-1 is encoded by the *PARK 7* gene. Although the function of DJ-1 is less studied than other *PARK* gene products, it is reported to play an important role in supporting mitochondrial function. DJ-1 binds directly to F_1Fo ATP synthase and the antiapoptotic protein Bcl-xL, and this interaction promotes mitochondrial energy metabolism and survival of dopaminergic neurons [37]. The depletion of DJ-1 increases the vulnerability of mitochondria to neurotoxic insults which mimic PD pathology [38,39], whereas overexpression of DJ-1 improves intracellular antioxidants and protects neurons [38,40,41]. DJ-1 plays an important role in sensing intracellular redox status during oxidative stress [42–44]. Under oxidative stress, DJ-1 undergoes post-translational oxidation at its Cys106 residue to form cysteine-sulfonic acid and cysteine-sulfinic acid [42,45,46], and oxidative stress also enhances translocation of DJ-1 to mitochondria. Thus, it is possible that oxidation of Cys106 may act as the signal for DJ-1 to prevent mitochondrial dysfunction during ROS production in PD. In addition, DJ-1 regulates the expression of antioxidant genes by promoting nuclear translocation of Nrf2, a transcription factor that binds to genes containing an antioxidant response element (ARE) [41,47].

LRRK2, also known as dardarin, is a kinase with guanosine triphosphatase (GTPase) and scaffolding domains [48]. LRRK2 is found in the mitochondrial membrane and interacts with other *PARK* gene products including Parkin, PINK1, and DJ-1 [49,50]. LRRK2 is encoded by the *LRRK2* *(PARK8)* gene. Mutation of LRRK2 is associated with the gain of kinase activity, and this is common among patients with late-onset autosomal-dominant PD [51]. Mutation of the kinase domain of LRRK2, G2019S, exacerbates ROS-induced dopaminergic neuronal death, and application of truncated LRRK2 reverses ROS accumulation and prevents morphological alteration of these neurons [52]. In the same way, the depletion of LRRK2 or application of LRRK2 inhibitors decreases ROS, restores mitochondrial function, prevents mitochondrial fragmentation, and blocks increases in proapoptotic proteins including caspase 3, Bax, and apoptotic-inducing factor [53–55].

3. Oxidative Stress and Mitochondrial Dysfunction

Oxidative stress and mitochondrial dysfunction eventually lead to neuronal apoptosis during PD. Neurotoxic stimulation and ROS exposure increase the abundance of proapoptotic Bcl-2 protein Bax and Bak in the mitochondrial membrane (Figure 1). Oligomerization of proapoptotic proteins increases the permeability of the mitochondrial membrane causing the release of cytochrome c. Cytochrome c forms apoptosomes and activates executor caspases like caspase 3. Antiapoptotic proteins Bcl-2 and Bcl-xL are reported to block apoptosis by directly binding proapoptotic Bcl-2 proteins. Upregulation of proapoptotic proteins such as Bax and Bim as well as of other mechanisms including caspase activation and cytoplasmic release of cytochrome c have been reported in various PD models [54,56–60]. Transgenic mice lacking Bax are resistant to MPTP-induced neuronal death in the SNpc [56], and application of microRNA (miR) including miR216a and miR7 targeting Bax are protective against MPTP treatment in an in vitro and in vivo PD models [61,62]. Bcl-xL is an antiapoptotic protein that binds to DJ-1 and regulates energy metabolism in dopaminergic neurons [37,63]. A recent study shows that Bcl-xL undergoes post-translational cleavage during oxidative stress, and the accumulation of truncated Bcl-xL leads to mitochondrial dysfunction [64]. Approaches that inhibit proteolytic cleavage of Bcl-xL are reported to be protective against neurotoxicity. Treatment with antioxidants prevents the accumulation of truncated Bcl-xL and rescues neurons from oxidative stress [64]. SH-SY5Y cells derived from human bone marrow that overexpress PINK1 show decreased proteolytic cleavage of Bcl-xL by enhancing phosphorylation of Bcl-xL [65]. Bcl-xL Cre-lox knockout mice show decreased tyrosine hydroxylase-positive cells indicating loss of dopaminergic neurons in the SNpc [66]; thus, maintaining functional Bcl-xL may be critical in preventing PD-associated neuronal death.

The association between neuronal death and opening of mitochondrial permeability transition pore (mtPTP), a large less-selective mitochondrial inner membrane death channel, has been documented in PD models [24,67,68]. The opening of mtPTP allows the passage of ions and small molecules less than 1.5KDa and depolarizes the mitochondrial inner membrane. mtPTP also enhances calcium release [24] which can trigger apoptosis (Figure 1) [69]. Loss of the mitochondrial electrochemical gradient impairs ATP production by the F_1Fo ATP synthase and impairs neuronal energy metabolism [70–72]. The F_1Fo ATP synthase plays a key role in ATP production and mPTP formation [72–74]. The F_1Fo ATP synthase interacts with *PARK* gene products DJ-1 and α-synuclein [24,37]. Interaction between DJ-1 and F_1Fo ATP synthase enhances neuronal energy metabolism and promotes elongation and arborization of dopaminergic neurons [37]. On the other hand, oligomeric α-synuclein co-localizes with the F_1Fo ATP synthase and causes oxidative modification of its β subunit, the key subunit that interacts with ADP and ATP [24]. This oxidative modification increases the opening of mtPTP. Similarly, treatment with α-synuclein, known to form insoluble fibrils during PD pathology, favors mtPTP opening in both in vitro and in vivo models, and application of the mPTP inhibitor cyclosporin A reverses α-synuclein-induced mitochondrial dysfunction [60,75]. The depletion of PINK1 decreases mitochondrial inner membrane potential and increases the opening of mtPTP, and this leads to mitophagy and neuronal death [76,77].

4. Neuroprotective Dietary Antioxidants

Neurodegeneration at the cellular level develops years before patients exhibit clinical manifestations of PD. Therefore, finding strategies that can be applied over a lifetime seems of logical importance in fighting against PD. An increasing number of studies have addressed neuroprotective roles of nutrients and functional foods against neurodegeneration [78–80]. In particular, certain vitamins, minerals, and phytochemicals exhibit their antioxidant properties by directly scavenging ROS, binding to antioxidant enzymes as cofactors, and by regulating genes that control intracellular antioxidant systems (Figure 1). Advancing technologies in liquid chromatography and mass spectrometry such as LC/MS/MS and MALDI-TOF allow quantitative analysis of these nutrients and application of molecular approaches including sequencing, polymerase chain reaction, and electrophoresis to elucidate the association between *PARK* genes and dietary antioxidants. Here, we discuss dietary antioxidants that may potentially prevent or delay the progression of PD (Table 1).

Table 1. List of studies investigating the roles of antioxidant nutrients in PD models.

	Vit C	Vit E	Vit A & Car	Se	GSH & NAC	Cur	Res	Cat	Ole
α-synuclein	[81,82]		[83]		[84]	[85–87]	[88,89]	[90–96]	[97,98]
Oxidative stress and antioxidant	[99]	[99]	[100]	[101]	[102]	[87,103–107]	[108–114]	[93,115–119]	[97,98,120–124]
Electron transport chain					[125]	[103,126]	[109,110,113]		
Neuronal death and apoptotic pathway	[127]	[128]	[83,100,129–133]		[102,112,134,135]	[87,103,104,107,126,136–138]	[88,89,108,111,113]	[95,116,118,119,139,140]	[97,121–123,141,142]
Behavioral or motor function	[127]	[128]	[130]	[101]		[105,136,143–146]	[88,108,110,113,147]	[92,115–118,139,148]	[123]

Vitamin C (Vit C), vitamin E (Vit E), vitamin A (Vit A), carotenoids (Car), selenium (Se), glutathione (GSH), N-acetylcysteine (NAC), curcumin (Cur), resveratrol (Res), catechin (Cat), oleuropein (Ole).

4.1. Vitamin C

Vitamin C, also called ascorbic acid or ascorbate, is abundant in fruits and vegetables. Although most mammals are able to synthesize vitamin C endogenously, humans lack the necessary enzyme L-gulonolactone oxidase, so humans must ingest this essential nutrient in food or supplements [149]. Vitamin C acts as an antioxidant by donating electrons to neutralize the toxic effect of free radicals. Depending on available in vivo concentration, at high doses (≥500 mg/d), vitamin C has been shown to exhibit prooxidant properties [150]. In addition to its role in regulating cellular redox status, vitamin C supports the actions of hydroxylases involved in neurotransmitter synthesis including dopamine β-hydroxylase. Neural tissue including the brain contains high levels of vitamin C relative to other tissues, and neuroprotective roles of vitamin C have been discussed in various neurodegenerative disease models [151]. Treatment with divalent metal cations like copper and iron augment oligomerization of α-synuclein during challenge with DOPAL, a neurotoxic byproduct of dopamine metabolism [81], and treatment with vitamin C prevents α-synuclein oligomerization by inhibiting the oxidation of DOPAL [81] or interaction with copper [82]. A *Drosophila* model of PD shows increased oxidative stress with subsequent loss of dopaminergic neurons and locomotor deficits; treatment with vitamin C increased antioxidant enzyme activity and alleviated the PD-associated phenotype [99,127,152,153]. This model of PD is based on depletion of ubiquitin c-terminal hydrolase (UCH), an antioxidant enzyme, that thus enhances aging-associated degeneration of dopaminergic neurons and decreases dopamine content in the brain. The application of vitamin C (0.5 mM) compensates for these effects of UCH knockdown in *Drosophila* [152]. Vitamin C activates ten-eleven-translocation 1-3 (Tet1-3) enzymes and Jumonji C-domain-containing histone demethylases (Jmjds) [154]. These enzymes catalyze the formation of 5-hydroxymethylcytosine in DNA [155] and demethylation of lysine residues in histone, respectively. Tets and JmJds are required during the early stages of dopaminergic neuron differentiation, and treatment with vitamin C advances the development of neural stem cells derived from the embryonic midbrain [154]. Despite the protective roles of vitamin C found in in vitro and animal models, the efficacy of vitamin C against PD in humans is still controversial. Blood samples collected from PD patients show increased lipid peroxidation coupled with significantly lower levels of vitamin C compared to healthy controls [156], but some studies have also reported negligible effects of vitamin C on PD in human subjects [157]. Despite controversial results in human subjects, vitamin C may improve the therapeutic capacity of levodopa by enhancing its bioavailability and alleviating its toxic side effects [158,159].

4.2. Vitamin E

Vitamin E encompasses the tocopherols and tocotrienols found in plant sources including grains, legumes, vegetables, and seeds. Both tocopherols and tocotrienols have a chromanol ring and a hydrocarbon chain. Tocopherols have a saturated chain whereas tocotrienols contain double bonds. Vitamin E exhibits strong antioxidant properties by acting as a ROS scavenger, attenuating mitochondrial dysfunction, and preventing neuronal apoptosis during neurotoxic insults that mimic neurodegenerative disease [64,160]. Both tocopherol and tocotrienol bind to α-tocopherol transfer protein (TTP), a critical regulator of vitamin E movement and metabolism. α-tocopherol has an 8.5-fold higher affinity for TTP than α-tocotrienol [161], thus α-tocopherol is generally considered to have better bioavailability. However, studies are increasingly demonstrating that tocopherols and tocotrienols have varying roles in different tissues and microenvironments. For example, tocotrienols exhibit a stronger antioxidant capacity in lipid-rich biological membranes [162], thus tocotrienols may be effective in protecting lipid-rich organs like the brain [64,163]. Long-term intraperitoneal injection of α-tocopherol and the water-soluble analog Trolox improved long-term potentiation (LTP) and long-term depression (LTD) in PINK1 knockout mice [164]. Martella et al. report that chronic treatment with low concentration rotenone does not alter ATP production or viability of dopaminergic neurons in heterozygous PINK1 knockout (PINK1 $^{+/-}$) mice [165]. Despite this seemingly insignificant outcome, this treatment also completely impairs both LTP and LTD, and intraperitoneal injection of α-tocopherol (100 mg/kg) and Trolox (5 mg/kg) reverse this synaptic plasticity impairment [165]. DJ-1 mutant flies show altered redox homeostasis as evidenced by high levels of global ROS and hydrogen peroxide production and decreased activity of catalase and superoxide dismutase [99]. However, supplementation with α-tocopherol decreases global ROS levels in DJ-1 mutant flies [99]. In addition to tocopherols, tocotrienols protect neurons against oxidative stress-associated damage. Primary hippocampal neurons treated with α-tocotrienol show a decrease in total and mitochondrial ROS accumulation, and α-tocotrienol attenuates glutamate-induced post-translational cleavage of Bcl-xL to enhance the functions of antiapoptotic Bcl-xL [166,167]. In this study, α-tocotrienol was suggested to exert its effect by blocking the oligomerization of proapoptotic Bcl-2 proteins [167]. Oral administration of 100 μg/kg δ-tocotrienol prevents the loss of dopaminergic neurons in the SNpc and improves motor behavior in a mouse model of PD [128]. δ-tocotrienol binds to the estrogen receptor β and activates PI3K/Akt signaling pathways including phosphorylation of protein kinase B (PKB, Akt) and extracellular signal-regulated kinase (ERK) 1/2 [128,168]. Akt activates Nrf2 [169,170], and Nrf2-mediated upregulation of antioxidant and prosurvival genes is an important mechanism for the neuroprotective properties of many antioxidant nutrients [171–173]. Clinical studies with PD patients show that higher consumption of dietary vitamin E is inversely related to PD occurrence [157,164,174,175]. However, contrary reports have also been published on PD in human subjects [176,177]. Data from randomized controlled trials with vitamin E are limited. However, in a randomized double-blind placebo-controlled trial, Taghizadeh et al. reported significant improvement in clinical symptoms as assessed by the Unified Parkinson's Disease Rating Scale (UPDRS) among PD patients who received 400 IU of vitamin E in combination with 1000 mg of omega-3 fatty acids [178]. These researchers also reported increases in circulating glutathione and total antioxidant capacity along with decreased high-sensitivity C-reactive protein with treatment compared to placebo. Although promising, further investigation into the specific roles of vitamin E subgroups will be important to clarify the efficacy of vitamin E in clinical disease.

4.3. Vitamin A and Carotenoids

Vitamin A is a fat-soluble vitamin found in both animal (e.g., liver) and plant sources and can also be produced from provitamin A carotenoids. Vitamin A exists as multiple forms: retinol (alcohol), retinal (aldehyde), retinoic acid (carboxylic acid), and retinyl ester (ester form). Retinal binds to opsin and activates rhodopsin, a G-protein coupled receptor that senses light in the eye. Retinoic acid binds to nuclear receptors including retinoic acid receptor (RAR) and retinoid X receptor (RXR) and regulates transcription of genes that control growth and differentiation [179]. In addition to these roles, vitamin A exhibits neuroprotective properties against neurodegeneration. Retinoic acid promotes differentiation of GABAergic neurons expressing dopamine receptors [132,133,179], and changes in PD include inhibition of retinoic acid-mediated neuronal differentiation [180]. Oral supplementation with retinoic acid upregulates the μ-type opioid receptor (MOR1), a G-protein-coupled receptor that mediates inhibitory signaling, in the dorsal striatum and attenuates repetitive dyskinetic movements in PD mice [181].

Carotenoids include the yellow, orange, and red pigments found in fruits and vegetables like carrots, tomatoes, watermelons, and pumpkins, and are also found in algae, salmon, and shrimp. Examples of carotenoids include carotene, lycopene, lutein, and astaxanthin. Serum α-carotene, β-carotene, and lycopene levels are significantly decreased in PD patients, and decreased serum carotenoid levels are also associated with poorer motor function [174,182]. However, a meta-analysis that examined the association between PD and vitamin A and carotenoids (lutein, α-carotene, β-carotene, lycopene, β-cryptoxanthin, zeaxanthin and canthaxanthin) concluded that the evidence was insufficient to make an epidemiological association between vitamin A/carotenoids and risk of developing PD [183]. In an in vivo animal model, oral administration of lycopene (5–20 mg/kg) attenuates oxidative stress induced by intraperitoneal injection of MPTP in mice, and lycopene also inhibits apoptosis by decreasing Bax and caspases while increasing Bcl-2 [129]. Treatment with lutein prevents MPTP-induced Bax and caspase increases, and lutein also improves motor function in MPTP challenged mice [130]. Astaxanthin lowers intracellular ROS and improves superoxide dismutase and catalase activity, and treatment with astaxanthin prevents apoptotic death in MPTP challenged SH-SY5Y cells [100]. Astaxanthin attenuates MPTP-induced neuronal injury via the downregulation of α-synuclein [83]. miR-7 directly binds to the 3' UTR of α-synuclein mRNA and decreases the translation of α-synuclein [184]. Treatment with astaxanthin prevents the loss of miR-7 to lower the toxic effects of α-synuclein in SH-SY5Y cells [83]. Although clinical trials are lacking, oral supplementation with astaxanthin prevents loss of neurons in the SNpc and tyrosine hydroxylase-positive cells in the striatum from intraperitoneally injected MPTP in mice [131].

4.4. Selenium

Selenium is an essential trace mineral-rich in Brazil nuts, seafood, and organ meats and is also found in water and soil. The selenium content of plants is directly related to the selenium content of the soil [185]. Enzymes that regulate intracellular redox status likes glutathione peroxidase and thioredoxin reductase are selenoproteins that require selenium at their active sites, and mutations of the selenocysteine residues impair enzyme activity [186]. Microarray investigation reveals that rotenone treatment downregulates the *SELENBP1* gene which encodes selenium binding protein 1, along with other genes that control apoptosis and mitochondrial function [187]. Neuroprotective functions of the selenium-containing quinoline derivative, 7-chloro-4-(phenylselanyl) quinoline, against the rotenone challenge highly correlates with selenium content in the brain of fruit flies [188]. Intraperitoneal delivery of selenium selenite (0.1, 0.2, and 0.3 mg/kg) increases glutathione peroxidase activity, alleviates lipid peroxidation, and improves motor function of the 6-hydroxydopamine challenged striatum in rats [101]. Interestingly, selenium treatment also shows dose-dependent protection of other antioxidant enzymes including glutathione reductase, glutathione transferase, and catalase [101]. Intraperitoneal injection of selenium partially improves dopamine metabolism during the MPTP challenge [189]. Analysis of soil samples from 4856 sites in the US demonstrates that higher selenium content inversely correlates with mortality from PD [190]. Human studies investigating selenium supplementation for PD are lacking. However, low plasma selenium concentrations are associated with decreased performance in neurological tests among older adults [191]. Conversely, increased levels of selenium in cerebrospinal fluid and plasma have been reported in PD patients [192,193]. Chronic exposure to selenium enhances oxidative stress in the brain and leads to cognitive impairment in animal models [194,195]. The underlying mechanism for these findings is unclear; however, evidence suggests that either a deficiency or excess of selenium may contribute to neurodegeneration or conversely PD pathology may impair mobilization of selenium in neurons. The Recommended Dietary Allowance for selenium is 55 mg/day, and the Institute of Medicine has established a Tolerable Upper Intake Level for selenium at 400 mg/day. Therefore, meeting the RDA without excess may be prudent [196].

4.5. Glutathione

Glutathione is a tripeptide of glycine, cysteine, and glutamate that is widely present in both plant and animal foods. In particular, avocados, asparagus, spinach, and amino acid-rich meat, fish and poultry are good sources of glutathione. Glutathione is a major intracellular antioxidant that reduces reactive oxygen species by being oxidized to glutathione disulfide. Glutathione is required by glutathione peroxidase during the conversion of hydrogen peroxide to water. The depletion of glutathione leads to oxidative stress-induced mitochondrial dysfunction and degeneration of dopaminergic neurons [125,134,197]. Interestingly, excess of glutathione also causes neuronal damage [134], and this may be due to the overproduction of glutathione disulfide, an oxidized form of glutathione responsible for mitochondrial dysfunction and neuronal death [198]. Strategies to support glutathione homeostasis by preventing loss of glutathione or facilitating clearance of glutathione disulfide protect the brain [163,198]. Treatment with glutathione's precursor N-acetylcysteine (NAC) prevents oxidative stress and calcium overload and rescues neurons and other brain cells during PD-like stress [102,112,135]. Consistently, a protective effect of intravenous and oral delivery of NAC has been reported in PD patients [199–201]; NAC is naturally found in onions and garlic, and it is available in various dosages as an over-the-counter dietary supplement [202]. However, the best duration and concentration of supplementation to consistently show a therapeutic effect in humans has not been established [200,203]. Therefore, further investigation is required. Additionally, since oral glutathione is less bioavailable, finding nutrients that enhance the body's ability to synthesize glutathione may also be of benefit.

5. Polyphenols

Polyphenols are characterized by the presence of multiple phenol groups and a six-membered hydrocarbon ring structure. Based on the arrangement of phenol groups, hydrocarbon chain and additional functional groups, polyphenols are further classified into subgroups including flavonoids, isoflavonoids, curcuminoids, tannins, and stilbenoids. There are estimated to be over 8000 different polyphenols present in nature [204]. We will describe four well-investigated polyphenols—curcumin, resveratrol, catechin, and oleuropein—and their role in PD models.

5.1. Curcumin

Curcumin, 1,7-bis(4-hydroxy-3-methoxyphenyl)-1,6-heptadiene-3,5-dione is a polyphenol found in turmeric. Curcumin scavenges biological radicals including superoxide anion, hydrogen peroxide, 1,1-diphenyl-2-picryl-hydrazyl free radical, 2,2′-azino-bis (3-ethylbenzthiazoline-6-sulfonic acid) radical, and N,N-dimethyl-p-phenylenediamine dihydrochloride radical [205]. In addition, treatment with curcumin (10 µM) decreases oxidation-associated protein modification including carbonylation and nitrotyrosine formation to rescue dopaminergic cells [106]. Curcumin effectively protects mitochondria from oxidative stress-associated damage [206]. Curcumin (2 µM) prevents loss of mitochondrial membrane potential and electron transfer system capacity in SH-SY5Y cells depleted with PINK1 [126]. Similarly, treatment with curcumin monoglucoside (0.25–5 µM) restores mitochondrial complex I and IV activity by decreasing the accumulation of hydroperoxides and increasing glutathione levels [103]. Curcumin exhibits antiapoptotic properties. Treatment with curcumin (5 µM) decreases ROS-induced calcium influx, lowering activation of caspase 3 and caspase 9 [104]. In addition, curcumin interferes with prodeath JNK signaling to prevent downstream apoptotic pathways including the release of cytochrome c and cleavage of procaspase 3 [103,138]. In vivo studies demonstrated antioxidant [105,144] and antiapoptotic [87,136] effects of curcumin to improve PD-associated neurobehavior [103,105,107,143–146]. Intraperitoneal injection of curcumin (200 mg/kg) attenuates rotenone-induced motor impairment in rats [143]. Male Wistar rat orally administered 5–20 mg/kg demethoxycurcumin, a derivative of curcumin, show concentration-dependent protection against rotenone challenge [105]. Demethoxycurcumin attenuates rotenone-induced oxidative stress and prevents loss of dopamine in the brain [105], and animals treated with demethoxycurcumin show improved motor function [105]. Dietary supplementation with 0.5% and 2% curcumin also show similar effects on MPTP-induced mouse PD models [137]. In addition to neuroprotection, curcumin may regulate cell differentiation and proliferation. C57BL mice transplanted with curcumin-activated mesenchymal stem cells have increased antiapoptotic Bcl-2, decreased proapoptotic Bax and caspases, and avoided the loss of dopaminergic neurons during MPTP challenge [136]. Curcumin prevents α-synuclein aggregation [87] and attenuates α-synuclein-induced cytotoxicity [85]. Curcumin derivative increases the nuclear translocation of transcription factor EB, a regulator of autophagy, potentially promoting degradation of α-synuclein [86].

5.2. Resveratrol

Resveratrol, 3,5,4′-trihydroxy-$trans$-stilbene is a nonflavonoid polyphenol with two aromatic ring structures. Resveratrol is found in grapes and berries, and it is also commonly consumed in red wine. Resveratrol promotes brain cell differentiation and proliferation during normal physiology [207], and it is well-described to attenuate oxidative stress-associated damage during the progression of PD pathology [108–112,114]. Intraperitoneally administered resveratrol (20 mg/kg) decreases lipid peroxidation, increases glutathione levels, and prevents deterioration of rat SNpc against 6-hydroxydopamine, an oxidant that causes degeneration of dopaminergic neurons [108]. Various research groups have shown that resveratrol effectively protects mitochondria by decreasing the accumulation of mitochondrial ROS, preventing mitochondrial inner membrane potential loss, restoring mitochondrial respiratory enzyme activity, regulating mitochondrial fission and fusion, and protecting mitochondrial DNA in *PARK2* mutation [109–111,113]. Wang et al. showed that resveratrol treatment (25 µM) increases phosphorylation of Akt and prevents rotenone-induced death of PC12 cells [111]. Akt upregulates genes containing cAMP response element (CRE) including Bcl-2 [208,209], and it inactivates proapoptotic Bad and proteolytic caspases [210]. Thus resveratrol-mediated Akt phosphorylation may hinder apoptotic death during PD-like challenges. In addition, resveratrol may alleviate *PARK* gene-associated PD pathology. Male C57BL/6 mice subjected to intragastric gavage of 100 mg/kg resveratrol attenuate the loss of dopaminergic neurons and have improved motor behavior during the MPTP challenge [88]. This same study also shows that resveratrol significantly increases protein levels of LC3-II, a key protein found in the membrane of autophagosomes, and thereby facilitates degradation of α-synuclein [88]. Resveratrol also increases microRNA-214 which potentially inhibits translation of α-synuclein [89]. Fibroblasts isolated from patients with *PARK2* mutations have increased production of whole-cell ROS and mitochondrial ROS, and treatment with resveratrol protects mitochondria and improves respiration and ATP production in these cells [109].

5.3. Catechin

Catechins are flavonoids containing two benzene rings and one dihydropyran heterocycle. Catechins are found in various herbs and fruits. Tea in particular is a good source of catechins. Four major catechins include (−)-epicatechin (EC), (−)-epicatechin-3-gallate (ECG), (−)-epigallocatechin (EGC), and (−)-epigallocatechin-3-gallate (EGCG) [211]. Catechins donate an electron from a phenolic hydroxyl group and to scavenge free radicals and thus exhibit direct antioxidant properties [212–214]. Catechins also improve intracellular redox status by preventing the loss of other antioxidants [116]. Treatment with 10 µM EGCG lowers the accumulation of ROS and prevents activation of caspases during hydrogen peroxide challenge and protects N27 dopaminergic cells from apoptotic death [119]. Koch et al. show that a longer brewing time tends to enhance antiradical activity in teas [215] indicating that catechins retain antioxidant properties after exposure to high temperature. Although further investigation is needed, orally supplemented catechins are shown to be delivered to the brain (0.5 nmol/g) in rats [216] and an in vitro blood–brain barrier system (BBB) shows that <10% of catechins are BBB permeable [217,218]. Various research groups have demonstrated that EGCG prevents neurotoxicity associated with α-synuclein [91,92,94,95]. EGCG chelates metal ions including Cu(II) and Fe(III) to inhibit fibrillation of α-synuclein [90,93]. EGCG (350µM) enhances the formation of stable oligomers (a less-toxic form) thus prevents the accumulation of pathological fibril [95] EGCG immobilizes α-synuclein and interferes with its oligomerization in biological membranes [96], thus EGCG helps to maintain membrane integrity [95,96]. EGCG suppresses fibrillation of γ-synuclein, a type of synuclein also found in Lewy bodies [91]. EGCG improves motor behavior in *Drosophila* by preventing mitochondrial dysfunction caused by abnormalities of LRRK2 and Parkin genes [148]. Chemically induced rodent PD models produced by injection with MPTP and 6-hydroxydopamine demonstrate PD-like symptoms like bradykinesia, and administration of 10-50 mg catechin (both oral and intraperitoneal injection) improves locomotor behavior in these animals [115,116,139]. Intraperitoneal injection of 10 or 30 mg/kg catechin restores glutathione levels and increases dopamine in the rat brain [116]. Oral supplementation with 25 mg EGCG reduces oxidative stress and preserves striatal dopamine in C57BL/6J mice challenged with MPTP [115]. C57BL/6J mice intraperitoneally injected with MPTP demonstrate PD-like symptoms including bradykinesia due to loss of SNpc dopaminergic neurons, and oral administration of EGCG (25 and 50 mg/kg) in these animals lowers proinflammatory cytokines, rescues dopaminergic neurons from death, and improves motor behavior [139]. In addition to catechins' role inhibiting PD pathology, catechins may also support existing PD treatments. Orally administered EGCG (100 and 400 mg/kg) inhibits methylation of levodopa to improve bioavailability [219].

5.4. Oleuropein

Oleuropein contains hydroxytyrosol, elenolic acid, and glucose. It is a major phenolic compound found in olive oil. Although oleuropein is predominant, other oleuropein derivatives such as oleuropein aglycon and oleuroside are also found in olive oil [220]. Oleuropein acts as a scavenger of superoxide, nitric oxide, 2,2′-azinobis-(3-ethylbenzothiazoline-6-sulfonic acid, and 2,2-diphenyl-1-picrylhydrazyl radicals [221,222]. Various research groups have demonstrated that treatment with oleuropein and its derivatives inhibit the accumulation of ROS and prevent the progression of PD pathology [97,98,120]. Palazzi et al. demonstrated that in vitro incubation with oleuropein aglycone stabilizes α-synuclein monomers to prevent pathological aggregation [97]. Similarly, Mohammad-Beigi et al. show that olive fruit extracts containing oleuropein and oleuropein aglycone inhibit α-synuclein fibril elongation, decreasing cytotoxicity caused by α-synuclein oligomers [98]. In addition, oleuropein activates redox-sensitive transcription factors like Nrf2 to potentially improve intracellular antioxidant capacity via the upregulation of antioxidant genes [120,223]. Oleuropein protects mitochondria by mitigating mitochondrial superoxide production [121]. PC12 cells treated with 1-50 µM oleuropein retain mitochondrial membrane potential during the 6-hydroxydopamine challenge, and oleuropein also alleviates endoplasmic reticulum stress to protect PC12 cells from apoptotic death [141]. Oleuropein increases mitochondrial antiapoptotic Bcl-2 and decreases proapoptotic Bax and apoptotic-inducing factor [121,142]. Furthermore, oleuropein regulates phosphorylation of dynamin-related protein 1 (Drp1) [142] and LC3-II [121], key proteins that control mitochondrial fission and mitophagy, respectively. Thus, oleuropein potentially supports an optimal mitochondrial population in cells. Oral supplementation with olive leaf extract (75–300 mg/kg) significantly increases antioxidant enzymes including superoxide dismutase and glutathione peroxidase in the rat brain [123]. Rats fed with olive leaf extract are protected from loss of dopaminergic neuron during rotenone-induced mitochondrial damage, and showed improved neurobehavior [123]. Similarly, rats supplemented with extra virgin olive oil extract show decreased lipid peroxidation and increased antioxidant enzyme activities [124]. Oral administration of oleuropein is distributed to the brain 2h after ingestion [224], so oleuropein may be a key component in olive leaf and olive oil-mediated neuroprotection.

6. Conclusions

Although increasing numbers of studies performed in vitro and using animal models demonstrate a potential role in dietary prevention of PD, the efficacy of nutritional intervention to do so in humans remains controversial. Epidemiological studies examining dietary intake of antioxidant micronutrients and the risk of developing PD have yielded equivocal results, and there is a paucity of data from randomized controlled trials among people with pre-existing PD. Dietary antioxidants exhibit multiple effects rather than targeting a single specific process. Vitamin C, vitamin E, and polyphenols directly interact with ROS and terminate oxidative chain reactions. Other minerals like selenium act as cofactors to support the activity of antioxidant enzymes. Many antioxidant nutrients are involved in signaling transduction and protect downstream targets of oxidative stress to alleviate the damage that promotes the development of PD. Nutrients also regulate genes that control the development, growth, and survival of dopaminergic neurons. Polyphenols like curcumin, resveratrol, catechin, and oleuropein inhibit the formation of Lewy bodies. In this review, we have described the complex cellular and molecular mechanisms of these dietary antioxidants as an important step in developing a therapeutic strategy against PD. Future clinical studies with data safety and monitoring are warranted to determine whether these antioxidant micronutrients may act individually or in synergy as a nonpharmacological means of prevention and treatment.

Author Contributions: Writing and editing: H.-A.P. and A.C.E. All authors have read and agreed to the published version of the manuscript.

Funding: This research received no external funding.

Conflicts of Interest: The authors declare no conflict of interest.

References

1. Armstrong, M.J.; Okun, M.S. Diagnosis and treatment of parkinson's disease: A review. *JAMA* **2020**, *323*, 548–560. [CrossRef]
2. Goldman, J.G.; Guerra, C.M. Treatment of nonmotor symptoms associated with Parkinson's disease. *Neurol. Clin.* **2020**, *38*, 269–292. [CrossRef] [PubMed]
3. Blesa, J.; Trigo, D.I.; Quiroga, V.A.; Jackson, L.V.R. Oxidative stress and Parkinson's disease. *Front Neuroanat.* **2015**, *9*, 91. [CrossRef] [PubMed]
4. Dias, V.; Junn, E.; Mouradian, M.M. The role of oxidative stress in Parkinson's disease. *J. Parkinsons Dis.* **2013**, *3*, 461–491. [CrossRef] [PubMed]
5. Puspita, L.; Chung, S.Y.; Shim, J.W. Oxidative stress and cellular pathologies in Parkinson's disease. *Mol. Brain* **2017**, *10*, 53. [CrossRef]
6. Park, J.S.; Davis, R.L.; Sue, C.M. Mitochondrial dysfunction in parkinson's disease: New mechanistic insights and therapeutic perspectives. *Curr. Neurol. Neurosci. Rep.* **2018**, *18*, 21. [CrossRef]
7. Winklhofer, K.F.; Haass, C. Mitochondrial dysfunction in Parkinson's disease. *Biochim. Biophys. Acta* **2010**, *1802*, 29–44. [CrossRef]
8. Keeney, P.M.; Xie, J.; Capaldi, R.A.; Bennett, J.P.J. Parkinson's disease brain mitochondrial complex I has oxidatively damaged subunits and is functionally impaired and misassembled. *J. Neurosci.* **2006**, *26*, 5256–5264. [CrossRef]
9. Parker, W.D.J.; Parks, J.K.; Swerdlow, R.H. Complex I deficiency in Parkinson's disease frontal cortex. *Brain Res.* **2008**, *1189*, 215–218. [CrossRef]
10. Valdez, L.B.; Zaobornyj, T.; Bandez, M.J.; Lopez-Cepero, J.M.; Boveris, A.; Navarro, A. Complex I syndrome in striatum and frontal cortex in a rat model of Parkinson's disease. *Free Radic. Biol. Med.* **2019**, *135*, 274–282. [CrossRef]
11. Perier, C.; Bove, J.; Vila, M.; Przedborski, S. The rotenone model of Parkinson's disease. *Trends Neurosci.* **2003**, *26*, 345–346. [CrossRef]
12. Sriram, K.; Pai, K.S.; Boyd, M.R.; Ravindranath, V. Evidence for generation of oxidative stress in brain by MPTP: In vitro and in vivo studies in mice. *Brain Res.* **1997**, *749*, 44–52. [CrossRef]
13. Meiser, J.; Weindl, D.; Hiller, K. Complexity of dopamine metabolism. *Cell Commun. Signal* **2013**, *11*, 34. [CrossRef] [PubMed]
14. Coelho, E.-C.; de Araujo, C.C.; Follmer, C. Formation of large oligomers of DOPAL-modified alpha-synuclein is modulated by the oxidation of methionine residues located at C-terminal domain. *Biochem. Biophys. Res. Commun.* **2019**, *509*, 367–372. [CrossRef] [PubMed]
15. Plotegher, N.; Berti, G.; Ferrari, E.; Tessari, I.; Zanetti, M.; Lunelli, L. DOPAL derived alpha-synuclein oligomers impair synaptic vesicles physiological function. *Sci. Rep.* **2017**, *7*, 40699. [CrossRef] [PubMed]
16. Sarafian, T.A.; Yacoub, A.; Kunz, A.; Aranki, B.; Serobyan, G.; Cohn, W. Enhanced mitochondrial inhibition by 3,4-dihydroxyphenyl-acetaldehyde (DOPAL)-oligomerized alpha-synuclein. *J. Neurosci. Res.* **2019**, *97*, 1689–1705. [CrossRef] [PubMed]
17. Kristal, B.S.; Conway, A.D.; Brown, A.M.; Jain, J.C.; Ulluci, P.A.; Li, S.W. Selective dopaminergic vulnerability: 3,4-dihydroxyphenylacetaldehyde targets mitochondria. *Free Radic. Biol. Med.* **2001**, *30*, 924–931. [CrossRef]
18. Burbulla, L.F.; Song, P.; Mazzulli, J.R.; Zampese, E.; Wong, Y.C.; Jeon, S. Dopamine oxidation mediates mitochondrial and lysosomal dysfunction in Parkinson's disease. *Science* **2017**, *357*, 1255–1261. [CrossRef]
19. Klein, C.; Westenberger, A. Genetics of Parkinson's disease. *Cold Spring Harb. Perspect. Med.* **2012**, *2*, a008888. [CrossRef]
20. Thomas, B.; Beal, M.F. Parkinson's disease. *Hum. Mol. Genet.* **2007**, *16*, R183–R194. [CrossRef] [PubMed]
21. Lesage, S.; Brice, A. Parkinson's disease: From monogenic forms to genetic susceptibility factors. *Hum. Mol. Genet.* **2009**, *18*, R48–R59. [CrossRef] [PubMed]

22. Cheng, F.; Vivacqua, G.; Yu, S. The role of alpha-synuclein in neurotransmission and synaptic plasticity. *J. Chem. Neuroanat.* **2011**, *42*, 242–248. [CrossRef]
23. Hsu, L.J.; Mallory, M.; Xia, Y.; Veinbergs, I.; Hashimoto, M.; Yoshimoto, M. Expression pattern of synucleins (non-Abeta component of Alzheimer's disease amyloid precursor protein/alpha-synuclein) during murine brain development. *J. Neurochem.* **1998**, *71*, 338–344. [CrossRef] [PubMed]
24. Ludtmann, M.H.R.; Angelova, P.R.; Horrocks, M.H.; Choi, M.L.; Rodrigues, M.; Baev, A.Y. Alpha-synuclein oligomers interact with ATP synthase and open the permeability transition pore in Parkinson's disease. *Nat. Commun.* **2018**, *9*, 2293. [CrossRef] [PubMed]
25. Perni, M.; Galvagnion, C.; Maltsev, A.; Meisl, G.; Muller, M.B.; Challa, P.K. A natural product inhibits the initiation of alpha-synuclein aggregation and suppresses its toxicity. *Proc. Natl. Acad. Sci. USA* **2017**, *114*, E1009–E1017. [CrossRef]
26. Ding, H.; Xiong, Y.; Sun, J.; Chen, C.; Gao, J.; Xu, H. Asiatic acid prevents oxidative stress and apoptosis by inhibiting the translocation of alpha-synuclein into mitochondria. *Front Neurosci.* **2018**, *12*, 431. [CrossRef]
27. Scudamore, O.; Ciossek, T. Increased oxidative stress exacerbates alpha-synuclein aggregation in vivo. *J. Neuropathol. Exp. Neurol.* **2018**, *77*, 443–453. [CrossRef]
28. Kruger, R.; Kuhn, W.; Muller, T.; Woitalla, D.; Graeber, M.; Kosel, S. Ala30Pro mutation in the gene encoding alpha-synuclein in Parkinson's disease. *Nat. Genet.* **1998**, *18*, 106–108. [CrossRef]
29. Xiang, W.; Schlachetzki, J.C.; Helling, S.; Bussmann, J.C.; Berlinghof, M.; Schaffer, T.E. Oxidative stress-induced posttranslational modifications of alpha-synuclein: Specific modification of alpha-synuclein by 4-hydroxy-2-nonenal increases dopaminergic toxicity. *Mol. Cell Neurosci.* **2013**, *54*, 71–83. [CrossRef]
30. Lucking, C.B.; Durr, A.; Bonifati, V.; Vaughan, J.; De Michele, G.; Gasser, T. Association between early-onset Parkinson's disease and mutations in the parkin gene. *N. Engl. J. Med.* **2000**, *342*, 1560–1567. [CrossRef]
31. Koyano, F.; Okatsu, K.; Kosako, H.; Tamura, Y.; Go, E.; Kimura, M. Ubiquitin is phosphorylated by PINK1 to activate parkin. *Nature* **2014**, *510*, 162–166. [CrossRef] [PubMed]
32. Wang, X.; Winter, D.; Ashrafi, G.; Schlehe, J.; Wong, Y.L.; Selkoe, D. PINK1 and Parkin target Miro for phosphorylation and degradation to arrest mitochondrial motility. *Cell* **2011**, *147*, 893–906. [CrossRef]
33. Chen, Y.; Dorn, G.W., II. PINK1-phosphorylated mitofusin 2 is a Parkin receptor for culling damaged mitochondria. *Science* **2013**, *340*, 471–475. [CrossRef]
34. Barodia, S.K.; Creed, R.B.; Goldberg, M.S. Parkin and PINK1 functions in oxidative stress and neurodegeneration. *Brain Res. Bull.* **2017**, *133*, 51–59. [CrossRef]
35. Hwang, C.J.; Kim, Y.E.; Son, D.J.; Park, M.H.; Choi, D.Y.; Park, P.H. Parkin deficiency exacerbate ethanol-induced dopaminergic neurodegeneration by P38 pathway dependent inhibition of autophagy and mitochondrial function. *Redox Biol.* **2017**, *11*, 456–568. [CrossRef] [PubMed]
36. Rita, D.A.; D'Acunzo, P.; Simula, L.; Campello, S.; Strappazzon, F.; Cecconi, F. AMBRA1-Mediated mitophagy counteracts oxidative stress and apoptosis induced by neurotoxicity in human neuroblastoma SH-SY5Y cells. *Front Cell Neurosci.* **2018**, *12*, 92. [CrossRef] [PubMed]
37. Chen, R.; Park, H.A.; Mnatsakanyan, N.; Niu, Y.; Licznerski, P.; Wu, J. Parkinson's disease protein DJ-1 regulates ATP synthase protein components to increase neuronal process outgrowth. *Cell Death Dis.* **2019**, *10*, 469. [CrossRef] [PubMed]
38. Hao, L.Y.; Giasson, B.I.; Bonini, N.M. DJ-1 is critical for mitochondrial function and rescues PINK1 loss of function. *Proc. Natl. Acad. Sci. USA* **2010**, *107*, 9747–9752. [CrossRef]
39. Larsen, N.J.; Ambrosi, G.; Mullett, S.J.; Berman, S.B.; Hinkle, D.A. DJ-1 knock-down impairs astrocyte mitochondrial function. *Neuroscience* **2011**, *196*, 251–264. [CrossRef]
40. De Miranda, B.R.; Rocha, E.M.; Bai, Q.; Ayadi, E.A.; Hinkle, D.; Burton, E.A. Astrocyte-specific DJ-1 overexpression protects against rotenone-induced neurotoxicity in a rat model of Parkinson's disease. *Neurobiol. Dis.* **2018**, *115*, 101–114. [CrossRef]
41. Li, R.; Wang, S.; Li, T.; Wu, L.; Fang, Y.; Feng, Y. Salidroside protects dopaminergic neurons by preserving complex I activity via DJ-1/Nrf2-Mediated antioxidant pathway. *Parkinsons Dis.* **2019**, *2019*, 6073496. [CrossRef] [PubMed]
42. Canet-Aviles, R.M.; Wilson, M.A.; Miller, D.W.; Ahmad, R.; McLendon, C.; Bandyopadhyay, S. The Parkinson's disease protein DJ-1 is neuroprotective due to cysteine-sulfinic acid-driven mitochondrial localization. *Proc. Natl. Acad. Sci. USA* **2004**, *101*, 9103–9108. [CrossRef] [PubMed]

43. Mitsumoto, A.; Nakagawa, Y. DJ-1 is an indicator for endogenous reactive oxygen species elicited by endotoxin. *Free Radic. Res.* **2001**, *35*, 885–893. [CrossRef] [PubMed]
44. Saito, Y. Oxidized DJ-1 as a possible biomarker of Parkinson's disease. *J. Clin. Biochem. Nutr.* **2014**, *54*, 138–144. [CrossRef]
45. Kinumi, T.; Kimata, J.; Taira, T.; Ariga, H.; Niki, E. Cysteine-106 of DJ-1 is the most sensitive cysteine residue to hydrogen peroxide-mediated oxidation in vivo in human umbilical vein endothelial cells. *Biochem. Biophys. Res. Commun.* **2004**, *317*, 722–728. [CrossRef]
46. Blackinton, J.; Lakshminarasimhan, M.; Thomas, K.J.; Ahmad, R.; Greggio, E.; Raza, A.S. Formation of a stabilized cysteine sulfinic acid is critical for the mitochondrial function of the parkinsonism protein DJ-1. *J. Biol. Chem.* **2009**, *284*, 6476–6485. [CrossRef]
47. Narasimhan, K.K.S.; Jayakumar, D.; Velusamy, P.; Srinivasan, A.; Mohan, T.; Ravi, D.B. Morinda citrifolia and its active principle scopoletin mitigate protein aggregation and neuronal apoptosis through augmenting the DJ-1/Nrf2/ARE signaling pathway. *Oxid. Med. Cell Longev.* **2019**, *2019*, 2761041. [CrossRef]
48. Jaleel, M.; Nichols, R.J.; Deak, M.; Campbell, D.G.; Gillardon, F.; Knebel, A. LRRK2 phosphorylates moesin at threonine-558: Characterization of how Parkinson's disease mutants affect kinase activity. *Biochem. J.* **2007**, *405*, 307–317. [CrossRef]
49. Smith, W.W.; Pei, Z.; Jiang, H.; Moore, D.J.; Liang, Y.; West, A.B. Leucine-rich repeat kinase 2 (LRRK2) interacts with parkin, and mutant LRRK2 induces neuronal degeneration. *Proc. Natl. Acad. Sci. USA* **2005**, *102*, 18676–18681. [CrossRef]
50. Venderova, K.; Kabbach, G.; Abdel-Messih, E.; Zhang, Y.; Parks, R.J.; Imai, Y. Leucine-Rich Repeat Kinase 2 interacts with Parkin, DJ-1 and PINK-1 in a Drosophila melanogaster model of Parkinson's disease. *Hum. Mol. Genet.* **2009**, *18*, 4390–4404. [CrossRef]
51. Zimprich, A.; Biskup, S.; Leitner, P.; Lichtner, P.; Farrer, M.; Lincoln, S. Mutations in LRRK2 cause autosomal-dominant parkinsonism with pleomorphic pathology. *Neuron* **2004**, *44*, 601–607. [CrossRef]
52. Vermilyea, S.C.; Babinski, A.; Tran, N.; To, S.; Guthrie, S.; Kluss, J.H. In vitro CRISPR/Cas9-Directed gene editing to model LRRK2 G2019S Parkinson's disease in common marmosets. *Sci. Rep.* **2020**, *10*, 3447. [CrossRef] [PubMed]
53. Kim, J.; Pajarillo, E.; Rizor, A.; Son, D.S.; Lee, J.; Aschner, M. LRRK2 kinase plays a critical role in manganese-induced inflammation and apoptosis in microglia. *PLoS ONE* **2019**, *14*, e0210248. [CrossRef]
54. Mendivil, M.-P.; Velez, C.-P.; Jimenez-Del-Rio, M. Neuroprotective Effect of the LRRK2 kinase inhibitor PF-06447475 in human nerve-like differentiated cells exposed to oxidative stress stimuli: Implications for Parkinson's disease. *Neurochem. Res.* **2016**, *41*, 2675–2692. [CrossRef]
55. Saez-Atienzar, S.; Bonet-Ponce, L.; da Casa, C.; Perez-Dolz, L.; Blesa, J.R.; Nava, E. Bcl-xL-mediated antioxidant function abrogates the disruption of mitochondrial dynamics induced by LRRK2 inhibition. *Biochim. Biophys. Acta* **2016**, *1862*, 20–31. [CrossRef] [PubMed]
56. Vila, M.; Jackson-Lewis, V.; Vukosavic, S.; Djaldetti, R.; Liberatore, G.; Offen, D. Bax ablation prevents dopaminergic neurodegeneration in the 1-methyl-4-phenyl-1,2,3,6-tetrahydropyridine mouse model of Parkinson's disease. *Proc. Natl. Acad. Sci. USA* **2001**, *98*, 2837–2842. [CrossRef] [PubMed]
57. Perier, C.; Bove, J.; Wu, D.C.; Dehay, B.; Choi, D.K.; Jackson-Lewis, V. Two molecular pathways initiate mitochondria-dependent dopaminergic neurodegeneration in experimental Parkinson's disease. *Proc. Natl. Acad. Sci. USA* **2007**, *104*, 8161–8166. [CrossRef]
58. Shen, Y.F.; Zhu, Z.Y.; Qian, S.X.; Xu, C.Y.; Wang, Y.P. MiR-30b protects nigrostriatal dopaminergic neurons from MPP(+)-induced neurotoxicity via SNCA. *Brain Behav.* **2020**, *10*, e01567. [CrossRef]
59. Dionisio, P.A.; Oliveira, S.R.; Gaspar, M.M.; Gama, M.J.; Castro-Caldas, M.; Amaral, J.D. Ablation of RIP3 protects from dopaminergic neurodegeneration in experimental Parkinson's disease. *Cell Death Dis.* **2019**, *10*, 840. [CrossRef]
60. Gao, G.; Wang, Z.; Lu, L.; Duan, C.; Wang, X.; Yang, H. Morphological analysis of mitochondria for evaluating the toxicity of alpha-synuclein in transgenic mice and isolated preparations by atomic force microscopy. *Biomed. Pharmacother.* **2017**, *96*, 1380–1388. [CrossRef]
61. Yang, X.; Zhang, M.; Wei, M.; Wang, A.; Deng, Y.; Cao, H. MicroRNA-216a inhibits neuronal apoptosis in a cellular Parkinson's disease model by targeting Bax. *Metab. Brain Dis.* **2020**. [CrossRef] [PubMed]
62. Li, S.; Lv, X.; Zhai, K.; Xu, R.; Zhang, Y.; Zhao, S. MicroRNA-7 inhibits neuronal apoptosis in a cellular Parkinson's disease model by targeting Bax and Sirt2. *Am. J. Transl. Res.* **2016**, *8*, 993–1004. [PubMed]

63. Alavian, K.N.; Li, H.; Collis, L.; Bonanni, L.; Zeng, L.; Sacchetti, S. Bcl-xL regulates metabolic efficiency of neurons through interaction with the mitochondrial F1FO ATP synthase. *Nat. Cell Biol.* **2011**, *13*, 1224–1233. [CrossRef] [PubMed]
64. Park, H.A.; Mnatsakanyan, N.; Broman, K.; Davis, A.U.; May, J.; Licznerski, P. Alpha-Tocotrienol prevents oxidative stress-mediated post-translational cleavage of Bcl-xL in primary hippocampal neurons. *Int. J. Mol. Sci.* **2019**, *21*. [CrossRef] [PubMed]
65. Arena, G.; Gelmetti, V.; Torosantucci, L.; Vignone, D.; Lamorte, G.; De Rosa, P. PINK1 protects against cell death induced by mitochondrial depolarization, by phosphorylating Bcl-xL and impairing its pro-apoptotic cleavage. *Cell Death Differ.* **2013**, *20*, 920–930. [CrossRef] [PubMed]
66. Savitt, J.M.; Jang, S.S.; Mu, W.; Dawson, V.L.; Dawson, T.M. Bcl-x is required for proper development of the mouse substantia nigra. *J. Neurosci.* **2005**, *25*, 6721–6728. [CrossRef]
67. Martin, L.J.; Semenkow, S.; Hanaford, A.; Wong, M. Mitochondrial permeability transition pore regulates Parkinson's disease development in mutant alpha-synuclein transgenic mice. *Neurobiol. Aging* **2014**, *35*, 1132–1152. [CrossRef]
68. Rasheed, M.Z.; Tabassum, H.; Parvez, S. Mitochondrial permeability transition pore: A promising target for the treatment of Parkinson's disease. *Protoplasma* **2017**, *254*, 33–42. [CrossRef]
69. Pivovarova, N.B.; Nguyen, H.V.; Winters, C.A.; Brantner, C.A.; Smith, C.L.; Andrews, S.B. Excitotoxic calcium overload in a subpopulation of mitochondria triggers delayed death in hippocampal neurons. *J. Neurosci.* **2004**, *24*, 5611–5622. [CrossRef]
70. Jonas, E.; Porter, G.A.; Beutner, G.; Mnatsakanyan, N.; Park, H.A.; Mehta, N. The mitochondrial permeability transition pore: Molecular structure and function in health and disease. In *Molecular Basis for Mitochondrial Signaling*; Rostovtseva, T.K., Ed.; Springer: Cham, Germany, 2017; pp. 69–105.
71. Jonas, E.; Sacchetti, S.; Park, H.A.; Lazrove, E.; Beutner, G.; Porter, G.A. The C-Subunit of the ATP Synthase Forms the Pore of the PTP. *Biophys. J.* **2014**, *106*, 3a–4a. [CrossRef]
72. Alavian, K.N.; Beutner, G.; Lazrove, E.; Sacchetti, S.; Park, H.A.; Licznerski, P. An uncoupling channel within the c-subunit ring of the F1FO ATP synthase is the mitochondrial permeability transition pore. *Proc. Natl. Acad. Sci. USA* **2014**, *111*, 10580–10585. [CrossRef]
73. Mnatsakanyan, N.; Llaguno, M.C.; Yang, Y.; Yan, Y.; Weber, J.; Sigworth, F.J. A mitochondrial megachannel resides in monomeric F1FO ATP synthase. *Nat. Commun.* **2019**, *10*, 5823. [CrossRef] [PubMed]
74. Bonora, M.; Bononi, A.; De Marchi, E.; Giorgi, C.; Lebiedzinska, M.; Marchi, S. Role of the c subunit of the FO ATP synthase in mitochondrial permeability transition. *Cell Cycle* **2013**, *12*, 674–683. [CrossRef] [PubMed]
75. Ganguly, U.; Banerjee, A.; Chakrabarti, S.S.; Kaur, U.; Sen, O.; Cappai, R. Interaction of alpha-synuclein and Parkin in iron toxicity on SH-SY5Y cells: Implications in the pathogenesis of Parkinson's disease. *Biochem. J.* **2020**, *477*, 1109–1122. [CrossRef] [PubMed]
76. Gautier, C.A.; Giaime, E.; Caballero, E.; Nunez, L.; Song, Z.; Chan, D. Regulation of mitochondrial permeability transition pore by PINK1. *Mol. Neurodegener.* **2012**, *7*, 22. [CrossRef]
77. Cui, T.; Fan, C.; Gu, L.; Gao, H.; Liu, Q.; Zhang, T. Silencing of PINK1 induces mitophagy via mitochondrial permeability transition in dopaminergic MN9D cells. *Brain Res.* **2011**, *1394*, 1–13. [CrossRef]
78. Park, H.A.; Broman, K.; Stumpf, A.; Kazyak, S.; Jonas, E.A. Nutritional Regulators of Bcl-xL in the Brain. *Molecules* **2018**, *23*. [CrossRef]
79. Zhang, Y.J.; Gan, R.Y.; Li, S.; Zhou, Y.; Li, A.N.; Xu, D.P. antioxidant phytochemicals for the prevention and treatment of chronic diseases. *Molecules* **2015**, *20*, 21138–21156. [CrossRef]
80. Virmani, A.; Pinto, L.; Binienda, Z.; Ali, S. Food, nutrigenomics, and neurodegeneration–Neuroprotection by what you eat! *Mol. Neurobiol.* **2013**, *48*, 353–362. [CrossRef]
81. Jinsmaa, Y.; Sullivan, P.; Gross, D.; Cooney, A.; Sharabi, Y.; Goldstein, D.S. Divalent metal ions enhance DOPAL-induced oligomerization of alpha-synuclein. *Neurosci Lett.* **2014**, *569*, 27–32. [CrossRef]
82. Wang, C.; Liu, L.; Zhang, L.; Peng, Y.; Zhou, F. Redox reactions of the alpha-synuclein-Cu (2+) complex and their effects on neuronal cell viability. *Biochemistry* **2010**, *49*, 8134–8142. [CrossRef]
83. Shen, D.F.; Qi, H.P.; Ma, C.; Chang, M.X.; Zhang, W.N.; Song, R.R. Astaxanthin suppresses endoplasmic reticulum stress and protects against neuron damage in Parkinson's disease by regulating miR-7/SNCA axis. *Neurosci. Res.* **2020**. [CrossRef]

84. Wang, R.; Wang, Y.; Qu, L.; Chen, B.; Jiang, H.; Song, N. Iron-induced oxidative stress contributes to alpha-synuclein phosphorylation and up-regulation via polo-like kinase 2 and casein kinase 2. *Neurochem. Int.* **2019**, *125*, 127–135. [CrossRef]
85. Jha, N.N.; Ghosh, D.; Das, S.; Anoop, A.; Jacob, R.S.; Singh, P.K. Effect of curcumin analogs onalpha-synuclein aggregation and cytotoxicity. *Sci. Rep.* **2016**, *6*, 28511. [CrossRef]
86. Wang, Z.; Yang, C.; Liu, J.; Chun, K.; Tong, B.; Zhu, Z.; Malampati, S. A curcumin derivative activates TFEB and protects against parkinsonian neurotoxicity in vitro. *Int. J. Mol. Sci.* **2020**, *21*. [CrossRef]
87. Sharma, N.; Nehru, B. Curcumin affords neuroprotection and inhibits alpha-synuclein aggregation in lipopolysaccharide-induced Parkinson's disease model. *Inflammopharmacology* **2018**, *26*, 349–360. [CrossRef]
88. Guo, Y.J.; Dong, S.Y.; Cui, X.X.; Feng, Y.; Liu, T.; Yin, M. Resveratrol alleviates MPTP-induced motor impairments and pathological changes by autophagic degradation of alpha-synuclein via SIRT1-deacetylated LC3. *Mol. Nutr. Food Res.* **2016**, *60*, 2161–2175. [CrossRef]
89. Wang, Z.H.; Zhang, J.L.; Duan, Y.L.; Zhang, Q.S.; Li, G.F.; Zheng, D.L. MicroRNA-214 participates in the neuroprotective effect of Resveratrol via inhibiting alpha-synuclein expression in MPTP-induced Parkinson's disease mouse. *Biomed. Pharmacother.* **2015**, *74*, 252–256. [CrossRef]
90. Teng, Y.; Zhao, J.; Ding, L.; Ding, Y.; Zhou, P. Complex of EGCG with Cu(II) suppresses amyloid aggregation and Cu(II)-Induced cytotoxicity of alpha-Synuclein. *Molecules* **2019**, *24*. [CrossRef]
91. Roy, S.; Bhat, R. Suppression, disaggregation, and modulation of gamma-Synuclein fibrillation pathway by green tea polyphenol EGCG. *Protein Sci.* **2019**, *28*, 382–402. [CrossRef] [PubMed]
92. Li, Y.; Chen, Z.; Lu, Z.; Yang, Q.; Liu, L.; Jiang, Z. "Cell-addictive" dual-target traceable nanodrug for Parkinson's disease treatment via flotillins pathway. *Theranostics* **2018**, *8*, 5469–5481. [CrossRef] [PubMed]
93. Zhao, J.; Xu, L.; Liang, Q.; Sun, Q.; Chen, C.; Zhang, Y. Metal chelator EGCG attenuates Fe(III)-induced conformational transition of alpha-synuclein and protects AS-PC12 cells against Fe(III)-induced death. *J. Neurochem.* **2017**, *143*, 136–146. [CrossRef]
94. Ponzini, E.; De Palma, A.; Cerboni, L.; Natalello, A.; Rossi, R.; Moons, R. Methionine oxidation in alpha-synuclein inhibits its propensity for ordered secondary structure. *J. Biol. Chem.* **2019**, *294*, 5657–5665. [CrossRef]
95. Yang, J.E.; Rhoo, K.Y.; Lee, S.; Lee, J.T.; Park, J.H.; Bhak, G. EGCG-mediated Protection of the Membrane Disruption and Cytotoxicity Caused by the 'Active Oligomer' of alpha-Synuclein. *Sci. Rep.* **2017**, *7*, 17945. [CrossRef]
96. Lorenzen, N.; Nielsen, S.B.; Yoshimura, Y.; Vad, B.S.; Andersen, C.B.; Betzer, C. How epigallocatechin gallate can inhibit alpha-synuclein oligomer toxicity in vitro. *J. Biol. Chem.* **2014**, *289*, 21299–21310. [CrossRef]
97. Palazzi, L.; Bruzzone, E.; Bisello, G.; Leri, M.; Stefani, M.; Bucciantini, M. Oleuropein aglycone stabilizes the monomeric alpha-synuclein and favours the growth of non-toxic aggregates. *Sci. Rep.* **2018**, *8*, 8337. [CrossRef]
98. Mohammad, H.-B.; Aliakbari, F.; Sahin, C.; Lomax, C.; Tawfike, A.; Schafer, N.P. Oleuropein derivatives from olive fruit extracts reduce alpha-synuclein fibrillation and oligomer toxicity. *J. Biol. Chem.* **2019**, *294*, 4215–4232. [CrossRef]
99. Casani, S.; Gomez-Pastor, R.; Matallana, E.; Paricio, N. Antioxidant compound supplementation prevents oxidative damage in a Drosophila model of Parkinson's disease. *Free Radic. Biol. Med.* **2013**, *61*, 151–160. [CrossRef] [PubMed]
100. Lee, D.H.; Kim, C.S.; Lee, Y.J. Astaxanthin protects against MPTP/MPP+-induced mitochondrial dysfunction and ROS production in vivo and in vitro. *Food Chem. Toxicol.* **2011**, *49*, 271–280. [CrossRef]
101. Zafar, K.S.; Siddiqui, A.; Sayeed, I.; Ahmad, M.; Salim, S.; Islam, F. Dose-dependent protective effect of selenium in rat model of Parkinson's disease: Neurobehavioral and neurochemical evidences. *J. Neurochem.* **2003**, *84*, 438–446. [CrossRef]
102. Botsakis, K.; Theodoritsi, S.; Grintzalis, K.; Angelatou, F.; Antonopoulos, I.; Georgiou, C.D. 17beta-Estradiol/N-acetylcysteine interaction enhances the neuroprotective effect on dopaminergic neurons in the weaver model of dopamine deficiency. *Neuroscience* **2016**, *320*, 221–229. [CrossRef] [PubMed]
103. Pandareesh, M.D.; Shrivash, M.K.; Naveen, K.H.N.; Misra, K.; Srinivas, B.M.M. curcumin monoglucoside shows improved bioavailability and mitigates rotenone induced neurotoxicity in cell and drosophila models of Parkinson's disease. *Neurochem. Res.* **2016**, *41*, 3113–3128. [CrossRef] [PubMed]

104. Oz, A.; Celik, O. Curcumin inhibits oxidative stress-induced TRPM2 channel activation, calcium ion entry and apoptosis values in SH-SY5Y neuroblastoma cells: Involvement of transfection procedure. *Mol. Membr. Biol.* **2016**, *33*, 76–88. [CrossRef] [PubMed]
105. Ramkumar, M.; Rajasankar, S.; Gobi, V.V.; Janakiraman, U.; Manivasagam, T.; Thenmozhi, A.J. Demethoxycurcumin, a natural derivative of curcumin abrogates rotenone-induced dopamine depletion and motor deficits by its antioxidative and anti-inflammatory properties in parkinsonian rats. *Pharmacogn Mag.* **2018**, *14*, 9–16. [CrossRef]
106. Buratta, S.; Chiaradia, E.; Tognoloni, A.; Gambelunghe, A.; Meschini, C.; Palmieri, L. Effect of Curcumin on Protein Damage Induced by Rotenone in Dopaminergic PC12 Cells. *Int. J. Mol. Sci.* **2020**, *21*. [CrossRef]
107. Wang, Y.L.; Ju, B.; Zhang, Y.Z.; Yin, H.L.; Liu, Y.J.; Wang, S.S. Protective effect of curcumin against oxidative stress-induced injury in rats with Parkinson's disease through the Wnt/beta-catenin signaling pathway. *Cell Physiol. Biochem.* **2017**, *43*, 2226–2241. [CrossRef]
108. Khan, M.M.; Ahmad, A.; Ishrat, T.; Khan, M.B.; Hoda, M.N.; Khuwaja, G. Resveratrol attenuates 6-hydroxydopamine-induced oxidative damage and dopamine depletion in rat model of Parkinson's disease. *Brain Res.* **2010**, *1328*, 139–151. [CrossRef]
109. Ferretta, A.; Gaballo, A.; Tanzarella, P.; Piccoli, C.; Capitanio, N.; Nico, B. Effect of resveratrol on mitochondrial function: Implications in parkin-associated familiar Parkinson's disease. *Biochim. Biophys. Acta* **2014**, *1842*, 902–915. [CrossRef]
110. Palle, S.; Neerati, P. Improved neuroprotective effect of resveratrol nanoparticles as evinced by abrogation of rotenone-induced behavioral deficits and oxidative and mitochondrial dysfunctions in rat model of Parkinson's disease. *Naunyn. Schmiedebergs Arch. Pharmacol.* **2018**, *391*, 445–453. [CrossRef]
111. Wang, H.; Dong, X.; Liu, Z.; Zhu, S.; Liu, H.; Fan, W. Resveratrol suppresses rotenone-induced neurotoxicity through activation of SIRT1/Akt1 signaling pathway. *Anat. Rec. (Hoboken)* **2018**, *301*, 1115–1125. [CrossRef]
112. Sun, Y.; Sukumaran, P.; Selvaraj, S.; Cilz, N.I.; Schaar, A.; Lei, S. TRPM2 promotes neurotoxin MPP(+)/MPTP-Induced cell death. *Mol. Neurobiol.* **2018**, *55*, 409–420. [CrossRef] [PubMed]
113. Peng, K.; Tao, Y.; Zhang, J.; Wang, J.; Ye, F.; Dan, G. Resveratrol regulates mitochondrial biogenesis and fission/fusion to attenuate rotenone-induced neurotoxicity. *Oxid. Med. Cell Longev.* **2016**, *2016*, 6705621. [CrossRef] [PubMed]
114. Vergara, D.; Gaballo, A.; Signorile, A.; Ferretta, A.; Tanzarella, P.; Pacelli, C. Resveratrol modulation of protein expression in parkin-mutant human skin fibroblasts: A proteomic approach. *Oxid. Med. Cell Longev.* **2017**, *2017*, 2198243. [CrossRef] [PubMed]
115. Xu, Q.; Langley, M.; Kanthasamy, A.G.; Reddy, M.B. Epigallocatechin gallate has a neurorescue effect in a mouse model of Parkinson's disease. *J. Nutr.* **2017**, *147*, 1926–1931. [CrossRef] [PubMed]
116. Teixeira, M.D.; Souza, C.M.; Menezes, A.P.; Carmo, M.R.; Fonteles, A.A.; Gurgel, J.P. Catechin attenuates behavioral neurotoxicity induced by 6-OHDA in rats. *Pharmacol. Biochem. Behav.* **2013**, *110*, 1–7. [CrossRef]
117. Martinez-Perez, D.A.; Jimenez-Del-Rio, M.; Velez-Pardo, C. Epigallocatechin-3-Gallate protects and prevents paraquat-induced oxidative stress and neurodegeneration in knockdown dj-1-beta drosophila melanogaster. *Neurotox. Res.* **2018**, *34*, 401–416. [CrossRef] [PubMed]
118. Bitu, P.N.; da Silva, A.B.; Neves, K.R.; Silva, A.H.; Leal, L.K.; Viana, G.S. Neuroprotective properties of the standardized extract from camellia sinensis (green tea) and its main bioactive components, epicatechin and epigallocatechin gallate, in the 6-OHDA model of Parkinson's disease. *Evid. Based Complement. Alternat. Med.* **2015**, *2015*, 161092. [CrossRef]
119. Xu, Q.; Kanthasamy, A.G.; Reddy, M.B. Epigallocatechin gallate protects against TNFalpha- or H_2O_2- induced apoptosis by modulating iron related proteins in a cell culture model. *Int. J. Vitam. Nutr. Res.* **2018**, *88*, 158–165. [CrossRef]
120. Lambert, D.M.M.; Courtel, P.; Sleno, L.; Abasq, M.L.; Ramassamy, C. Synergistic properties of bioavailable phenolic compounds from olive oil: Electron transfer and neuroprotective properties. *Nutr. Neurosci.* **2019**, 1–14. [CrossRef]
121. Achour, I.; Arel-Dubeau, A.M.; Renaud, J.; Legrand, M.; Attard, E.; Germain, M. Oleuropein prevents neuronal death, mitigates mitochondrial superoxide production and modulates autophagy in a dopaminergic cellular model. *Int. J. Mol. Sci.* **2016**, *17*. [CrossRef] [PubMed]

122. Pasban-Aliabadi, H.; Esmaeili-Mahani, S.; Sheibani, V.; Abbasnejad, M.; Mehdizadeh, A.; Yaghoobi, M.M. Inhibition of 6-hydroxydopamine-induced PC12 cell apoptosis by olive (Olea europaea L.) leaf extract is performed by its main component oleuropein. *Rejuvenation Res.* **2013**, *16*, 134–142. [CrossRef] [PubMed]
123. Sarbishegi, M.; Charkhat, G.E.A.; Khajavi, O.; Komeili, G.; Salimi, S. The neuroprotective effects of hydro-alcoholic extract of olive (Olea europaea L.) leaf on rotenone-induced Parkinson's disease in rat. *Metab. Brain Dis.* **2018**, *33*, 79–88. [CrossRef]
124. Amel, N.; Wafa, T.; Samia, D.; Yousra, B.; Issam, C.; Cheraif, I. Extra virgin olive oil modulates brain docosahexaenoic acid level and oxidative damage caused by 2,4-Dichlorophenoxyacetic acid in rats. *J. Food Sci. Technol.* **2016**, *53*, 1454–1464. [CrossRef] [PubMed]
125. Liang, L.P.; Kavanagh, T.J.; Patel, M. Glutathione deficiency in Gclm null mice results in complex I inhibition and dopamine depletion following paraquat administration. *Toxicol. Sci.* **2013**, *134*, 366–373. [CrossRef] [PubMed]
126. van der Merwe, C.; van Dyk, H.C.; Engelbrecht, L.; van der Westhuizen, F.H.; Kinnear, C.; Loos, B. Curcumin Rescues a PINK1 Knock Down SH-SY5Y Cellular Model of Parkinson's Disease from Mitochondrial Dysfunction and Cell Death. *Mol. Neurobiol.* **2017**, *54*, 2752–2762. [CrossRef] [PubMed]
127. Man, A.H.; Linh, D.M.; My, D.V.; Phuong, T.; Thao, D. Evaluating dose- and time-dependent effects of Vitamin C Treatment on a Parkinson's disease fly model. *Parkinsons Dis.* **2019**, *2019*, 9720546. [CrossRef]
128. Nakaso, K.; Horikoshi, Y.; Takahashi, T.; Hanaki, T.; Nakasone, M.; Kitagawa, Y. Estrogen receptor-mediated effect of delta-tocotrienol prevents neurotoxicity and motor deficit in the MPTP mouse model of Parkinson's disease. *Neurosci. Lett.* **2016**, *610*, 117–122. [CrossRef]
129. Prema, A.; Janakiraman, U.; Manivasagam, T.; Thenmozhi, A.J. Neuroprotective effect of lycopene against MPTP induced experimental Parkinson's disease in mice. *Neurosci. Lett.* **2015**, *599*, 12–19. [CrossRef]
130. Nataraj, J.; Manivasagam, T.; Thenmozhi, A.J.; Essa, M.M. Lutein protects dopaminergic neurons against MPTP-induced apoptotic death and motor dysfunction by ameliorating mitochondrial disruption and oxidative stress. *Nutr. Neurosci.* **2016**, *19*, 237–246. [CrossRef]
131. Grimmig, B.; Daly, L.; Subbarayan, M.; Hudson, C.; Williamson, R.; Nash, K. Astaxanthin is neuroprotective in an aged mouse model of Parkinson's disease. *Oncotarget* **2018**, *9*, 10388–10401. [CrossRef]
132. Lopes, F.M.; da Motta, L.L.; De Bastiani, M.A.; Pfaffenseller, B.; Aguiar, B.W.; de Souza, L.F. RA differentiation enhances dopaminergic features, changes redox parameters, and increases dopamine transporter dependency in 6-Hydroxydopamine-Induced neurotoxicity in SH-SY5Y cells. *Neurotox. Res.* **2017**, *31*, 545–559. [CrossRef] [PubMed]
133. Avola, R.; Graziano, A.C.E.; Pannuzzo, G.; Albouchi, F.; Cardile, V. New insights on Parkinson's disease from differentiation of SH-SY5Y into dopaminergic neurons: An involvement of aquaporin4 and 9. *Mol. Cell Neurosci.* **2018**, *88*, 212–221. [CrossRef] [PubMed]
134. Garrido, M.; Tereshchenko, Y.; Zhevtsova, Z.; Taschenberger, G.; Bahr, M.; Kugler, S. Glutathione depletion and overproduction both initiate degeneration of nigral dopaminergic neurons. *Acta Neuropathol.* **2011**, *121*, 475–485. [CrossRef] [PubMed]
135. Gil-Martinez, A.L.; Cuenca, L.; Sanchez, C.; Estrada, C.; Fernandez-Villalba, E.; Herrero, M.T. Effect of NAC treatment and physical activity on neuroinflammation in subchronic Parkinsonism; is physical activity essential? *J. Neuroinflamm.* **2018**, *15*, 328. [CrossRef]
136. Wang, Y.L.; Liu, X.S.; Wang, S.S.; Xue, P.; Zeng, Z.L.; Yang, X.P. Curcumin-activated mesenchymal stem cells derived from human umbilical cord and their effects on mptp-mouse model of Parkinson's disease: A new biological therapy for Parkinson's disease. *Stem. Cells Int.* **2020**, *2020*, 4636397. [CrossRef]
137. He, X.J.; Uchida, K.; Megumi, C.; Tsuge, N.; Nakayama, H. Dietary curcumin supplementation attenuates 1-methyl-4-phenyl-1,2,3,6-tetrahydropyridine (MPTP) neurotoxicity in C57BL mice. *J. Toxicol Pathol.* **2015**, *28*, 197–206. [CrossRef]
138. Pan, J.; Li, H.; Ma, J.F.; Tan, Y.Y.; Xiao, Q.; Ding, J.Q. Curcumin inhibition of JNKs prevents dopaminergic neuronal loss in a mouse model of Parkinson's disease through suppressing mitochondria dysfunction. *Transl. Neurodegener.* **2012**, *1*, 16. [CrossRef]
139. Zhou, T.; Zhu, M.; Liang, Z. (-)-Epigallocatechin-3-gallate modulates peripheral immunity in the MPTP-induced mouse model of Parkinson's disease. *Mol. Med. Rep.* **2018**, *17*, 4883–4888. [CrossRef]

140. Zhou, W.; Chen, L.; Hu, X.; Cao, S.; Yang, J. Effects and mechanism of epigallocatechin-3-gallate on apoptosis and mTOR/AKT/GSK-3beta pathway in substantia nigra neurons in Parkinson's rats. *Neuroreport* **2019**, *30*, 60–65. [CrossRef]
141. Elmazoglu, Z.; Ergin, V.; Sahin, E.; Kayhan, H.; Karasu, C. Oleuropein and rutin protect against 6-OHDA-induced neurotoxicity in PC12 cells through modulation of mitochondrial function and unfolded protein response. *Interdiscip Toxicol.* **2017**, *10*, 129–141. [CrossRef]
142. Kim, M.H.; Min, J.S.; Lee, J.Y.; Chae, U.; Yang, E.J.; Song, K.S. Oleuropein isolated from Fraxinus rhynchophylla inhibits glutamate-induced neuronal cell death by attenuating mitochondrial dysfunction. *Nutr. Neurosci.* **2018**, *21*, 520–528. [CrossRef] [PubMed]
143. Darbinyan, L.V.; Hambardzumyan, L.E.; Simonyan, K.V.; Chavushyan, V.A.; Manukyan, L.P.; Badalyan, S.A. Protective effects of curcumin against rotenone-induced rat model of Parkinson's disease: In vivo electrophysiological and behavioral study. *Metab. Brain Dis.* **2017**, *32*, 1791–1803. [CrossRef]
144. Song, S.; Nie, Q.; Li, Z.; Du, G. Curcumin improves neurofunctions of 6-OHDA-induced parkinsonian rats. *Pathol. Res. Pract.* **2016**, *212*, 247–251. [CrossRef] [PubMed]
145. Abbaoui, A.; Chatoui, H.; El Hiba, O.; Gamrani, H. Neuroprotective effect of curcumin-I in copper-induced dopaminergic neurotoxicity in rats: A possible link with Parkinson's disease. *Neurosci. Lett.* **2017**, *660*, 103–108. [CrossRef] [PubMed]
146. Laabbar, W.; Elgot, A.; Elhiba, O.; Gamrani, H. Curcumin prevents the midbrain dopaminergic innervations and locomotor performance deficiencies resulting from chronic aluminum exposure in rat. *J. Chem. Neuroanat.* **2019**, *100*, 101654. [CrossRef] [PubMed]
147. Sur, M.; Dey, P.; Sarkar, A.; Bar, S.; Banerjee, D.; Bhat, S. Sarm1 induction and accompanying inflammatory response mediates age-dependent susceptibility to rotenone-induced neurotoxicity. *Cell Death Discov.* **2018**, *4*, 114. [CrossRef]
148. Ng, C.H.; Guan, M.S.; Koh, C.; Ouyang, X.; Yu, F.; Tan, E.K. AMP kinase activation mitigates dopaminergic dysfunction and mitochondrial abnormalities in Drosophila models of Parkinson's disease. *J. Neurosci.* **2012**, *32*, 14311–14317. [CrossRef]
149. Nishikimi, M.; Yagi, K. Molecular basis for the deficiency in humans of gulonolactone oxidase, a key enzyme for ascorbic acid biosynthesis. *Am. J. Clin. Nutr.* **1991**, *54*, 1203S–1208S. [CrossRef]
150. Podmore, I.D.; Griffiths, H.R.; Herbert, K.E.; Mistry, N.; Mistry, P.; Lunec, J. Vitamin C exhibits pro-oxidant properties. *Nature* **1998**, *392*, 559. [CrossRef]
151. Kocot, J.; Luchowska-Kocot, D.; Kielczykowska, M.; Musik, I.; Kurzepa, J. Does Vitamin C influence neurodegenerative diseases and psychiatric disorders? *Nutrients* **2017**, *9*. [CrossRef]
152. Tran, H.H.; Dang, S.N.A.; Nguyen, T.T.; Huynh, A.M.; Dao, L.M.; Kamei, K. Drosophila ubiquitin C-terminal hydrolase knockdown model of Parkinson's disease. *Sci. Rep.* **2018**, *8*, 4468. [CrossRef] [PubMed]
153. Khan, S.; Jyoti, S.; Naz, F.; Shakya, B.; Rahul, A.M. Effect of L-ascorbic Acid on the climbing ability and protein levels in the brain of Drosophila model of Parkinson's disease. *Int. J. Neurosci.* **2012**, *122*, 704–709. [CrossRef] [PubMed]
154. He, X.B.; Kim, M.; Kim, S.Y.; Yi, S.H.; Rhee, Y.H.; Kim, T. Vitamin C facilitates dopamine neuron differentiation in fetal midbrain through TET1- and JMJD3-dependent epigenetic control manner. *Stem. Cells* **2015**, *33*, 1320–1332. [CrossRef]
155. Shen, L.; Wu, H.; Diep, D.; Yamaguchi, S.; D'Alessio, A.C.; Fung, H.L. Genome-wide analysis reveals TET- and TDG-dependent 5-methylcytosine oxidation dynamics. *Cell* **2013**, *153*, 692–706. [CrossRef] [PubMed]
156. Medeiros, M.S.; Schumacher, S.A.; Cardoso, A.M.; Bochi, G.V.; Baldissarelli, J.; Kegler, A. Iron and oxidative stress in Parkinson's disease: An observational study of injury biomarkers. *PLoS ONE* **2016**, *11*, e0146129. [CrossRef] [PubMed]
157. Etminan, M.; Gill, S.S.; Samii, A. Intake of vitamin E, vitamin C, and carotenoids and the risk of Parkinson's disease: A meta-analysis. *Lancet Neurol.* **2005**, *4*, 362–365. [CrossRef]
158. Nagayama, H.; Hamamoto, M.; Ueda, M.; Nito, C.; Yamaguchi, H.; Katayama, Y. The effect of ascorbic acid on the pharmacokinetics of levodopa in elderly patients with Parkinson's disease. *Clin. Neuropharmacol.* **2004**, *27*, 270–273. [CrossRef]
159. Nikolova, G.; Karamalakova, Y.; Gadjeva, V. Reducing oxidative toxicity of L-dopa in combination with two different antioxidants: An essential oil isolated from Rosa Damascena Mill., and vitamin C. *Toxicol. Rep.* **2019**, *6*, 267–271. [CrossRef]

160. Numakawa, Y.; Numakawa, T.; Matsumoto, T.; Yagasaki, Y.; Kumamaru, E.; Kunugi, H. Vitamin E protected cultured cortical neurons from oxidative stress-induced cell death through the activation of mitogen-activated protein kinase and phosphatidylinositol 3-kinase. *J. Neurochem.* **2006**, *97*, 1191–1202. [CrossRef]
161. Hosomi, A.; Arita, M.; Sato, Y.; Kiyose, C.; Ueda, T.; Igarashi, O. Affinity for alpha-tocopherol transfer protein as a determinant of the biological activities of vitamin E analogs. *FEBS Lett.* **1997**, *409*, 105–108. [CrossRef]
162. Suzuki, Y.J.; Tsuchiya, M.; Wassall, S.R.; Choo, Y.M.; Govil, G.; Kagan, V.E. Structural and dynamic membrane properties of alpha-tocopherol and alpha-tocotrienol: Implication to the molecular mechanism of their antioxidant potency. *Biochemistry* **1993**, *32*, 10692–10699. [CrossRef] [PubMed]
163. Park, H.A.; Kubicki, N.; Gnyawali, S.; Chan, Y.C.; Roy, S.; Khanna, S. Natural vitamin E alpha-tocotrienol protects against ischemic stroke by induction of multidrug resistance-associated protein 1. *Stroke* **2011**, *42*, 2308–2314. [CrossRef] [PubMed]
164. Schirinzi, T.; Martella, G.; Imbriani, P.; Di Lazzaro, G.; Franco, D.; Colona, V.L. Dietary Vitamin E as a protective factor for Parkinson's disease: Clinical and experimental evidence. *Front. Neurol.* **2019**, *10*, 148. [CrossRef] [PubMed]
165. Martella, G.; Madeo, G.; Maltese, M.; Vanni, V.; Puglisi, F.; Ferraro, E. Exposure to low-dose rotenone precipitates synaptic plasticity alterations in PINK1 heterozygous knockout mice. *Neurobiol. Dis.* **2016**, *91*, 21–36. [CrossRef] [PubMed]
166. Park, H.A.; Jonas, E.A. DeltaN-Bcl-xL, a therapeutic target for neuroprotection. *Neural. Regen. Res.* **2017**, *12*, 1791–1794. [CrossRef] [PubMed]
167. Park, H.A.; Licznerski, P.; Mnatsakanyan, N.; Niu, Y.; Sacchetti, S.; Wu, J. Inhibition of Bcl-xL prevents pro-death actions of DeltaN-Bcl-xL at the mitochondrial inner membrane during glutamate excitotoxicity. *Cell Death Differ.* **2017**, *24*, 1963–1974. [CrossRef]
168. Nakaso, K.; Tajima, N.; Horikoshi, Y.; Nakasone, M.; Hanaki, T.; Kamizaki, K. The estrogen receptor beta-PI3K/Akt pathway mediates the cytoprotective effects of tocotrienol in a cellular Parkinson's disease model. *Biochim. Biophys. Acta* **2014**, *1842*, 1303–1312. [CrossRef]
169. Sotolongo, K.; Ghiso, J.; Rostagno, A. Nrf2 activation through the PI3K/GSK-3 axis protects neuronal cells from Abeta-mediated oxidative and metabolic damage. *Alzheimers Res. Ther.* **2020**, *12*, 13. [CrossRef]
170. Wang, L.; Chen, Y.; Sternberg, P.; Cai, J. Essential roles of the PI3 kinase/Akt pathway in regulating Nrf2-dependent antioxidant functions in the RPE. *Invest. Ophthalmol. Vis. Sci.* **2008**, *49*, 1671–1678. [CrossRef]
171. Niture, S.K.; Jaiswal, A.K. Nrf2-induced antiapoptotic Bcl-xL protein enhances cell survival and drug resistance. *Free Radic. Biol. Med.* **2013**, *57*, 119–131. [CrossRef]
172. Liu, Q.; Jin, Z.; Xu, Z.; Yang, H.; Li, L.; Li, G. Antioxidant effects of ginkgolides and bilobalide against cerebral ischemia injury by activating the Akt/Nrf2 pathway in vitro and in vivo. *Cell Stress Chaperones* **2019**, *24*, 441–452. [CrossRef] [PubMed]
173. Hu, L.; Chen, W.; Tian, F.; Yuan, C.; Wang, H.; Yue, H. Neuroprotective role of fucoxanthin against cerebral ischemic/reperfusion injury through activation of Nrf2/HO-1 signaling. *Biomed. Pharmacother.* **2018**, *106*, 1484–1789. [CrossRef] [PubMed]
174. Yang, F.; Wolk, A.; Hakansson, N.; Pedersen, N.L.; Wirdefeldt, K. Dietary antioxidants and risk of Parkinson's disease in two population-based cohorts. *Mov. Disord.* **2017**, *32*, 1631–1636. [CrossRef] [PubMed]
175. Ghani, H.; Stevens, D.; Weiss, J.; Rosenbaum, R. Vitamins and the risk for Parkinson's disease. *Neurology* **2002**, *59*, E8–E9. [CrossRef] [PubMed]
176. Hughes, K.C.; Gao, X.; Kim, I.Y.; Rimm, E.B.; Wang, M.; Weisskopf, M.G. Intake of antioxidant vitamins and risk of Parkinson's disease. *Mov. Disord.* **2016**, *31*, 1909–1914. [CrossRef] [PubMed]
177. King, D.; Playfer, J.R.; Roberts, N.B. Concentrations of vitamins A, C and E in elderly patients with Parkinson's disease. *Postgrad. Med. J.* **1992**, *68*, 634–637. [CrossRef]
178. Taghizadeh, M.; Tamtaji, O.R.; Dadgostar, E.; Daneshvar, K.R.; Bahmani, F.; Abolhassani, J. The effects of omega-3 fatty acids and vitamin E co-supplementation on clinical and metabolic status in patients with Parkinson's disease: A randomized, double-blind, placebo-controlled trial. *Neurochem. Int.* **2017**, *108*, 183–189. [CrossRef]
179. Podlesny, A.-D.; Sobska, J.; de Lera, A.R.; Golembiowska, K.; Kaminska, K.; Dolle, P. Distinct retinoic acid receptor (RAR) isotypes control differentiation of embryonal carcinoma cells to dopaminergic or striatopallidal medium spiny neurons. *Sci. Rep.* **2017**, *7*, 13671. [CrossRef]

180. Kim, S.; Lim, J.; Bang, Y.; Moon, J.; Kwon, M.S.; Hong, J.T. Alpha-Synuclein suppresses retinoic Acid-Induced neuronal differentiation by targeting the glycogen synthase Kinase-3beta/beta-Catenin signaling pathway. *Mol. Neurobiol.* **2018**, *55*, 1607–1619. [CrossRef]
181. Pan, J.; Yu, J.; Sun, L.; Xie, C.; Chang, L.; Wu, J. ALDH1A1 regulates postsynaptic mu-opioid receptor expression in dorsal striatal projection neurons and mitigates dyskinesia through transsynaptic retinoic acid signaling. *Sci. Rep.* **2019**, *9*, 3602. [CrossRef]
182. Kim, J.H.; Hwang, J.; Shim, E.; Chung, E.J.; Jang, S.H.; Koh, S.B. Association of serum carotenoid, retinol, and tocopherol concentrations with the progression of Parkinson's Disease. *Nutr. Res. Pract.* **2017**, *11*, 114–120. [CrossRef] [PubMed]
183. Takeda, A.; Nyssen, O.P.; Syed, A.; Jansen, E.; Bueno-de-Mesquita, B.; Gallo, V. Vitamin A and carotenoids and the risk of Parkinson's disease: A systematic review and meta-analysis. *Neuroepidemiology* **2014**, *42*, 25–38. [CrossRef] [PubMed]
184. Junn, E.; Lee, K.W.; Jeong, B.S.; Chan, T.W.; Im, J.Y.; Mouradian, M.M. Repression of alpha-synuclein expression and toxicity by microRNA-7. *Proc. Natl. Acad. Sci. USA* **2009**, *106*, 13052–13057. [CrossRef] [PubMed]
185. Zhao, C.; Ren, J.; Xue, C.; Lin, E. Study on the relationship between soil selenium and plant selenium uptake. *Plant Soil* **2005**, *277*, 197–206. [CrossRef]
186. Zhong, L.; Holmgren, A. Essential role of selenium in the catalytic activities of mammalian thioredoxin reductase revealed by characterization of recombinant enzymes with selenocysteine mutations. *J. Biol. Chem.* **2000**, *275*, 18121–18128. [CrossRef]
187. Cabeza, Y.-A.; Schiestl, R.H. Transcriptome analysis of a rotenone model of parkinsonism reveals complex I-tied and -untied toxicity mechanisms common to neurodegenerative diseases. *PLoS ONE* **2012**, *7*, e44700. [CrossRef]
188. de Freitas, C.S.; Araujo, S.M.; Bortolotto, V.C.; Poetini, M.R.; Pinheiro, F.C.; Santos, M.E.A. 7-chloro-4-(phenylselanyl) quinoline prevents dopamine depletion in a Drosophila melanogaster model of Parkinson's-like disease. *J. Trace Elem. Med. Biol.* **2019**, *54*, 232–243. [CrossRef]
189. Khan, H.A. Selenium partially reverses the depletion of striatal dopamine and its metabolites in MPTP-treated C57BL mice. *Neurochem. Int.* **2010**, *57*, 489–491. [CrossRef]
190. Sun, H. Association of soil selenium, strontium, and magnesium concentrations with Parkinson's disease mortality rates in the USA. *Environ. Geochem. Health* **2018**, *40*, 349–357. [CrossRef]
191. Shahar, A.; Patel, K.V.; Semba, R.D.; Bandinelli, S.; Shahar, D.R.; Ferrucci, L. Plasma selenium is positively related to performance in neurological tasks assessing coordination and motor speed. *Mov. Disord.* **2010**, *25*, 1909–1915. [CrossRef]
192. Maass, F.; Michalke, B.; Leha, A.; Boerger, M.; Zerr, I.; Koch, J.C. Elemental fingerprint as a cerebrospinal fluid biomarker for the diagnosis of Parkinson's disease. *J. Neurochem.* **2018**, *145*, 342–351. [CrossRef] [PubMed]
193. Zhao, H.W.; Lin, J.; Wang, X.B.; Cheng, X.; Wang, J.Y.; Hu, B.L. Assessing plasma levels of selenium, copper, iron and zinc in patients of Parkinson's disease. *PLoS ONE* **2013**, *8*, e83060. [CrossRef] [PubMed]
194. Naderi, M.; Salahinejad, A.; Jamwal, A.; Chivers, D.P.; Niyogi, S. Chronic Dietary Selenomethionine Exposure Induces Oxidative Stress, Dopaminergic Dysfunction, and Cognitive Impairment in Adult Zebrafish (Danio rerio). *Environ. Sci. Technol.* **2017**, *51*, 12879–12888. [CrossRef] [PubMed]
195. Naderi, M.; Salahinejad, A.; Ferrari, M.C.O.; Niyogi, S.; Chivers, D.P. Dopaminergic dysregulation and impaired associative learning behavior in zebrafish during chronic dietary exposure to selenium. *Environ. Pollut.* **2018**, *237*, 174–185. [CrossRef]
196. *Dietary Reference Intakes for Vitamin C, Vitamin E, Selenium, and Carotenoids*; Institute of Medicine: Washington, DC, USA, 2000.
197. Chinta, S.J.; Andersen, J.K. Reversible inhibition of mitochondrial complex I activity following chronic dopaminergic glutathione depletion in vitro: Implications for Parkinson's disease. *Free Radic. Biol. Med.* **2006**, *41*, 1442–1448. [CrossRef] [PubMed]
198. Park, H.A.; Khanna, S.; Rink, C.; Gnyawali, S.; Roy, S.; Sen, C.K. Glutathione disulfide induces neural cell death via a 12-lipoxygenase pathway. *Cell Death Differ.* **2009**, *16*, 1167–1179. [CrossRef]
199. Monti, D.A.; Zabrecky, G.; Kremens, D.; Liang, T.W.; Wintering, N.A.; Bazzan, A.J. N-Acetyl cysteine is associated with dopaminergic improvement in Parkinson's disease. *Clin. Pharmacol. Ther.* **2019**, *106*, 884–890. [CrossRef]

200. Hauser, R.A.; Lyons, K.E.; McClain, T.; Carter, S.; Perlmutter, D. Randomized, double-blind, pilot evaluation of intravenous glutathione in Parkinson's disease. *Mov. Disord.* **2009**, *24*, 979–983. [CrossRef]
201. Monti, D.A.; Zabrecky, G.; Kremens, D.; Liang, T.W.; Wintering, N.A.; Cai, J. N-Acetyl cysteine may support dopamine neurons in Parkinson's disease: Preliminary clinical and cell line data. *PLoS ONE* **2016**, *11*, e0157602. [CrossRef]
202. Salamon, S.; Kramar, B.; Marolt, T.P.; Poljsak, B.; Milisav, I. Medical and dietary uses of N-Acetylcysteine. *Antioxidants* **2019**, *8*. [CrossRef]
203. Coles, L.D.; Tuite, P.J.; Oz, G.; Mishra, U.R.; Kartha, R.V.; Sullivan, K.M. Repeated-Dose oral N-Acetylcysteine in Parkinson's disease: Pharmacokinetics and effect on brain glutathione and oxidative stress. *J. Clin. Pharmacol.* **2018**, *58*, 158–167. [CrossRef] [PubMed]
204. Tsao, R. Chemistry and biochemistry of dietary polyphenols. *Nutrients* **2010**, *2*, 1231–1246. [CrossRef] [PubMed]
205. Ak, T.; Gulcin, I. Antioxidant and radical scavenging properties of curcumin. *Chem. Biol. Interact.* **2008**, *174*, 27–37. [CrossRef]
206. Zhu, Y.G.; Chen, X.C.; Chen, Z.Z.; Zeng, Y.Q.; Shi, G.B.; Su, Y.H. Curcumin protects mitochondria from oxidative damage and attenuates apoptosis in cortical neurons. *Acta Pharmacol. Sin.* **2004**, *25*, 1606–1612. [PubMed]
207. Namsi, A.; Nury, T.; Hamdouni, H.; Yammine, A.; Vejux, A.; Vervandier-Fasseur, D. Induction of neuronal differentiation of murine n2a cells by two polyphenols present in the mediterranean diet mimicking neurotrophins activities: Resveratrol and apigenin. *Diseases* **2018**, *6*. [CrossRef]
208. Almeida, A.; Heales, S.J.; Bolanos, J.P.; Medina, J.M. Glutamate neurotoxicity is associated with nitric oxide-mediated mitochondrial dysfunction and glutathione depletion. *Brain Res.* **1998**, *790*, 209–216. [CrossRef]
209. Pugazhenthi, S.; Nesterova, A.; Sable, C.; Heidenreich, K.A.; Boxer, L.M.; Heasley, L.E. Akt/protein kinase B up-regulates Bcl-2 expression through cAMP-response element-binding protein. *J. Biol. Chem.* **2000**, *275*, 10761–10766. [CrossRef]
210. Zhou, H.; Li, X.M.; Meinkoth, J.; Pittman, R.N. Akt regulates cell survival and apoptosis at a postmitochondrial level. *J. Cell Biol.* **2000**, *151*, 483–494. [CrossRef]
211. Reygaert, W.C. Green tea catechins: Their use in treating and preventing infectious diseases. *Biomed. Res. Int.* **2018**, *2018*, 9105261. [CrossRef]
212. Grzesik, M.; Naparlo, K.; Bartosz, G.; Sadowska-Bartosz, I. Antioxidant properties of catechins: Comparison with other antioxidants. *Food Chem.* **2018**, *241*, 480–492. [CrossRef]
213. Bors, W.; Heller, W.; Michel, C.; Saran, M. Flavonoids as antioxidants: Determination of radical-scavenging efficiencies. *Methods Enzymol.* **1990**, *186*, 343–355. [CrossRef]
214. Bernatoniene, J.; Kopustinskiene, D.M. The role of catechins in cellular responses to oxidative stress. *Molecules* **2018**, *23*. [CrossRef] [PubMed]
215. Koch, W.; Kukula-Koch, W.; Glowniak, K. Catechin composition and antioxidant activity of black teas in relation to brewing time. *J. AOAC Int.* **2017**, *100*, 1694–1699. [CrossRef] [PubMed]
216. Nakagawa, K.; Miyazawa, T. Absorption and distribution of tea catechin, (-)-epigallocatechin-3-gallate, in the rat. *J. Nutr. Sci. Vitaminol. (Tokyo)* **1997**, *43*, 679–684. [CrossRef] [PubMed]
217. Unno, K.; Pervin, M.; Nakagawa, A.; Iguchi, K.; Hara, A.; Takagaki, A. Blood-Brain barrier permeability of green tea catechin metabolites and their neuritogenic activity in human neuroblastoma SH-SY5Y Cells. *Mol. Nutr. Food Res.* **2017**, *61*. [CrossRef] [PubMed]
218. Pervin, M.; Unno, K.; Takagaki, A.; Isemura, M.; Nakamura, Y. Function of green tea catechins in the brain: Epigallocatechin gallate and its metabolites. *Int. J. Mol. Sci.* **2019**, *20*. [CrossRef]
219. Kang, K.S.; Wen, Y.; Yamabe, N.; Fukui, M.; Bishop, S.C.; Zhu, B.T. Dual beneficial effects of (-)-epigallocatechin-3-gallate on levodopa methylation and hippocampal neurodegeneration: In vitro and in vivo studies. *PLoS ONE* **2010**, *5*, e11951. [CrossRef]
220. Omar, S.H. Oleuropein in olive and its pharmacological effects. *Sci Pharm.* **2010**, *78*, 133–154. [CrossRef]
221. Visioli, F.; Bellomo, G.; Galli, C. Free radical-scavenging properties of olive oil polyphenols. *Biochem. Biophys. Res. Commun.* **1998**, *247*, 60–64. [CrossRef]

222. Lins, P.G.; Marina, P.P.S.; Scatolini, A.M.; de Melo, M.P. In vitro antioxidant activity of olive leaf extract (*Olea europaea* L.) and its protective effect on oxidative damage in human erythrocytes. *Heliyon* **2018**, *4*, e00805. [CrossRef]
223. Sun, W.; Wang, X.; Hou, C.; Yang, L.; Li, H.; Guo, J. Oleuropein improves mitochondrial function to attenuate oxidative stress by activating the Nrf2 pathway in the hypothalamic paraventricular nucleus of spontaneously hypertensive rats. *Neuropharmacology* **2017**, *113*, 556–566. [CrossRef] [PubMed]
224. Serra, A.; Rubio, L.; Borras, X.; Macia, A.; Romero, M.P.; Motilva, M.J. Distribution of olive oil phenolic compounds in rat tissues after administration of a phenolic extract from olive cake. *Mol. Nutr. Food Res.* **2012**, *56*, 486–496. [CrossRef] [PubMed]

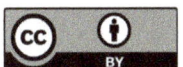 © 2020 by the authors. Licensee MDPI, Basel, Switzerland. This article is an open access article distributed under the terms and conditions of the Creative Commons Attribution (CC BY) license (http://creativecommons.org/licenses/by/4.0/).

MDPI
St. Alban-Anlage 66
4052 Basel
Switzerland
Tel. +41 61 683 77 34
Fax +41 61 302 89 18
www.mdpi.com

Antioxidants Editorial Office
E-mail: antioxidants@mdpi.com
www.mdpi.com/journal/antioxidants

www.ingramcontent.com/pod-product-compliance
Lightning Source LLC
LaVergne TN
LVHW070433100526
838202LV00014B/1592